TEXT BOOK OF MATERIA MEDICA

By
AD: LIPPE, M.D.
Professor of Materia Medica at the Homoeopathic College of Pennsylvania.

B. JAIN PUBLISHERS (P) LTD
NEW DELHI

Reprint Edition: 2001, 2005

© Copyright with the Publishers

All rights are reserved. No part of this publication may be reproduced, stored in a retrieval system or transmitted, in any form or by any means, mechanical, photocopying, recording or otherwise, without prior written permission of the publishers.

Published by :
Kuldeep Jain
For
B. Jain Publishers (P.) Ltd.
1921, Street No. 10, Chuna Mandi,
Paharganj, New Delhi 110 055 (INDIA)
Phones: 2358 0800, 2358 1100, 2358 1300. 2358 3100,
Fax: 011-2358 0471   Email: bjain@vsnl.com
Website: **www.bjainbooks.com**

Printed in India by:
J.J. Offset Printers
522, FIE, Patpar Ganj, Delhi - 110 092

Price. Rs. 179.00

ISBN : 81-7021-455-6
BOOK CODE: B-2357

PREFACE.

This work was originally prepared for the use of those attending the Lectures on the Materia Medica, in the Homœopathic Medical College of Pennsylvania, and at their request.

It contains the *characteristic* and *most prominent special symptoms* of the best proved and most used of our Medicines.

The distinction of symptoms, as the result of provings on the healthy (pathogenetic,) or as the result of clinical observations on the sick (curative,) or as belonging to both these classes, has not been retained in this work. Such distinctions belong exclusively to the complete Materia Medica, the study of which the present Text-book is intended to facilitate, not to supersede. And to a more thorough and satisfactory study and knowledge of Materia Medica than has been general of late years, it is sincerely hoped that this book may prove both an introduction and a guide.

So great is the multiplicity of symptoms, the result of provings, clinical corroborations and observations, with which our growing Materia Medica is overladen, that it seems little less than an impossibility to obtain a clear, discriminating view of each separate remedy.

The efforts previously made to overcome this difficulty, by *abridging* the Materia Medica, have proved but failures. Nor was it possible for them to have resulted otherwise, since they did not exhibit the essentially characteristic symptoms of the different medicines. They were attempts at mechanical sifting, weeding out, made without proper comprehension of the subject; which disappointed those who referred to them, and led them to demand a differently prepared and more reliable guide.

It is with the greatest reluctance that I have yielded to the requests of my professional friends and of those whom I have the pleasure of instructing, and endeavored to meet this demand. As only those who have undertaken such a work can truly realize its arduous nature, so no one can be more thoroughly conscious of its imperfections than is the author himself.

PREFACE.

Those who have mastered the Materia Medica, the author is well aware, may be acquainted with characteristic symptoms unknown to him or overlooked by him; and he will thankfully receive and acknowledge such supplementary, characteristic and especial symptoms, for incorporation in the present work.

In presenting this Text-book to his colleagues, the author relies as well upon the intelligence as upon the charity of those most conversant with the subject; since while they will undoubtedly notice many omissions and much room for improvement, they will, at the same time, appreciate the formidable nature of the task which he has been induced to undertake.

The method and object of the work are different from those of any before published on the Homœopathic Materia Medica; but its arrangement is simple, varying but little from that originally adopted by Hahneman.

The first symptoms given are those of the mind, followed by those of the different parts of the body, beginning with the head,—which also includes giddiness,—and concluding with the feet. Then come the generalities, comprising the symptoms relating to the Nervous Systems and to the Circulation; these belonging to Sleep, Fever and the Skin; and finally, the most prominent conditions of Aggravation and Amelioration, from time, place and circumstance.

The usefulness of this book can only be determined by the practical test, to which it is respectfully submitted by

THE AUTHOR.

PHILADELPHIA, *December* 30th, 1865.

ACONITUM NAPELLUS.

Mind and Disposition.
Great, inconsolable anxiety.
Complaining fear of approaching death; predicts the day he is to die.
Sensitive irritability.
Sadness.
5. Maliciousness.
Fitful mood, changing from one thing to another; now he is full of mirth, whistles and warbles a song; and then he is disposed to weep.
Delirium, especially at night—with ecstasy.
Fear of ghosts.

Head.
Vertigo when rising, with nausea; vanishing of sight; bleeding of the nose.
10. Congestion to the head, especially towards evening, with fullness and pulsation in the head, vanishing of sight, singing in the ears, red-hot face.
Inflammation of the brain—sensation of fulness and heaviness in the forehead, with the sensation as if the whole brain would start out of the eyes, with nausea and giddiness, aggravated by talking and from motion.
Burning head-ache, as if the brain was moved by boiling water.
Crampy sensation in the forehead over the root of the nose: it feels as if he would lose his senses.
Sensation of heat in the head, which perspires, with pale face.

Eyes.
15. Aversion to, or great desire for, light.
Ophthalmia, very painful, with blear-eyedness, or from foreign bodies having come into the eyes, (dust, sparks.)
Red, hard swelling of the eyelids.

Ears.
Tearing (left ear.)
Roaring in the ears.
20. Hearing very sensitive, noise is intolerable.

Nose.
Bleeding of the nose, especially in plethoric persons.

Face.
Red and hot.
Yellow.
Red and pale, alternately.
25. Redness of one cheek and paleness of the other.
When raising himself up, the red face becomes pale.
Perspiration on the side of the face on which he lies.
Tingling in the cheeks.
Lips dry and black, peeling off.

Teeth.
30. Toothache from cold, with throbbing in one side of the face, intense redness of the cheek, congestion of blood to the head, and great restlessness.

Mouth.
Dryness of the mouth and of the tongue.
Pricking and burning on the tongue.
Tongue coated white.
Trembling and stammering speech.

Throat.
35. Tingling in the œsophagus.
Acute inflammation of the throat (palate, tonsils and fauces) with high fever, dark redness of the parts, burning and stinging in the fauces.
Stinging in the throat when swallowing and coughing.
Almost entire inability to swallow, with hoarseness.

Appetite and Taste.
Taste bitter.
40. Every thing tastes bitter, except water.
Aversion to food.
Burning, unquenchable thirst.

Stomach.
Vomiting, with nausea and thirst, heat, profuse perspiration and increased micturition.
Vomiting of bloody mucus, or of what has been drunk, followed by thirst.
45. Pressure in the stomach and pit of the stomach, as from a weight or a hard stone.

Abdomen.

Tension, heaviness and pressure in the hypochondria.
Inflammation and sensation of soreness in the liver.
Pressure in the region of the liver, with obstruction of breathing.
Inflammation of the peritoneum, with restlessness, sleeplessness and thirst.
50. Inflammation of the bowels, with burning, tearing pain.
Inflammation of the hernial stricture, with vomiting of bile.

Stool and Anus.

Frequent small stools with tenesmus.
Watery diarrhœa.
Stools, white with dark red urine.

Urinary Organs.

55. Enuresis, with thirst.
Scanty, red, hot urine, without sediment.

Sexual Organs.

Men. Sexual desire either increased or decreased, with relaxed parts.
Testicles pain, as if bruised.
Women. Catamenia too profuse and too protracted.
60. Suppressed menstruation from fright.
After pains, too painful and too protracted.
Milk fever (with delirium.)
Puerperal peritonitis.

Larynx and Trachea.

Inflammation of Larynx and Bronchia.
65. Angina membranacea, with dry cough and quick breathing.
Short dry cough from titillation in the larynx.
Cough with stitches in the chest or small of the back.
Expectoration of bloody mucus.
Hæmoptysis.

Chest.

70. Shortness of breathing, especially when sleeping or raising one's self.
Anxious, labored, sobbing breathing.
Stitches through the chest and side, especially when breathing and coughing.
Pleurisy and Pneumonia, especially with great heat, much thirst, dry cough and great nervous excitability, only somewhat relieved when lying on the back.
Asthma of Millar.
75. Oppression of the chest preventing deep breathing.
Palpitation of the heart, with great anguish.

ACONIT.

Inflammation of the heart.
Chronic diseases of the heart, with continuous pressure in the left side of the chest, oppressed breathing when moving fast and ascending steps, stitches in the region of the heart, congestions to the head; attacks of fainting and tingling in the fingers.

Back.

Pain, as if bruised in the small of the back.
80. Tingling in the back.

Upper Extremities.

Tingling in the fingers, even while writing.
Icy coldness of the hands.
Hot hands with cold feet.
Numbness in the left arm;—he can scarcely move the hand.

Lower Extremities.

85. The hip-joint feels as if bruised.
Drawing, tearing pains in the knee-joint.
Unsteadiness of the knees.
Coldness of the feet up to the ankles, or only of the toes, with perspiration of the toes and soles of the feet.

Generalities.

Fainting, especially when rising, with paleness of the cheeks, which were red when lying.
90. Sudden great sinking of strength.
Lameness (paralysis) (left side.)
Cataleptic attacks, with rigor of the body, loud lamentations and grinding of the teeth.
Burning in internal parts.
Congestions (head, chest, heart.)
95. Inflammations (serous membranes.)
Stinging pains in internal organs.
Tearing in external parts (Rheumatism.)
Tingling (fingers, œsophagus, cheeks, back.)
Painful sensitiveness of the body to contact: he does not wish to be touched.
100. Attacks of pain, with thirst and redness of the face.

Sleep.

Sleeplessness, with restlessness (eyes closed) and constant tossing about.
Anxious dreams, with much talking and moving while sleeping.
Nightmare.

ACONIT.

Fever.

Pulse. Hard, full, frequent; sometimes intermitting; when slow, almost imperceptible (thread like.)

105. *Fever.* Sensation of coldness in the blood-vessels.
Chilliness. From being uncovered and from being touched.
Chilliness, with thirst.
Shuddering runs up from the feet to the chest.
Chill, with internal heat, anxiety and red cheeks.
110. *Heat*, with agonized tossing about.
Dry burning heat, generally extending from the head and face, with much thirst for cold drinks.
Heat, with inclination to uncover.
Heat, with chilliness at the same time.
Inflammatory fevers and inflammations, with much heat, dry burning skin, violent thirst, red face, or alternate red and pale face, nervous excitability, groaning and agonized tossing about, shortness of breath, and congestion to the head.
115. *Perspiration* over the whole body, especially the covered parts, smelling sour.

Skin.

Red, hot, swollen and shining skin, with violent pain.
Rash of children.
Burning in the skin.
Yellow face.

Conditions.

120. While at rest, he is better; but during the night, in bed, the pain is insupportable.
Bad effects from dry cold air, suppressed perspiration, from fright, with fear and anger.
Aggravation in the evening (chest symptoms) when lying on the (left) side; when rising; in the warm room.
Amelioration. In the open air (nervous symptoms); when sitting still (rheumatism.)

ÆTHUSA CYNAPIUM.

Mind and Disposition.
Bad humor, irritability, especially in the afternoon, and in the open air.
Anxiety.
Delirium.

Head.
Giddiness, with sleepiness.
5. Stitches and pulsations in the head.
Heaviness in the forehead.
Heat rises to the head; the body becomes warmer; the face becomes red and the giddiness ceases.
Sensation, as if both sides of the head were in a vice.

Eyes.
Eyes brilliant and protruding.
10. Pupils dilated and insensible.

Ears.
Stitches in the ears, especially in the right ear, as if something hot were streaming from it.

Face.
Tearing in the face, in the malar bones.

Throat.
Sensation of constriction, preventing deglutition.
Stinging in the throat, between the acts of deglutition.

Taste.
15. Taste sweetish, especially in the morning, when awaking.

Stomach.
Violent vomiting (in children) of curdled milk; of green mucus.
Violent vomiting, with diarrhœa—green mucus, or (in children) bloody substances.

Abdomen.
Sensation of coldness in the abdomen.
Black bluish swelling of the abdomen.

Stool.

20. Loose stools, preceded by cutting in the abdomen, with tenesmus in the morning, after rising.
Diarrhœa—discharges green, thin, bilious, with violent tenesmus.
Bloody stools.

Back.

Sensation, as if the small of the back were in a vice.

Generalities.

Epileptic spasms, with clenched thumb, red face, eyes turned downwards, pupils fixed, dilated, foam at the mouth, jaws locked, small, hard and quick pulse.
25. Spasms, with stupor and delirium.

Sleep.

Sleepiness all day; sometimes better in the open air.

Conditions.

Coldness, stiffness and rigor of the limbs.
Sensation of parts, as if they were in a vice (head, small of back.)

AGARICUS MUSCARIUS.

Mind and Disposition.

Indisposed to talk.
Indisposed to perform any kind of labor, especially mental.
Exuberant fancy.
Ecstasy.
5. Prophecy.
He makes verses.

Head.

Vertigo, giddiness, as from intoxication, especially in the morning, in the open air, and caused by the bright rays of the sun.
Sensation of heaviness, in the morning, as after intoxication.
Drawing head-ache in the morning, extending into the root of the nose.
10. Pressing in the (right) side of the head, as if a nail had been

thrust in; worse when sitting quietly; relieved by slowly moving about.

Great sensitiveness of the scalp, as from subcutaneous ulceration.

Itching of the hairy scalp, especially early in the morning, after rising.

Eyes.

Burning in the corners of the eyes.

Twitching of the eyelids and eyeballs.

15. A viscid yellow humor glues the eyelids together.

Narrowing of the intervals between the eyelids.

Muscæ volitantes.

Short-sightedness.

Black mote before the left eye.

20. He sees things double.

Ears.

Itching, burning and redness of the ears, as if they had been frozen.

Nose.

Bleeding of the nose in the morning, after blowing it.

Face.

Tearing in the face and jaw bones.

Twitching in the (right) cheek.

25. Pulsation in the cheeks.

Itching in the face, with redness and burning, as if frozen.

Teeth.

Tearing in the lower molar teeth, worse from cold air.

Gums painful and bleeding.

Mouth.

Smell from the mouth offensive, as from horse-radish.

30. Soreness of the tongue.

Tongue coated white.

Stool and Anus.

Stools pappy, with violent cutting in the abdomen, and discharge of much flatulency.

Itching in the anus, as from worms.

Chest.

Short breath and dyspnœa, making it very difficult to walk.

Back.

35. Sensation of soreness and great weakness in the back.

Upper Extremities.
Trembling of the hands.
Lower Extremities.
Heaviness of the legs.
Generalities.
Great debility, with trembling of the limbs.
Trembling.
40. Twitchings in the eyeballs, eyelids, cheeks, posteriorly in the chest, in the abdomen.
Epilepsy (with great exertions of strength.)
Great sensitiveness of the body to pressure and cold air.
Tearing pains, face, legs, continuous while at rest, disappearing while moving about.
Soreness and sensation of rawness, (nose, mouth.)
45. Itching, burning, and redness, (as if frost-bitten,) ears, nose, cheeks, fingers, toes.
Sleep.
Sleepiness in the day-time, especially after eating.
Fever.
Pulse. Accelerated in the morning, slower during the day, uneven, and sometimes intermitting.
Chilliness. Great chilliness in the open air.
Chilliness, with natural heat of the skin.
50. *Perspiration,* from the least exertion.
Skin.
Burning, itching, and redness, as if frost-bitten.
Miliary eruptions, close and white, with burning and itching.
Conditions.
Symptoms often appear diagonally, (right arm, left leg.)

AGNUS CASTUS.

Mind and Disposition.
Low-spirited, he fears approaching death.
Melancholic and hypochondriac mood.
Absent-minded.

Head.

Pain in the temple, as from a blow.
5. Heaviness in the head, and pressure, as if the head would fall forward.
Pain in the vertex, as from staying in a room filled with a thick and smoky atmosphere.
Tension and chilliness in the scalp, which is warm to the touch.

Eyes.

Corrosive itching over and on the eyebrows, on the eyelids and under the eyes.
Dilated pupils.

Ears.

10. Roaring in the ears.
Hardness of hearing.

Nose.

Odor before the nose, like herrings or musk.
Hard, aching pressing on the dorsum of the nose, relieved by pressure.

Face.

Corrosive itching of the cheeks, under the eyes, and on the chin.
15. Formication in the cheeks.

Mouth.

Ulcers in the mouth, and on the gums.
The teeth are painful, when touched by warm food or drink.

Appetite and Taste.

Thirstlessness and aversion to drink.
Metallic, coppery taste.

Stomach.

20. Nausea first in the pit of the stomach, later in the stomach, with the sensation as if all the intestines were pressing downwards.

Abdomen.

Swelling and induration of the spleen.
Ascites.
Rumbling of flatulence during sleep.

Stool and Anus.

Difficulty of passing soft stools.
25. When pressing at stool, discharge of prostatic fluid.
Sensation as of subcutaneous ulceration near the anus, only when walking.
Corrosive itching of the perineum.
Rhagades at the anus.

AGNUS CASTUS.

Urine.
Frequent micturition.

Sexual Organs.
30. *Men.* Diminution of sexual powers, the penis is small and flaccid, the testicles are cold.
Yellow discharges from the urethra.
Gonorrhœa, with suppressed sexual desire.
Drawing along the spermatic cords.
Itching of the genital organs.
35. *Women.* Suppression of the menses, with drawing pain in the abdomen.
Sterility, with suppressed menses, and want of sexual desire.
Deficient secretion of milk in lying-in women.

Chest.
Hard pressure in the region of the sternum, especially during a deep inspiration.
Cough in the evening in bed, before going to sleep.

Upper Extremities.
40. Hard pressure in the (right) axilla and upper arm, increased by motion and contact.
Swelling of the finger joints, with arthritic, tearing pains.

Lower Extremities.
Lancinating pain in the right hip-joint.
Stitches in the legs, (left big toe.)
The feet easily turn, when walking on a stone pavement.

Generalities.
45. Great debility.
Inflammatory, rheumatic swelling of the joints.
Gouty nodosities.

Fever.
Pulse. Small, slow, imperceptible.
Chilliness, internal with trembling, the external skin is warm.
50. Much chilliness, with cold hands.
Heat. Flushes of burning heat, principally in the face, with cold knees in the evening in bed.
Perspiration. Almost only on the hands, when walking in the open air.

Skin.
Corrosive itching on different parts of the body, relieved by scratching, but it soon returns.
Itching around the ulcers, in the evening.

ALLIUM CEPA.

Mind and Disposition.
Melancholy.
Fear that the pains would become unbearable.

Head.
Dulness.
Dull head-ache, with coryza; worse in the evening; better in the open air; but aggravated when returning to a warm room.

Eyes.
5. Flow of (mild) tears.
Redness of the eyes, with itching, burning and stinging, with inclination to rub them.
Swelling around the eyes.
Dulness of the eyes, with aversion to light and coryza.

Ears.
Earache.
10. Discharge of pus from the ear.
Hardness of hearing.

Nose.
Profuse watery discharge from the nose, with sneezing, acrid burning, excoriating the nose and upper lip.
Fluent coryza, with running of water from the eyes, headache, heat, thirst, cough, trembling of the hands; worse in the evening and in a room; better in the open air.
Bleeding of the nose.

Throat.
15. Sensation as of a lump in the throat.
Expectoration of a lumpy mucus through the posterior nares.

Abdomen.
Violent cutting pain in the left lower abdomen, with frequent desire to micturate, and burning micturition.

Stool and Anus.
Diarrhœa after midnight and in the morning.
Stitches in the rectum.
20. Rhagades at the anus.
Itching at the anus (worms.)

Urinary Organs.
Pressure and other pains in the region of the bladder.
Sensation of weakness in the bladder and urethra.
Increased secretion of urine with coryza.
Urine red, with much pressure and burning in the urethra.

Chest.
25. Oppressed breathing, from pressure in the middle of the chest; worse in the evening.
Cough, when inhaling cold air.

Upper Extremities.
Trembling of the right hand.
Panaritium.

Lower Extremities.
Soreness; the skin is rubbed off by the shoes, especially on the heel.

Generalities.
30. Inflammation and increased secretions of the mucous membranes.
Stitches (head, eyes, ears, rectum, skin.)
Burning (eyelids, throat, nose, mouth, bladder, skin.)
Bad effects from wet feet.

Fever.
Pulse full and accelerated.
35. *Heat*, with rumbling in the abdomen, coryza and thirst.

ALOE.

Mind and Disposition.
Anxiety and ebullition.
Restlessness, fear, fear of man.
Bad humor, especially in cloudy weather.
He is dissatisfied and angry about himself; more so when he is constipated or when he suffers from pain; better in the open air.
5. Aversion to labor.
Children chat and laugh.

Head.

Giddiness and starts.
Giddiness, with anxiety when moving; he feels as if he were sitting too high (after dinner.)
Dulness in the forehead, with chilliness.
10. Pressure in the forehead and vertex, as from a weight.
Pressing pain above the eyes.
Congestions to the head, compelling one to sit up.
Stitches above the eyebrows.
Pressing out of the temples, with flickering before the eyes and heat in the face.
15. Stitches in the temples at every step.
Headache after pain in the abdomen; after (an insufficient) stool; worse from heat, better from cold.
Sensitiveness of the scalp (in small spots.)
With the pain in the forehead the eyes become small.

Eyes.

Congestion to the eyes; pressure in the orbits.
20. Lachrymation.

Ears.

Earache.
Stitches in the ears; first in the left ear, afterwards in the right ear.
Internal and external heat of the ears.
Cracking in the ears when reading aloud.

Nose.

25. Redness of the nose in the open, cold air.
Coldness of the point of the nose.
Bleeding of the nose in bed after awaking.
Dryness of the nose in the morning, in bed.

Face.

Heat of the face when excited, or during headache.
30. Face pale during cloudy weather.

Mouth.

Lips dry, peeling off, cracked, bleeding.
Yellow ulcers on the tongue.
Tongue painful.
When moving the tongue, stitches from below to the tip.
35. Dry tongue and mouth, with increased thirst and greater redness of the lips.
Tongue red and dry.

Teeth.

Great sensitiveness of a decayed molar tooth (lower) right side.

Throat.

Throat rough, scraped, hot, as if burnt.
Pain, when yawning, masticating solid food; worse in the evening, and in the morning, when awaking.
40. Thick lumps of tough mucus in the throat.

Appetite and Taste.

Taste bitter, sour, like ink.
Aversion to meat; desire for juicy things (fruits.)
Hunger unusually keen in the evening.
Thirst while eating, after eating, and during the night.
45. After eating flatulency, pulsations in the rectum, and sexual irritation.

Stomach.

Pain in the stomach after drinking water.
Sour things disagree with him.
Vomiting of blood.
Eructations; tasteless, bitter, sour.
50. Pain in the pit of the stomach from a mis-step.

Abdomen.

Tension in the region of the liver.
Pain in the liver, when standing; stitches in the liver, when drawing a long breath.
Congestion to the abdomen, (portal system.)
Sensation of fulness, heaviness, heat and inflammation.
55. The whole abdomen is painfully sensitive to the touch.
Bloated abdomen, more on the left side, or along the colon, worse after eating.
Pulsation in the region of the navel.
Pain around the navel, worse from pressure.
Rumbling in the abdomen.
60. Discharge of much flatulency, burning, smelling offensive, relieving the pain in the abdomen, after each meal, in the evening and morning, before stools.
Cutting in the abdomen, with disinclination to go into the open air, which relieves the pain.
The abdominal walls are painful when rising, pressing to stool, when touched, and when standing erect.
Heaviness, fulness, and pressing downwards in the pelvis.

Stool and Anus.

Sudden or continued desire to go to stool.
65. Continuous desire to go to stool.
Desire for a stool after each meal.
Rumbling and cramp in the abdomen, before and during stool.
The hard stool falls out without being noticed.

Involuntary soft stool, while passing wind.
70. With the diarrhœa, flatulency, pinching in the abdomen, pain in the back and rectum, and chilliness.
Stools like mush—thin, bright yellow, gray, hot, undigested.
During the stool, congestion to the head and red face, or hunger.
Heaviness, heat, pressing, burning in the rectum.
Mucus and blood in the fæces.
75. Itching, burning, pulsations, pain as from fissures, at the anus.
Hæmorrhoidal tumors protrude like bunches of grapes, very painful, sore, tender, hot, relieved by cold water.

Urine.

Increased secretion of urine, especially at night.

Sexual Organs.

Men. Increased sexual desire. Worse after awaking, after eating, in the evening.
Erections in the morning, and after passing water.
80. Involuntary emissions during the siesta, towards morning, followed by sexual excitement, micturition and stool, and restless sleep.
Penis shrunk, and testicles cold.
Women. Fulness and heaviness in the region of the uterus.
Labor-like pains drawing into the legs.
Catamenia too early, and too profuse.
85. During menstruation, headache, which is relieved by the application of cold water; ear-ache, pain in the small of the back, pressing down in the rectum.
Fulness in the pelvis.
Fluor albus.

Chest.

Congestion to the chest.
Breathing impeded by stitches in the left side of the chest.
90. Expectoration of blood.

Back.

Pain in the small of the back, worse when sitting, or when awaking at night, better when moving about.

Extremities.

Cold hands, with warm feet.

Generalities.

Great weakness, and weak pulse after vomiting.
Lameness in all the limbs.

ALUMINA.

95. Pricking, dull twitching, drawing pain in the joints, (fingers, knees, elbows.)
Sensation of weakness in the joints of the hands and feet.
Pains of short duration, as if bruised or dislocated, (left forearm, right shoulder-blade, left ribs.)
Bad effects from sedentary habits.
Especially suitable for persons of a lymphatic or hypochondriac temperament.

Conditions.

100. *Aggravation.* When standing erect, or from sitting still, (small of the back.) Drinking vinegar, (colic.)
From motion, (nausea, pain in the abdomen.)
In the afternoon, especially the symptoms of the mucous membranes.
Amelioration, from cold water, (head.)
When walking.

ALUMINA.

Mind and Disposition.

Easily offended.
Disposition to shed tears.
Anxious and full of fears.
Alternate vivacity and thoughtfulness.
5. Great weakness of memory and inability to think coherently.

Head.

Reeling vertigo, as if he would fall over, with a faint feeling or nausea early in the morning, disappearing after breakfast.
Vertigo, with white stars before the eyes.
Pressing headache in the forehead, over the eyes, with congestion of blood to the eyes and nose, with a chill when walking in the open air; better after lying or eating.
Pulsations in the head (vertex) with congestions to the eyes and nose.
10. Stitches in the brain, with nausea.
The headache is worse in the evening and when walking in the open air; better after lying down and after eating.

ALUMINA.

Eyes.

Stitches in the eyes.
Sensation of coldness in the eyes and eyelids.
Swelling of the eyelids.
15. Inclination to stare.
Squinting.
Spasmodic contraction of the eyelids at night, with violent pain on opening the eyes.
Dim-sightedness, as from a mist, compelling him to rub the eyes.
The eyes water during the day, agglutination at night.

Ears.

20. Stitches in the (left) ear (evening.)
One ear hot and red (in the evening.)

Nose.

Soreness and scabs in the nose, with discharge of thick yellow mucus.
Swelling and redness.
Frequent attacks of coryza.
25. Ozæna.

Face.

Tension on the face, as if the white of an egg had dried on the skin.
Bulbous swellings and blood-boils on the face and nose.

Mouth.

Sensation of soreness in the mouth when eating.

Throat.

Sensation of constriction in the œsophagus when swallowing.
30. Sensation, as if the œsophagus were contracted when swallowing a small morsel of food;—it is felt until it enters into the stomach.
Great dryness of the throat.
The pains in the throat are worse *in* the evening and at night, and are relieved by warm food and drinks.

Stomach.

Sour eructations.
Nausea, with faintness.
35. Constriction of the Stomach, extending to the œsophagus.

Abdomen.

Painter's colic.

Stool and Anus.

Difficult evacuations from want of peristaltic motion of the

ALUMINA.

intestines; even the soft stool can only be passed by great pressing.
Constipation of pregnant women, children and painters.
Diarrhœa, with tenesmus.
40. Discharges of dark blood when walking, or in typhus fever, or with a hard stool.
Humidity of hæmorrhoidal tumors.
Itching at the anus.

Urinary Organs.

Frequent ineffectual desire to urinate: the urine can only be passed during a stool.
Increased secretion and frequent discharge of pale, water-colored urine.

Sexual Organs.

45. *Women.* Menstruation too early, too short and too scanty; blood pale.
Before and during menstruation, pain in the abdomen.
Fluor albus acrid, excoriating, transparent mucus before and after menstruation.

Larynx and Trechea.

Dry, short cough, especially in the morning, with dyspnœa.
Cough, with expectoration, in the morning.
50. Hoarseness, especially in the afternoon and evening.

Chest.

Pressing pain in the chest, at night.
Constriction in the chest, when stooping.

Back.

Pain in the back, as if a hot iron were thrust through the lower vertebræ.
Stitches in the back.

Upper Extremities.

55. Paralytic lameness of the arms.
Pain in the arm, down to the fingers, as if a hot iron were thrust through it.
Rhagades on the hands.

Lower Extremities.

The legs feel numb, as if asleep, especially at night.

Generalities.

Great debility and weakness, especially when talking (a short walk fatigues him much.)
60. Spasms, with attacks of laughing and weeping.
Involuntary motions (jerks of the head and other parts.)

Unpleasant want of animal heat.
Illusive sensations; some parts of the body feel as if they had become larger.
While sitting, frequent stretching of the limbs (as from drowsiness.)
65. Sensation of constriction in internal organs (œsophagus, stomach, rectum, bladder.)
Great heaviness in the legs and arms.

Fever.
Pulse full and accelerated.
Chill, generally in the evening, in bed, or near the warm stove; often with heat of the face.
During the day, chill; during the night, fever.
70. *Heat* in the evening, which spreads from the face; at times only over the right side of the body.
Perspiration at night, or more towards morning, in bed; mostly in the face, or on one side of the face.
Inability to perspire.

Skin.
Tetters itching in the evening.
Humid scabs.
75. Rhagades.
Brittle nails.
Chapped skin and bulbous eruptions.

Conditions.
Aggravation, on alternate days.
The skin symptoms at each full and new moon; periodically; in the afternoon; while sitting in a room; while urinating; from eating potatoes.
80. *Amelioration*, during moderate exercise; in the open air; on alternate days.

AMBRA GRISEA.

Mind and Disposition.
Great restlessness.
Hastiness and nervous excitement when talking.
The fancy is crowded with fantastic illusions.
Aversion to talking and laughing.

5. Embarrassed manner in society.
Despair, loathing of life.

Head.

Vertigo when walking in the open air, with weakness in the stomach.
Congestion of blood to the head, when listening to music.
Dartings in the head.
10. Pressing pain in the forehead and vertex, with heat in the head, with pale face on alternate days, with fear of losing his senses.
The hair is sensitive to the touch, it falls out.
The scalp feels sore in the morning, when awaking: this is followed by a sensation of numbness, extending over the whole body.

Face.

Flushes of heat to the face.
Yellow color of the face.
15. Spasmodic trembling and twitches of the facial muscles.
Cramp of the lower lip.

Mouth.

Offensive smell from the mouth, (in the morning.)

Appetite and Taste.

Entire thirstlessness.

Stomach.

Sour eructations.
20. Heartburn from drinking milk.

Abdomen.

Sensation of coldness in the abdomen, (on one side only.)
Pressure in the liver.
Pain in the spleen, as if something were torn off.

Stool and Anus.

Itching, smarting, and stinging at the anus.

Urinary Organs.

25. Frequent micturition during the night, and in the morning after rising.
Increased secretion of urine, much more than the amount of fluid drank.
Urine, when passing, is turbid, brown, smelling sour.

Sexual Organs.

Men. Violent erections in the morning without sexual desire, with numbness in the parts.
Women. Violent itching, with swelling of the external parts.
30. Menses too early, and too profuse.

Larynx and Trachea.
Hoarseness and roughness of the voice, with accumulation of thick, tough mucus, easily thrown off by coughing.
Itching, scraping, and soreness in the larynx and trachea.
Cough, with frequent eructations.
Spasmodic cough from tickling in the throat, with expectoration of yellowish, or grayish-white mucus, tasting salt or sour, in the morning; without expectoration in the evening.

Chest.
35. Itching in the chest, and in the thyroid gland.
Oppression felt in the chest, and between the scapulæ.
Asthma of old people, and of children.

Upper Extremities.
The arms go to sleep easily, especially when lying on them, or when carrying something in the hands.
Points of the fingers are shrivelled.
40. Cramps in the hands sometimes, only when taking hold of any thing.
Itching in the palms of the hands.

Lower Extremities.
Cramps in the calves at night.
Sensation of contraction in the (right) thigh, the limb seems to be shortened.

Generalities.
Numbness of the whole body (externally) in the morning.
45. Weakness in the morning, and at night, when awaking.
Spasms and twitches in the muscular parts.
Ebullitions and pulsations in the whole body, especially after walking in the open air.
Tearing in the muscles of the joints, often on one side, (from the small of the back through the right leg.)

Sleep.
Disturbed by coldness of the body and twitchings of the limbs.

Fever.
50. *Pulse*, accelerated with ebullitions.
Chill, in the forenoon, with weakness and sleepiness, better after eating.
Heat. Flushes of heat flying, returning every fifteen minutes, worse towards evening.
Perspiration, at night, more on the affected side, and after midnight.
Perspiration from slight exertion, especially on the abdomen and on the thighs.

Skin.

55. Dry, itching, burning.
Burning herpes.
Suppressed eruptions.

Conditions.

One-sided complaints, (perspiration, tearing, numbness, sensation of coldness in the abdomen.)
Especially suitable for lean or aged persons.
60. *Aggravation*, in the evening; while sleeping; while lying in a warm place; and on awaking.
Amelioration, when lying on the painful part; after rising from the bed; by slow motion in the open air.

AMMONIUM CARBONICUM.

Mind and Disposition.

Anxiety, with inclination to weep.
Forgetfulness, mistakes in writing and speaking.
Ill humor during wet, stormy weather.

Head.

Giddiness, especially in the morning, when sitting and reading; better when walking.
5. Pulsations, beating and pressing in the forehead, as if the head would burst; worse after eating and while walking in the open air; better from external pressure and in the warm room.

Eyes.

Burning of the eyes, with aversion to light.
Double vision.

Ears.

Hardness of hearing, with itching and suppuration of the ear.

Nose.

Discharge of sharp, burning water from the nose.
10. Stoppage of the nose, especially at night; he can only breathe through the mouth, with long-continued coryza.
Congestion of blood to the point of the nose, when stooping.

Face.

Pale, bloated face.
Itching eruptions, with soreness of the sub-maxillary glands.
Tetters around the mouth.
15. The corners of the mouth and lips are sore, cracked, and burn.
Hard swelling of the (right) parotid gland.

Teeth.

Pricking pain, especially in the molar teeth; worse when masticating or touching the decayed tooth with the tongue.
The edges of the teeth feel dull.
Aggravation from warm fluids, during the menses.
20. Looseness and rapid decay of the teeth.
Swollen, easily bleeding gums.

Mouth.

Vesicles on the tongue, at the tip, on the borders, burning, hindering eating and speaking.
Swelling of the internal mouth, especially the inside of the cheeks.
Great dryness of the mouth and throat.

Throat.

25. When swallowing, sensation as of a foreign body in the throat.
Scraping and soreness in the throat.

Appetite and Taste.

He must drink while eating.
Much thirst.
Bitter taste in the morning.
30. Longing for sugar.

Stomach.

Nausea and vomiting after each meal.
Heartburn after eating.
Sensitive painfulness of the stomach, even to the clothing.
Pressure in the stomach, and soreness at the pit of the stomach, after eating.
35. Burning and heat in the stomach.
Pain, as from constriction in the stomach, with nausea, waterbrash and chilliness (ameliorated by pressure and by lying down.)

Stool and Anus.

Stool difficult, hard, knotty.
Hæmorrhoidal tumors protruding before, during, and after stool.

AMMONIUM CARBONICUM.

Discharge of blood from the rectum, during and after stool.
40. Bleeding hæmorrhoids.
Itching at the anus.

Urinary Organs.

Frequent desire to urinate, with continued pressure on the bladder.
Involuntary micturition at night, during sleep (morning.)
Urine pale, with sandy sediment.

Sexual Organs.

45. *Men.* Choking pains in the relaxed testicles.
Frequent involuntary seminal emissions.
Itching at the genitals, especially the scrotum.
Women. Itching, burning and swelling of the pudendum.
Menstruation too early, too scanty, and of too short duration.
50. Menstruation too profuse, blood clotted, black, with colicky pains and hard, difficult stool.
During the menses, pain in the abdomen, toothache, backache, chilliness.
Fluor albus burning, acrid, watery.

Larynx and Trachea.

Hoarseness and inability to speak a loud word.
Cough at night; every morning, at 3 o'clock, dry from tickling in the throat, as of dust.
55. Cough, with spitting of blood, with previous sweet taste and with great dyspnœa.
Cough, with stitches in the small of the back.

Chest.

Dyspnœa, with palpitation of the heart, especially when moving.
Stitches in the left side of the chest; worse when lying on it.
Heaviness on the chest, as from congestion of blood to the chest.
60. Burning and heat in the chest (hydrothorax.)

Upper Extremities.

After washing in cold water, the hands look blue, and the veins are distended.
The fingers swell when the arm is hanging down.
Heaviness and loss of power of the right arm.
Pain in the wrist-joint, which had formerly been sprained.
65. The skin peels off from the palms of the hands.

Lower Extremities.

Pain, as if bruised in the thighs.
Swelling and pain of the big toe in the evening.

Cramp in the calf of the leg, when walking.
Cramps in the soles of the feet.

Generalities.

70. Debility, which compels one to lie down.
Great sensitiveness to cold, open air.
Drawing and tension, as from shortening of the muscles.
Inclination to stretch the limbs.
Pain, as from dislocation in the joints.
75. Tearing in the joints relieved by the heat of the bed.
Pain, as from subcutaneous ulceration.
Burning (chest.)

Sleep.

Sleepiness during the day.
Sleeplessness till 4, A.M., and when falling asleep, perspiration.

Fever.

80. *Pulse* hard, tense and frequent.
Chilliness. Attacks of chilliness in the evening.
Perspiration in the morning and during the day, mostly on the joints.

Skin.

Violent itching, and burning blisters after scratching.
The upper part of the body is red, and covered with scarlet rash.
85. Scarlet fever, with parotitis.
Desquamation of the skin (palms of the hands.)

Conditions.

Aversion to moving about.
The right side of the body is more affected.
Speaking, and hearing others speak, affects him much.
90. *Aggravation* in the evening, on bending down; from wet poultices; during wet weather; from pressing the teeth together; and re-appearance of some symptoms from washing (bleeding of the nose, blue hands, and swelling of the veins of the hands.)
Amelioration, when lying on the stomach; the right side; the painful side; from external pressure; in the room; from warmth; in dry weather.

AMMONIUM MURIATICUM.

Mind and Disposition.
Irritability and bad humor, especially in the morning, with disinclination to speak.

Head.
Giddiness, with fulness in the head.
Head feels too heavy and full; more in the forehead, and especially in the morning, after rising.

Eyes.
Burning in the eyes, at twilight: this disappears after lighting a candle.
5. Dimness of sight, as if obscured by a fog.
Flying spots and points before the eyes.
Yellow spots before the eyes, while sewing.

Ears.
Stitches in the ears.
Discharges of matter from the ears, with hardness of hearing.

Nose.
10. Coryza, with stoppage, great soreness and tenderness of the nose, and loss of smell.

Face.
The face is burning-hot in the room.
Dry, cracked lips, with blotches of the skin peeling off.

Mouth and Throat.
Stitches in the throat, when swallowing.
Burning blister on the tip of the tongue.
15. Swelling of the sub-maxillary glands, with pulsating pains.

Stomach.
Much thirst, especially in the evening.
Hiccough, with stitches in the chest.

Stool and Anus.
Constipation; stools hard, crumbling.
Diarrhœa, slimy, green.
20. Before the stool, pain around the navel.
During stool, stitches in the anus.

Urine.

Diminished secretion of urine.
Slow flow of urine; more abundant during stool.
Frequent urination, especially towards morning.
25. Sediment, like clay.

Sexual Organs.

Women. Menstruation too early and too profuse, with pain in the abdomen and small of the back; continuing during the night, when the menstrual discharge is more profuse.
During menstruation, vomiting and diarrhœa.
Fluor albus, like the white of an egg, preceded by pain around the navel.

Respiratory Organs.

Frequent hawking, with expectoration of mucus.
30. Hoarseness, with burning in the larynx.
Dry cough in the morning, from tickling in the throat.
Cough at night, when lying on the back.
Cough aggravated by eating, drinking any thing cold, and when lying down.
Pressure, heaviness and stitches in the chest, sensation, as if a swallowed morsel had lodged in the chest.
35. When breathing, stitches in the shoulder-blades.

Back.

Painful stiffness of the neck.
Intolerable pain in the small of the back, at night.
Coldness in the back, especially between the shoulders.

Upper Extremities.

Swelling and hardness of the axillary glands.
40. The right arm is heavy and stiff.
Blisters on the wrist, forming scabs.
The skin peels off between the fingers.
Stitches and pulsations in the tips of the fingers, or tingling in them.

Lower Extremities.

Pain in the left hip, as if the tendons were too short, causing limping or pain as from dislocation.
45. The muscles under the knee (hamstrings) feel too short when walking, with stiffness of the knee-joint.
Sensation of soreness and tearing in the heels.
The tips of the toes are very painful.
Coldness of the feet, especially in the evening, in bed.
Offensive perspiration of the feet.

50. Ebullitions, with anxiety and weakness, as if paralyzed.
Tension in the joints, as from shortening of the muscles.
Burning, stinging, throbbing, as from a boil.
Sensation of soreness in different parts of the body.

Sleep.
Sleeplessness after midnight, from cutting pain in the abdomen, at 2, A. M.; or from sneezing; pain in the small of the back.

Fever.
55. *Pulse* much accelerated, day and night.
Heat, with red, bloated face; worse in the warm room.
Frequent attacks of flushes of heat, followed by perspiration, which is more abundant on the face, palms of the hands and soles of the feet.
Perspiration most profuse after midnight and in the morning, in bed.

Skin.
Blisters, forming scabs.

Conditions.
60. Many groups of symptoms are accompanied by cough.
In the hours of the morning, sensation of stiffness, which is relieved by walking in the open air.
Aggravation, of the head and chest symptoms in the morning; of the abdominal symptoms in the afternoon; of the skin and fever symptoms in the evening.
Amelioration, in the open air.

ANACARDIUM.

Mind and Disposition.
Want of moral feeling.
Contradiction between reason and will; he feels as if he had two wills, one commanding him to do what the other tells him not to do.
Wickedness and cruelty.
Irresistible desire to curse and swear.
5. Loss of memory.

Head.
Pressing pain in the temple, as from a nail; worse after eating, in the cold air, and from exertions of the mind.

Congestion of blood to the head, with pain in the cerebellum
Stitches in the head.

Eyes.
Pressure in the eyes, as from a plug.
10. Dimness of sight.
Contraction of the pupils.

Ears.
Pressing in the ears, as from a plug.
Itching in the ear.
Hardness of hearing.

Nose.
15. Diminution of the sense of smell.
The sense of smell is too acute or illusory; smell like pigeon-dung or burning tinder.
Fluent coryza.
Frequent sneezing, and frequent inclination to sneeze.

Face.
Paleness of the face, with sunken eyes, surrounded by blue ridges.

Mouth and Throat.
20. Fetid odor from the mouth, without his perceiving it.
Heaviness and swelling of the tongue, which impedes speech.
White, rough tongue.
Taste lost.
Roughness and scraping in the throat.

Stomach.
25. Weak digestion, with fulness and distention of the abdomen and hypochondriacal humor.
Great thirst, with arrest of breathing while drinking.
1. Morning, nausea. 2. Vomiting of the ingesta, which gives relief.
Pressure in the pit of the stomach, when awaking in the morning.

Abdomen.
Hardness of the abdomen.
30. Pressure in the liver.
Pain, as if a blunt plug were pressed into the intestines.

Stool and Anus.
Ineffectual desire to go to stool.
The soft stool is passed with difficulty, on account of the inactivity of the bowels.
During stool he passes blood.
35. Painful hæmorrhoidal tumors at the anus.

Itching at the anus.
Moisture from the rectum.

Urinary Organs.

Frequent discharge of pale urine, in small quantities, with burning.

Sexual Organs.

Men. Involuntary erections during the day.
40. Discharge of prostatic fluid during hard and soft stool, and micturition.
Women. Leucorrhœa, with itching and soreness.

Respiratory Organs.

Oppression of the chest, with internal heat and anxiety, driving him into the open air.
Pressure in the chest, (right side,) as from a dull plug.
Rawness and scraping in the chest.
45. Violent convulsive cough, (hooping-cough,) caused by tickling in the pharynx; worse at night, and after eating; after the attacks, yawning and sleepiness.
Stitches in the region of the heart, extending to the small of the back.

Back.

Dull stitches in the left shoulder-blade.
Dull pressure in the shoulders, as from a weight.

Upper Extremities.

Sensation of weakness in the arms, with trembling.
50. Trembling (of the right hand.)

Lower Extremities.

Sensation of weakness in the knees, with trembling.
The legs feel stiff, as if bandaged, with painful restlessness in them.

Generalities.

Diminution of the senses, (smell, sight, hearing.)
Trembling, debility, and paralytic weakness.
55. Pain in different parts, as if a plug had entered.
Sensation, as of a hoop or band around the parts.
Cramp-like pains in the muscles.
Contraction of the joints.

Sleep.

Goes to sleep late.
60. Sleep disturbed by dreams of fire and corpses.
Heavy sleep till 9, A. M.

Fever.

Pulse, accelerated, with beating in the veins.
Chilliness, especially in the open air, relieved in the sunshine.
Heat. External heat, with internal chill.
65. Heat of the upper part of the body, with cold feet; internal chilliness and hot breath.
Perspiration, in the evening, on the head, abdomen and back, even when sitting still.
Clammy perspiration in the palms of the hands, (especially the left.)
Night-sweats on the abdomen and back.

Skin.

Burning, itching, worse from scratching.
70. Voluptuous itching, extending farther by scratching.
Itching of the skin, worse from scratching.
Often suitable for eruptions caused by poisoning with rhus tox.

Conditions.

Liability to take cold, and sensitiveness to a draught of air.
Symptoms appearing periodically.
75. Many symptoms appear after eating, while most of them disappear during dinner.
Aggravation. When lying on the side; from rubbing, and from taking hold of any thing.

ANGUSTURA.

Mind and Disposition.

Easily frightened, and starts.

Head.

Tension in the temporal muscles when opening the mouth.

Eyes.

The eyelids are spasmodically opened.
Dimness before the eyes from obscuration of the cornea, (in the morning.)

Face.

5. Heat and bluish redness of the face.

Tension in the muscles of the face.
Lockjaw; the lips are drawn back, showing the teeth.
After the attacks, the lips and cheeks remain blue for some time.

Stomach and Abdomen.
Aversion to solid food, but irresistible desire to drink coffee.
10. Thirst, without desire to drink.
Painful tension in the pit of the stomach and abdomen.

Sexual Organs.
Violent itching on the male organs, especially on the tip of the glans penis.

Respiratory Organs.
Intermitting spasmodic breathing.
Dry cough, with scraping and rattling of mucus in the chest.
15. Hoarseness from mucus in the trachea.
Painful spasm in the pectoral muscles.
Painful sensitiveness of the chest, even to the slightest touch.

Back.
Painful stiffness in the neck, and between the shoulder-blades.

Upper Extremities.
Cramp-like drawing, down the arm to the fingers.

Lower Extremities.
20. Drawing in the limbs, with soreness.
Pain on the inner side of the ankle, when walking, causing limping.

Generalities.
Weakness of the whole body, as if the marrow of the bone were stiff.
The spinal marrow and the exterior muscles are principally affected.
Stiffness and stretching of the limbs.
25. Twitching and jerking along the back, like electric shocks.
Spasmodic twitching.
Tetanic spasms, caused by contact, noise, or the drinking of lukewarm water; cheeks and lips become blue; the breathing is labored during the spasms, groaning and closing of the eyes, lips wide open, drawn up and down, exposing the teeth.
Paralysis.
30. Cracking of the joints.

Fever.
Pulse accelerated, spasmodic, irregular at times, intermitting.
Chill, in the morning and forenoon, preceded by thirst.

Violent chill every afternoon (at 3 o'clock.)
Repeated chilliness over the affected parts.
35. *Heat* in the evening, after entering a room, after supper, mostly in the face, at 3, A. M., disturbing sleep, followed by chilliness.
Perspiration only in the morning, and on the forehead.

Skin.
Caries and very painful ulcers, which affect the bones and pierce them to the marrow.

Conditions.
Aggravation, from touching the affected part.

ANTIMONIUM CRUDUM.

Mind and Disposition.
Ecstasy and exalted love, with great anxiety about his fate and inclination to shoot himself; worse when walking in the moonlight, and then his conduct is like that of an insane person.
The child cannot bear being touched or looked at.

Head.
Giddiness, with nausea, or bleeding of the nose.
Congestion of blood to the head, followed by bleeding of the nose.
5. Stupefying headache, with nausea; worse in the evening; after eating; and smoking tobacco; and better in the open air.
Headache, from bathing.

Eyes.
Stitches in the eyes.
Gum in the canthi of the eyes.
Moist place on the outer canthus.

Ears.
10. Redness, swelling and heat of the ears.
Continual roaring in the ears.
Deafness, as if a leaf were lying before the ears.

Nose.

Sensation of coldness in the nose, when inspiring air.
Soreness of the nostrils; nostrils cracked and full of crusts.
15. Bleeding of the nose (in the evening, after headache, with giddiness.)

Face.

Sad countenance.
Heat, especially on the cheeks, with itching.
Red, burning, suppurating eruptions, with yellow crusts.
Sore, cracked corners of the mouth.

Mouth and Teeth.

20. Bleeding of the teeth and gums.
Pain in decayed teeth, aggravated by cold water.
Bitter taste in the mouth.
Dryness of the mouth.
Ptyalism (tasting salty.)
25. Tongue coated white.

Stomach and Abdomen.

Aversion to all food.
Longing for acids.
Thirst at night.
Nausea and vomiturition, from overloading the stomach, or after drinking (sour) wine.
30. Vomiting of mucus and bile—with convulsions—with diarrhœa.
Cramp-like pains in the stomach.

Stool and Anus.

Difficult evacuations; the fæces are too large in size.
Alternate diarrhœa and constipation, especially in aged persons.
Watery diarrhœa, with cutting in the bowels.
35. Continuous discharge of mucus from the rectum.

Urinary Organs.

Increased and frequent discharge of urine at night, with discharge of mucus, burning in the urethra, and pain in the small of the back.

Upper Extremities.

Rheumatic pains in the arms.
Drawing (gouty) pains in the fingers and their joints.

Lower Extremities.

Rheumatic pains in the legs.
40. Painful stiffness of the knee (fungus of the knee.)
Large, horny corns on the soles of the feet.

The soles of the feet feel sore when walking.
Inflammatory redness of the heel.

Generalities.

Disposition to grow fat.
45. Dropsical swelling of the whole body.
Inflammation of the muscles.

Sleep.

Very sleepy during the day, especially in the forenoon

Fever.

Pulse very irregular, changing every few beats.
Chilliness predominating, even in the warm room.
50. Sensation of coldness in the nose when inhaling air.
Heat, especially during the night, before midnight, with cold feet.
Great heat from little exercise, especially in the sun.
Perspiration, when awaking in the morning, returning periodically, (every other morning.)
Intermittent fevers, with desire to sleep, and want of thirst.

Skin.

55. Horn-like excrescences, and disposition to abnormal organizations of the skin, (corns on the soles of the feet.)
Eruptions like boils and blisters; as from the bites of insects; like measles.
Fistulous ulcers.
Fungus of the joints.

Conditions.

When the symptoms re-appear, they change their locality, or go from one side of the body to the other.
60. *Aggravation*, from drinking sour wine; after eating (pork;) after bathing; in the heat of the sun; or at night.
Amelioration, during rest; or in the open air.

APIS MELLIFICA.

Mind and Disposition.

Restlessness, continually changing his occupation.
Delirium, (after suppressed scarlet eruption.)
Awkwardness, he breaks every thing.
Jealousy, (in women.)

Head.

5. Giddiness—when sitting, standing, lying, when closing the eyes, with nausea and headache.
Congestion to the head, with suppressed menstruation.
Pressing pain in the forehead and temples; worse when rising, and in a warm bed, relieved by pressing the forehead together.
The brain feels tired.
Hydrocephalus in children, and apoplexy in old persons.
10. Hydrocephalus, with copious perspiration of the head, torpor, delirium interrupted by sudden shrill cries, boring of the head deep into the pillows, squinting, grinding of the teeth, urine scanty, (milky,) twitching on one side of the body, while the other is paralyzed.

Eyes.

Sensation of mucus in the eyes.
Twitching of the eyeballs.
Inflammation of the eye, with intense photophobia and increased secretions.
Staphyloma.
15. Œdematous swelling of the eyelids.

Ears.

Redness and swelling of both ears.

Face.

Burning, stinging heat in the face, with purple color.
Erysipelas of the face.
Œdematous swelling of the face.

Mouth and Throat.

20. Swelling of the lips, especially the upper lip.
Dry, swollen, inflamed tongue, with inability to swallow.
White, dry tongue, (with diarrhœa.)
Fetid breath, (with paroxysms of headache.)
Tough, frothy saliva.
25. Dryness in the throat, without thirst.
Burning, stinging in the throat.
Inflammation of the throat, with swelling, redness, and stinging pains.
Ulcerated sore throat, (in scarlet fever, when the eruption does not come out.)

Appetite and Taste.

Thirstlessness, (with dropsy.)

Stomach and Abdomen.

30. Vomiting of bile.
    Vomiting, with inflammation of the stomach.
    Vomiting, with diarrhœa.
    Sensitiveness of the pit of the stomach to touch.
    Violent pain and sensitiveness in the region of the stomach.
35. Great sensitiveness of the abdomen to the touch.
    Sensation of fulness and distention of the abdomen.

Stool and Anus.

Diarrhœa, yellowish-green, with mucus, especially in the morning.
Stools smelling very offensively.
After stool, tenesmus and discharge of blood.
40. Diarrhœa and vomiting.
    Swelling of the anus.
    Hæmorrhoids, with stinging pains.

Urinary Organs.

Strangury.
Urine scanty and high-colored.
45. Too profuse discharge of urine.
    Burning and smarting in the urethra, as if it were scalded.
    Burning and stinging in the urethra.

Sexual Organs.

Men. Sexual desire increased.
Swelling of the testicles.
50. *Women.* Inflammation, induration, swelling and dropsy of the ovaries (right).
    Sharp, cutting, stinging pain in the swollen ovary; worse during menstruation.
    Pressing-down pain in the uterus.
    Dropsy of the uterus.
    Menstruation suppressed or diminished, with congestion to the head.
55. Abortion.

Respiratory Organs.

Hoarseness, in the morning.
Oppression of the chest, shortness of breath, especially when ascending; inability to remain in a warm room.
Asthma; worse in cold weather.
Sensation of soreness in the chest, as from a bruise.
60. Hydrothorax.
    Cough, after lying down and sleeping.

Extremities.

Upper. Hands bluish, and inclined to be cold.
Lower. Cold legs.
Œdematous swelling of the feet, ankles and legs.
Suppressed perspiration of the feet.

Generalities.

65. Great debility, as if he had worked hard; he is obliged to lie down.
Burning, stinging pains.
Great sensitiveness to touch and pressure (abdomen.)
Tension (over the eyes in the left side of the head) behind the ears, in the neck.
Sensation of soreness under the ribs.

Sleep.

70. Sleep disturbed by many dreams.
Sleep, late in the morning.
Awakens from sleep with a shrill shriek (child suffering from hydrocephalus.)

Fever.

Pulse full and rapid—small and trembling—intermitting.
Chill, mostly towards the evening (3–4 P. M.)
75. Chilliness from the least movement, with heat of the face and hands.
Dry heat towards the evening, with sleepiness.
The sensation of heat is more felt about the pit of the stomach and in the chest.
Perspiration, alternating with dryness of the skin.
After the fever paroxysm, sleep.

Skin.

80. Œdematous swellings.
Hives.
Carbuncles, with burning, stinging pains.
Erysipelas.
Scarlet eruptions.
85. Panaritium (burning, stinging.)

Conditions.

Aggravation. In the morning (restlessness, mucus in the mouth, diarrhœa.)
In the evening (giddiness, headache, pain in the eyes, toothache, hoarseness, cough, chills and fever.)
At night (eyes and chest.)
From heat, especially in the warm room.
Amelioration. Cold water relieves the pain, swelling and burning.
Pressing together relieves the headache.

ARGENTUM METALLICUM.

Mind and Disposition.
Restlessness, anxiety, which directs him from place to place.
Ill humor, with disinclination to talk.

Head.
Pressing, tearing pain in the skull, principally in the temporal bones, renewed every day at noon, with soreness of the external head, aggravated by pressure and contact, ameliorated in the open air.
Painful sensation of emptiness in the head.

Eyes.
5. Violent itching in the corners of the eyes.
Redness and swelling of the edges of the eyelids.

Ears.
Itching of the ears, he scratches them until they bleed.
Itching of the lobes of the ears.

Nose.
Violent fluent coryza, with much sneezing.

Face.
10. Redness of the face.
Swelling of the upper lip.

Throat.
The throat feels as if internally swollen.
The throat feels more sore from coughing than when swallowing, although the food passes with difficulty.
Accumulation of much gray, jelly-like mucus in the throat, which is easily hawked up.

Stomach.
15. Appetite much increased, he is hungry after eating a full meal.
Desire for wine.
Heartburn.
Burning in the stomach, ascending to the chest.

Abdomen.

Painful swelling of the abdomen.
20. Tension in the abdominal muscles.

Stool and Anus.

Frequent pressure in the lower part of the rectum, with discharge of small quantities of soft stool.
Dry stool, like sand, after dinner.

Urinary Organs.

Frequent desire to urinate, with profuse discharge of urine.

Sexual Organs.

Men. The testicles feel as if bruised.
25. Women. Prolapsus uteri, with pain in the left ovary.

Respiratory Organs.

When stooping, or ascending steps, mucus comes up into the larynx, which is easily expectorated by one cough.
Sensation of rawness or soreness of the larynx.
Laughing causes mucus in the trachea, and cough.
Cough, caused by stinging, cutting in the trachea, with mucus in the chest, and expectoration of transparent mucus, like boiled starch.
30. Rattling cough, only during the day in the room.
Stitches in the (right side) of the chest, when inhaling and exhaling.

Upper Extremities.

Tearing in the bones of the arms, especially of the hands and fingers.

Lower Extremities.

Tearing in the bones of the feet and toes.

Generalities.

Sensation of numbness in the limbs, as if asleep.
35. Sensation of soreness and rawness in internal organs.
Boring pain in the joints.
Sensation of soreness in the joints.
Strong effects on the secretions of the mucous membranes.

Fever.

Heat of the body, but none on the head, without thirst.
40. Perspiration only on the abdomen or chest.

Conditions.

Bad effects from the use of mercury.
Bad effects from onanism.
The symptoms are renewed at noon.

ARGENTUM NITRICUM.

Mind and Disposition.
Very impulsive; in continual motion; he walks fast.
Apathy.
Head.
Vertigo, with headache.
Morning headache, (when he awakens.)
5. Excessive congestion of blood to the head.
Stitches in the left frontal eminence.
Digging up, incisive motion, through the left hemisphere of the brain.
Headache, with chilliness.
Headache relieved by tying a handkerchief tightly around the head.
10. Headache worse in the open air.
Itching, creeping, crawling of the hairy scalp.
Sensation, as if the bones of the skull separated, with increase of temperature.
Eyes.
Mucus in the eyes drying up, and forming scurfs.
Vanishing of light; he is constantly obliged to wipe off the mucus, which obstructs the axis of vision.
15. Opacity of the cornea.
Ophthalmia, with intense pain; worse in the warm room, better in the open air.
Ears.
Ringing in the ears, and deafness, (left ear.)
Nose.
Violent itching of the nose.
Coryza, with chilliness, lachrymation, sneezing, and stupefying headache.
20. Discharge of pus, with clots of blood.
Face.
Sunken, pale, bluish countenance.
Hard blotches in the vermilion border of the upper lip, paler than the lip, and sore to the touch.

ARGENTUM NITRICUM.

The lips are dry and viscid, without thirst.
The gums are swollen, inflamed, bleed easily, and are painful when touched.
25. Sensitiveness of the teeth to cold water.

Mouth.
Dryness of the tongue. with thirst.
Papillæ prominent, erect, feeling sore.
Painful red tip of the tongue.
Fetid odor from the mouth.
30. Ptyalism.

Throat.
Dark redness of the uvula and fauces.
Sensation, as if a splinter were lodged in the throat when swallowing.
Thick, tenacious mucus in the throat.

Appetite and Taste.
Irresistible desire for sugar in the evening.
35. Sweetish-bitter taste.

Stomach.
Violent belching.
Violent vomiting, with anxiety in the præcordial region.
Black vomit.
Vomiting and diarrhœa, with violent colicky pains.
40. Gnawing pain in the left side of the stomach.
Pressure, with heaviness and nausea in the stomach.

Abdomen.
Stitches through the abdomen, like electric shocks, (left side.)

Stool and Anus.
Diarrhœa of green, fetid mucus, with very noisy emission of flatulence at night.
Bloody stools.
45. Constipation, fæces dry.
Itching at the anus.

Urinary Organs.
Frequent and copious emission of pale urine.
Inflammation, and violent burning or shooting pains in the urethra, with increased gonorrhœa.
Priapism, bleeding of the urethra.
50. Stricture of the urethra.

Sexual Organs.
Men. Chancre-like ulcer on the prepuce.
Sexual desire wanting, the genital organs having become shrivelled.

Chest.
Palpitation of the heart in paroxysms, with nausea.
Back.
Pain in the small of the back relieved when standing or walking.
Lower Extremities.
55. Heaviness and debility of the legs.
Great debility and weariness in the calf of the leg, as after a long journey.
Generalities.
Staggering gait.
Great debility and weariness, (lower limbs.)
Convulsions.
60. Epileptic attacks caused by fright, or during menstruation, (at night, or in the morning when rising.)
Sensation of expansion, (face and head.)
Sleep.
Soporous condition.
Nightly nervousness, with heat in the head.
Restless sleep, with stupefaction and headache.
Fever.
65. Chilliness, with nausea.
Morning perspiration.
Skin.
Wart-shaped excrescences on the skin.
Discoloration of the skin—blue-gray, violet or bronze-colored tinges, to real black.

ARNICA MONTANA.

Mind and Disposition.
Depression of spirits and absence of mind.
Shedding of tears and exclamations after rage.
Great sensitiveness of the mind, with anxiety and restlessness.
Unconsciousness, (like fainting after mechanical injuries.)
5. Declines to answer any questions.
Quarrelsome.

Head.

Giddiness, with nausea, when moving and rising; better when lying.
Burning and heat in the head, the rest of the body is cool, (night and morning, worse from motion, better when at rest.)
Pressure on one temple, as if a nail had been driven into it.
10. Cutting through the head, as with a knife, followed by a sensation of coldness.
Stitches in the head, especially in the temples and forehead.
Effects from concussion of the brain.

Eyes.

Inflammation of the eyes with suggillation after mechanical injuries.

Ears.

Stitches in and behind the ears.
15. Pains in the ears, as from a bruise.

Nose.

Tingling in the nose, and bleeding.

Face.

Heat of the face, the body being cool.
Sunken, pale face.
Redness of one cheek.
20. Hot, red, shining swelling of one cheek.
Burning, hot, cracked lips.

Mouth.

Toothache, with swollen face.
Dryness of the mouth, with much thirst.
Tongue coated white.
25. Putrid smell from the mouth.

Throat.

Burning in the throat.

Appetite and Taste.

Bitter taste, especially in the morning.
Putrid taste.
Aversion to food, especially to meat.
30. Desire for vinegar.
Thirst for cold water, without fever.
Longing for alcoholic drinks.

Stomach.

Frequent eructations, especially in the morning, empty, bitter, putrid, as from rotten eggs.

Nausea, and empty vomiturition.
35. After drinking, vomiting of what has been drunk.
Vomiting of blood, (dark, clotted.)

Abdomen.

Cutting, colicky pain in the abdomen.
Tympanitis.
Colic, with strangury.

Stool and Anus.

40. Flatus, smelling like rotten eggs.
Frequent stools—small, consisting of mucus.
Involuntary stool during sleep—thin, brown, or white.
Stools of undigested matter, or of blood, or pus.
Diarrhœa, with tenesmus.

Urinary Organs.

45. Tenesmus from spasms of the neck of the bladder.
Involuntary discharge of urine at night, when asleep, and during the day, when running.
Urine brown-red, with brick-dust sediment.
Bloody urine.
Frequent micturition of pale urine.

Sexual Organs.

50. *Men.* Purple-red swelling of the penis and testicles, after mechanical injuries.
Painful swelling of the spermatic cords, with stitches into the abdomen.
Women. Soreness of the parts after a severe labor.
Violent after-pains.
Erysipelatous inflammation of the mammæ and nipples.

Respiratory Organs.

55. Breath fetid, short, and panting.
Excessive difficulty of breathing.
Burning or rawness in the chest.
Sensation of soreness of the ribs.
Hooping-cough, after crying; from tickling in the œsophagus; with expectoration generally of foaming blood, mixed with clots of blood; sometimes in the evening with putrid mucus, which cannot be expectorated, but must be swallowed again.
60. Cough worse in the evening till midnight, from motion, in the warm room, and after drinking.
Stitches in the chest, (left side,) aggravated from a dry cough, with oppression of breathing; worse from motion, better from external pressure.

Back.
Tingling in the back.
Great soreness of the back.
Upper Extremities.
Tingling in the arms.
65. Sensation of soreness of the arms.
Sensation, as if the joints of the arms and wrists were sprained.
Lower Extremities.
Sensation of soreness in the legs.
Tingling in the legs.
White swelling of the knee.
70. Hot erysipelatous inflammation and painfulness of the foot.
Gout.
Generalities.
Over-sensitiveness of the whole body.
Pain, as if beaten or bruised in outer parts.
Pain, as if sprained in outer parts, and in the joints.
75. Tearing, drawing, in outer parts.
Pricking, from without, inward.
Pressing, in inner parts.
Tingling, in outer parts.
Twitching of the muscles.
80. Ebullitions, and burning of the upper part of the body, with coldness of the lower part of the body.
Bleeding of internal and external parts (vomiting of blood.)
Sleep.
Sleepiness during the day, with inability to sleep.
Drowsiness, with delirium.
Fever.
Pulse very variable, mostly hard, full and quick.
85. *Chilliness*, internally, with external heat.
Great chilliness, with heat and redness of one cheek.
Chilliness as soon as he lifts the cover of the bed.
Chilliness of the side on which he lays.
Heat. Dry heat over the whole body, or only in the face and on the back.
90. *Perspiration* smelling sour or offensive—sometimes cold.
Intermittent fever; chill in the morning or forenoon; drawing pains in the bones before the fever; changes his position continually; breath and perspiration offensive.
Skin.
Petechiæ.
Many small blood-boils.

Hot, hard, shining swelling (from the stings of insects.)
Suggillation.

Conditions.

95. *Aggravation.* Bad effects, even inflammations, from mechanical injuries, falls, bruises and contusions.
Amelioration, in the evening at at night; from contact and motion; even from noise.

ARSENICUM ALBUM.

Mind and Disposition.

Anguish, driving one out of bed at night, and from one place to another in the day-time.
Restlessness.
Great fear of death, and of being left alone.
Despair. He finds no rest, especially at night, with anguish.
5. Anger, with anxiety, restlessness and sensation of coldness.
Madness; loss of mind (from the abuse of alcoholic drinks.)
Delirium.

Head.

Tearing in the head, with vomiting, when raising up the head.
Headache (after meals) relieved by applying cold water, or by walking in the open air.
10. Periodical headaches.
The scalp is tender to the touch.
Eruptions, white, dry, like bran; burning, itching on the forepart of the head; when scratching it burns and bleeds violently.
Burning, biting boils on the scalp, with sensitiveness to touch and cold.
Erysipelatous burning, swelling of the head (face and genitals) with great weakness and coldness; worse at night.

Eyes.

15. Inflammation of the eyes and lids, with severe burning pains.
Inflammation of the inner surface of the eyelids, preventing the opening of the eye.
Excessive photophobia.
Specks or ulcers on the cornea.

Ears.

Hardness of hearing—he cannot hear the human voice.
20. Roaring in the ears (accompanying every attack of pain.)

Nose.

Swelling of and burning in the nose.
Ulcers in the nose (cancer of the nose.)
Profuse, fluent coryza of sharp, burning, excoriating water, with hoarseness and sleeplessness.
Peeling off of the epidermis.

Face.

25. Puffiness of the face, especially around the eyes.
Color pale, like earth, yellowish, (blue rings around the eyes.)
Distorted features; death-like countenance.
Drawing stitches here and there in the face.
Burning face-ache.
30. Crusta lactea.
Cancer of the face and lips, with burning pain.
Exanthema around the mouth.
Lips black, dry, and cracked.

Teeth.

Toothache at night, extending to the ear and temple, worse when lying on the affected side, better from the heat of the stove.
35. Grinding of the teeth.
Gums bleeding.

Mouth and Throat.

The mouth is reddish-blue, inflamed, burning.
Secretion of abundant tough, fetid, bloody saliva.
Aphthæ, stomacace.
40. Tongue dry, brown, black, cracked.
Swelling, inflammation, or gangrene of the tongue.
Ulceration of the tongue, with blue color.
Painful, difficult deglutition (constriction) of the œsophagus.
Burning in the throat.
45. Angina gangrenosa, (with aphthæ.)

Appetite and Taste.

Violent, unquenchable, burning thirst, with frequent drinking, with but little at a time.
Longing for cold water, acids, or alcoholic drinks.
Aversion to food, loathing the thought of eating.
Bitter taste in the mouth after eating and drinking.

Stomach.

50. Vomiting of the ingesta, (after each meal,) after drinking; of a brown substance with violent pain in the stomach; of

a black substance; of blood; of a green substance; with diarrhœa after drinking the least quantity.

Great painfulness and anxiety in the pit of the stomach and stomach.

Burning in the pit of the stomach and stomach.

Inflammation or induration of the stomach.

Cramp in the stomach, (2, A. M.)

Abdomen.

55. Hard, bloated abdomen,

Burning pains, with anguish.

Sensation of coldness, (upper part.)

Induration of the mesenteric glands.

Painful swelling and induration of the inguinal glands.

60. Ulcers about the navel.

Ascites.

Stool and Anus.

Burning stools, with violent pains in the bowels, with tenesmus, thirst, worse after eating.

Stools acrid, burning, consisting of mucus; black, bloody, offensive, watery and painless, involuntary.

In the rectum and anus, burning and soreness.

65. Prolapsus ani.

Hæmorrhoidal tumors, with burning pain.

Urinary Organs.

Suppressed or difficult micturition. (Paralysis of the bladder.)

Urine bloody, burning.

Involuntary discharge of burning urine.

Sexual Organs.

70. *Men.* Painful swelling of the genitals, and gangrene.

Blue-red swelling of the glans, with rhagades.

Erysipelatous inflammation of the scrotum.

Women. Catamenia too early, and too profuse.

Leucorrhœa acrid, corroding.

75. Scirrhus uteri.

Respiratory Organs.

Dryness, burning, and constriction in the larynx.

Bronchitis, with difficult secretion of mucus.

Respiration oppressed, anxious, short.

Oppressed, labored breathing, especially when ascending a height; in cold air; when turning in bed.

80. Suffocating spells in the evening, when lying down.

Constriction of the chest, with anguish; worse when moving.

Chilliness or coldness in the chest.

Heat, burning, itching in the chest.
Stitches and pressing in the sternum.
85. Cough, without expectoration, especially after drinking or eating; when lying down; during a walk in the cold air.
Cough, with arrest of breathing; with tough mucus in the chest; with expectoration of frothy mucus in lumps, or tasting salty; in day-time, without expectoration at night.
Periodically returning cough, (hooping-cough,) from burning-tickling in the pharynx.
Hæmoptysis at night, with burning heat over the whole body.
Palpitation of the heart, especially at night, with great anguish.

Back.

90. Burning in the back.
Sensation of weakness, as if bruised in the small of the back.

Extremities.

Upper. Rheumatic pains from the elbow up to the shoulder, worse at night.
Swelling of the arm, with putrid smelling, black blisters.
Burning ulcers on the tips of the fingers.
95. Sensation of swelling and fulness in the palms of the hands at night.
Soreness between the fingers.
Nails discolored.
Lower. Tearing and stinging in the hips, legs, and loins.
Tearing in the tibia.
100. Old ulcers on lower limbs, with burning and lancinating pains.
Ulcers on the soles of the feet and toes.
Swelling of the feet, hard, burning, shining, with red spots, or blue-black blisters.
Itching herpes in the bends of the knee.
Varices.

Generalities.

105. Paralysis, especially of the lower extremities.
Trembling of the limbs (in drunkards.)
Sudden sinking of strength.
Fainting, from weakness, with scarcely perceptible pulse.
Burning pains of inner or exterior parts (glands.)
110. Tearing pains in the arms and legs, which do not permit one to lie on the painful side, but which are relieved by moving the affected part.
Dropsy of internal and external parts.
Emaciation.

Sleep.

Starting of the limbs when on the point of falling asleep.
Sleeplessness, from anguish and restlessness, with tossing about (after midnight.)
115. Sleep anxious, unquiet.

Fever.

Pulse frequent in the morning, slower in the evening.
Pulse small, contracted, frequent, weak, tremulous or intermittent.
General coldness, with parchment-like dryness of the skin, or with profuse, cold, clammy perspiration.
Chilliness, without thirst; worse after drinking; with stretching of the limbs and restlessness; with external heat at the same time; when walking in the open air.
120. Internal heat, burning, dry, with anxiousness at night.
Intermittent fever, chill (in the afternoon) followed by dry, evening heat, and later sweat.
Thirst only during the hot stage, drinks often, but little at a time.
During the fever, great restlessness and anxiety, pain in the bones, small of the back, forehead; nausea, difficulty of breathing.
Perspiration at the beginning of sleep, or all night; cold, clammy, smelling sour or offensive.
125. During perspiration, unquenchable thirst; after the fever, attack of headache.
The concomitant complaints are more developed during the chill and fever.

Skin.

Dry, burning heat—dryness—like parchment.
Swelling—blue-black—dropsical.
130. Petechiæ.
White miliary eruptions.
Urticaria.
Red pustules, changing to ichorous, crusty, burning and spreading ulcers.
Vesicular eruptions.
135. Exanthema, black, pock-shaped, gangrenous.
Carbuncles (burning.)
Herpes, with vesicles, and violently burning, especially at night, or with coverings like fish-scales.
Ulcers, hard on the edges, stinging, burning, spongy; with proud flesh; turning black; flat; pus thin, ichorous (cancers.)
Sphacelus.

Conditions.

140. Cannot rest in any place; changing his position continually; wants to go from one bed to another, and lies now here, and now there.
Attacks of pains, with chilliness.
Periodical complaints.
Attacks of pain, driving one to despair, and even to madness.
The pains are felt during sleep.
145. Bad effects from poisoning, with anthrax, and other noxious substances (dissecting wounds.)
Aggravation, at night, after midnight, (1, A. M.)
From cold in general.
After drinking (wine or alcoholic drinks.)
From cold food, (ice-cream.)
From milk.
While lying on the affected side, or with the head low.
Amelioration. From heat in general.
From lying with the head high.

ARUM TRYPHYLLUM.

Eyes.
Aversion to light.

Nose.
Sore; discharge of burning, ichorous fluid from the nose, excoriating the nostrils and upper lip.
Nose stopped up; can only breathe with mouth open.

Face and Mouth.
Tongue sore, red, papillæ elevated.
5. Lips swollen, cracked; corners of the mouth sore, bleeding, cracked.
The mouth burns, and is so sore that he refuses to drink, and cries when any thing is offered.
Face swollen.
Swelling of the sub-maxillary glands.
Throat sore; feels as if excoriated; cannot swallow.
10. Excessive salivation—saliva acrid.

Urine.
Frequent discharge of abundant pale urine.

ASA FŒTIDA.

Respiratory Organs.
Hoarseness (clergymen's sore throat) worse from talking.
Voice uncertain, and changing continually.
Accumulation of mucus in the trachea.

Sleep.
15. Sleeplessness, from soreness of mouth and throat, or itching of the skin.

Fever.
Dry heat of the skin.

Skin.
Exanthema like scarlet rash, the skin peels off afterwards.
Itching of the scarlet eruption.

Conditions.
Amelioration in Scarlet fever, as soon as the urine becomes more abundant and watery.

ASA FŒTIDA.

Mind and Disposition.
Hysterical restlessness and anxiety.

Head.
The pains in the head cease, or change from touch.

Eyes.
Sensation of dryness in the eyes.

Ears.
Hardness of hearing, with discharge of pus from the ears.

Nose.
5. Ozæna, discharge of very offensive matter from the nose.

Face.
Sensation of numbness in the bones of the face.

Mouth and Throat.
Sensation of dryness in the mouth and throat.
Sensation of a ball rising in the throat.

Abdomen.
Pulsation in the pit of the stomach.
10. Sensation of fulness in the stomach.

Stool and Anus.
Diarrhœa, very offensive, with pain in the abdomen and discharge of fetid flatus.

Urine.
Urine brown, and of pungent smell.
Spasm in the bladder during and after urination.

Respiratory Orgns.
Spasmodic dyspnœa, as if the lungs could not be sufficiently expanded.
15. Stitches in the chest from within outwards.

Extremities.
Twitching of the muscles of the arms and legs.
Ulcer on the tibia.
Swelling and caries of the bones of the feet.
Stitches and pulsation in the big toe.

Generalities.
20. Sense of rigor.
Body heavy and bloated.
Hysterical attacks.
Twitching and jerking in the muscles.
Dull stitches (periodically) from within outwards, changed or relieved by touch.
25. Pains in the inside of the joints and limbs.
St. Vitus' dance.

Sleep.
Much against his habit, he is much inclined to sleep.

Fever.
Pulse small, rapid, and unequal.
Heat in the face after dinner, with anxiety or drowsiness, without thirst.

Skin.
30. Ulcers, very painful to contact, especially in the circumference, gangrenous.
Inflammation and caries of the bones, with thin, fetid pus.

Conditions.
Bad effects from the abuse of mercury, especially in syphilis.
Most pains are accompanied by numbness in the affected parts.
Many symptoms appear while sitting, and are relieved in the open air.

ASARUM EROPÆUM.

Mind and Disposition.
Nervous irritability and exaltation.

Head.
Pain, as from contraction in the forehead, temples, and behind the ears, with watering and burning of the eyes, worse in the afternoon, (5, P.M.,) relieved when sitting, and by washing.

Eyes.
Inflamed eyes, blear-eyedness.
The eyes stare.
5. The cold air is pleasant to the eyes; sunshine, light, and wind, are intolerable.

Ears.
Pressure and tension in the region of the orifice of the meatus auditorius.

Mouth.
Accumulation of cold, watery saliva in the mouth.

Stomach.
Eructations putrid or sour, setting the teeth on edge.
Violent, empty retching, which increases all the symptoms, only relieving the head.
10. Vomiting, with great anguish, under violent exertion, with chilliness.
Vomiting, with diarrhœa and violent colic.

Stool and Anus.
Diarrhœa, consisting of tenacious mucus.
During stool, discharge of thick, black blood.
Prolapsus ani during stool.
15. After stool, pressing and straining, and discharge of white, viscid, bloody mucus.

Generalities.
Over-sensitiveness of the nerves, the scratching of linen or silk is insupportable.

Sensation of lightness in the limbs, when she walks she thinks she is gliding through the air.

Fever.

Pulse full and accelerated.
Chilliness and coldness, after eating and drinking, with heat of the head.
20. Heat, especially in the face, and in the palms of the hands.
Perspiration smelling sour at night, in the arm-pits.
Easily excited perspiration, especially on the upper part of the body.

Conditions.

Aggravation in the evening, and in cold and dry weather.
Amelioration. Many symptoms disappear from washing the face in cold water, and from wetting the affected part.

AURUM FOLIATUM.

Mind and Disposition.

Melancholy mood, dejected, inclined to weep, and longing to die.
Excessive anguish, increasing even to self-destruction.
The least contradiction excites his wrath.
Alternate peevishness and cheerfulness.

Head.

5. Congestions to and heat in the head, with sparks before the eyes, and glossy bloatedness of the face, aggravated from every mental exertion.
Sensation, as if a current of air were rushing through the head, if it be not kept warm.
The bones of the skull are painful, especially when lying down.
Exostosis on the head.

Eyes.

Protruded eyes.
10. Vertical half-sight.
Fiery sparks before the eyes.

Ears.

Caries of the mastoid process.
Fetid otorrhœa.
Roaring in the ears.

Nose.

15. Caries of the nose.
    Discharge of fetid pus from the nose.
    Fetid odor from the nose.
    Very sensitive smell.

Face.

Bloated, shining face.
20. Swelling of the cheeks.
    Inflammation of the bones of the face.
    Painful swelling of the sub-maxillary glands.

Mouth and Throat.

Putrid smell from the mouth, as of old cheese.
Caries of the palate, especially after the abuse of mercury.

Stomach.

25. Immoderate appetite and thirst, with qualmishness in the stomach.

Stool and Anus.

Constipation; stool very large in size, or very hard or knotty.
Nightly diarrhœa, with burning in the rectum.

Urinary Organs.

Painful retention of urine, with pressure in the bladder.
He passes more urine than corresponds to the quantity he drinks.

Sexual Organs.

30. *Men.* Induration of the testes.
    Swelling of the (lower part) of the testicle (right.)
    Sexual desire increased.
    Women. Prolapsus and induration of the uterus.

Chest.

Suffocative attacks, with suffocative oppression of the chest.
35. Anxious palpitation of the heart, from congestion to the chest.

Generalities.

Over-sensitiveness to all pain, and to the cold air.
Hysterical spasms, with laughing and crying, alternately.
Great ebullitions, with congestions to the head and chest, and palpitation of the heart.

Sleep.

Sleepiness after dinner.
40. Frightful dreams—he sobs aloud when asleep.

Fever.

Pulse small, but accelerated.

BARYTA.

Chilliness predominates—coldness of the hands and feet, sometimes lasting all night.
Heat, only in the face.
Perspiration in the morning-hours; the strongest on and around the genitals.

Skin.

45. Ulcers (after the abuse of mercury) which attack the bones.
Inflammation of the bones—caries (palate and nasal bones.)

Conditions.

Bad effects from the misuse of mercury.
Paralytic drawing-in of the limbs in the morning, when awaking; and on getting cold.
Pain in the bones, at night.
50. Aggravation in the morning; on getting cold; while reposing.
Amelioration, from moving; while walking; and on getting warm.

BARYTA.

Mind and Disposition.

Mistrust; want of self-confidence, and aversion to strangers (the child does not want to play.)
Deficient memory (children cannot remember and learn.)

Head.

Pricking headache near the warm stove.
Baldness.
5. The scalp is very sensitive to the touch, especially on the side on which he lies, with the sensation of suggillation, worse from scratching.
Dry or humid scurf on the head.

Eyes.

The light hurts the eyes, and in the dark he sees sparks before them.
Burning and pressing in the eyes, if he looks attentively at any thing.
Inflammation of the eyes, with sensation of dryness.

Ears.

10. Cracking in the ears when swallowing, sneezing, and when walking fast.

Face.

Dark redness of the face, with congestions to the face.
Tension on the face, as if it were covered by spider webs.
Swelling of the submaxillary glands, with induration.

Mouth and Throat.

Tongue cracked, feels very sore.
15. Inflammation of the throat, with swollen, inflamed tonsils.
Sensation, as from a plug in the throat.

Stomach.

Weakness of the digestion after eating, pressing in the stomach; and pain in the hard, swollen abdomen.
Sensation of soreness of the stomach; while eating, it feels as if the food had to force itself through some raw places.

Stool and Anus.

Sudden, irresistible urging to stool, with painful soreness in the lumbar region, followed by frequent diarrhœtic stools.
20. Anus sore and humid.
Crawling in the rectum, (ascarides.)

Sexual Organs.

Erections (only) in the morning before rising.
Soreness and moistening between the scrotum and thighs.

Chest and Respiratory Organs.

Suffocative catarrh, and paralysis of the lungs in old people.
25. Sensation of soreness in the chest.
Sensation, as if something hard dropped down in the chest.
Sensation of smoke in the larynx.
Hoarseness and loss of voice from tough mucus in the larynx and trachea.
Palpitation and soreness of the heart, renewed by lying on the left side, and when thinking of it.
30. Spasmodic cough (like hooping-cough) from roughness and tickling in the throat and pit of the stomach.
Cough worse in the evening till midnight; after getting the feet cold; from exercise; when lying on the left side; in the cold air; from thinking of it.

Back and Neck.

Stiffness of the nape of the neck.
Sarcoma in the neck, with burning.

Beating and pulsation in the back.
35. Stiffness in the small of the back, in the evening, especially while sitting, which allows neither to rise nor to bend backwards.

Extremities.
Upper. Painfulness of the arms, with swelling of the axillary glands.
Lower. Fetid perspiration of the feet.
Corns, with burning and stinging.

Generalities.
Paralysis and palsy of aged persons.
40. Great weakness of mind and body of old men.
Emaciation, with bloated face, swelled abdomen, and difficult learning in children.
Tearing in the limbs, with chilliness.
Heaviness of the body.
Tension and shortening of the muscles.

Sleep.
45. Sleepiness day and night.

Fever.
Pulse accelerated, but weak.
Chilliness relieved by external heat.
Flushes of heat, more at night, with great restlessness.
Perspiration, one-sided, (left side,) every other evening.

Skin.
50. Burning prickings here and there.
Soreness and humid skin.
Swelling and induration of the glands.
Warts.

Conditions.
Especially suitable for old people, or scrofulous children, especially those who suffer from inflammation of the throat and swelling of the tonsils after the least cold.
55. Great liability to take cold, (sore throat,) stiffness of the neck, or diarrhœa.
The left side is most affected.
Aggravation while sitting, or when lying on the painful side, or when thinking of his disease.
Amelioration when walking in the open air.

BELLADONNA.

Mind and Disposition.

Nervous anxiety, restlessness, desire to escape.
Stupefaction, with congestion to the head; pupils enlarged—delirium.
Loss of consciousness.
Fantastic illusions (when closing the eyes.)
5. Rage, madness, disposition to bite, to spit, to strike and to tear things.
Disinclination to talk, or very fast talking.
Delirium, with frightful figures and images before the eyes.

Head.

Vertigo, with stupefaction, vanishing of sight and great debility.
Vertigo, with anguish, and falling insensibly on the left side, or backwards, with flickering before the eyes, especially when stooping, and when rising from a stooping posture.
10. Congestion of blood to the head, with external and internal heat; distended and pulsating arteries, stupefaction in the forehead, burning, red face; worse in the evening—when leaning the head forward, from the slightest noise, and from motion.
Stupefying, stunning headache, extending from the neck into the head, with heat and pulsation in it; worse in the evening, and from motion; better when laying the hand on the head, and when bending the head backward.
Boring headache in the right side of the head; changing to stitches in the evening.
Pressing headache, as if the head would split, pupils contracted, voice faint.
Periodical nervous headache, every day from 4, P.M., till 3, A.M., aggravated by the heat of the bed, and when lying down.
15. Jerks in the head, especially when walking fast, or when ascending steps; better from external pressure.
Inflammation of the brain, with burning and pulsation in the head; first in the cerebellum, then in the forehead, and

later in the whole head—blood-vessels on the head and neck enlarged, shaking with the head or boring in the pillows; worse in the evening, and when lying.

Hydrocephalus, with boring with the head in the pillows; sensation as if water were moving in the head; worse in the evening and when lying; better from external pressure, and from bending the head backwards.

Headache, from taking cold in the head, and from having the hair cut.

Headache, worse on the right side.

20. Headache, aggravated by moving the eyes, by shaking the head, when lying down, from a draft of air; relieved by sitting up, leaning the head backward, from pressing the head with the hands.

External heat and soreness of the head.

Smooth, erysipelatous, hot swelling, first of the face, then extending over the whole head, with stupefaction or delirium; violent headache, red, fiery eyes.

Stitches in the bones of the neck.

Convulsive shaking and bending of the head backwards.

25. Boring the head into the pillow.

Profuse, pungent-smelling perspiration, especially on the covered parts, while the body is burning hot.

Eyes.

Congestion of blood to the eyes, and redness of the veins.

Heat in the eyes—distention of the sclerotica.

Yellowness of the whites of the eyes.

30. Eyes sparkling, red, glistening, or dim.

Look, wild, unsteady, wavering.

Continued lachrymation (tears sharp and salty.)

Distortion, spasms, and convulsions of the eyes.

Photophobia, or photomania.

35. Ectropium.

Blindness at night (moon-blindness.)

Things look red.

He sees sparks of fire.

Diplopia.

40. Squinting.

Paralysis of the optic nerve.

Ears.

Inflammation of the external and internal (right) ear, with discharge of pus.

Stinging in and behind the ears.

Humming and roaring in the ears.

45. Paralysis of the auditory nerves.

Inflammatory swelling of the parotid glands—stitches in the parotid gland.

Nose.

Inflammatory swelling and redness of the external and internal nose.
Bleeding of the nose, with redness of the face.
Over-sensitiveness of the sense of smell.
50. Putrid smell from the nose.

Face.

Purple, red, hot face, or yellow color of the face.
Face pale, sunken, with distorted, anxious countenance.
Alternate redness and paleness of the face.
Convulsive motions of the muscles of the face and mouth.
55. Spasmodic distortion of the mouth (risus sardonicus.)
Erysipelatous swelling of the face.
Semilateral swelling of the face.
Nervous prosopalgia, with violent, cutting pains.
Lips dark red, swollen, indurated.
60. Swelling of the upper lip.
Ulcerated corners of the mouth.
Mouth half open, or spasmodically closed by lock-jaw.
Stitches in the articulations of the jaws.
Swelling and inflammation of the sub-maxillary glands.

Teeth.

65. Toothache, drawing and tearing up into the ear, with swelling of the cheek; worse in the evening and at night; aggravated by the cold air, by contact, while masticating, by mental exertion.
Grinding of the teeth.
Swelling of the gums, with burning heat and stinging.

Mouth.

Dryness of the mouth, without thirst.
Inflammatory swelling and redness of the inner mouth and soft palate.
70. Tongue hot, dry, red, cracked; or only red on the edges, with white coating on the middle; coated white or brown, or covered with mucus.
Inflammatory swelling of the tongue, painful to the touch.
Heaviness of the tongue, with difficulty in talking.
Stuttering.
Speaks through the nose, speechlessness.
75. Hemorrhage from the mouth.

Throat.

Inflammation of the throat, with sensation of a lump, which induces hawking, with dark redness and swelling of the velum palate, and pudendum.
Burning and dryness in the œsophagus.
Stinging in the œsophagus, in the tonsils; worse when swallowing, and when talking.
The œsophagus feels contracted, spasms in the throat not permitting one to swallow, the drink swallowed is discharged through the nostrils.
80. Continual inclination to swallow.
Tonsils inflamed, swollen, ulcers rapidly forming on them.

Appetite and Taste.

Loss of taste.
Taste bitter, insipid, sour (bread) or sticky, slimy taste in the mouth.
Excessive burning thirst, with constant desire to drink, drinks hastily; or aversion to drink, or inability to swallow.
85. Aversion to meat, acids, milk, beer.

Stomach and Abdomen.

Bitter eructations.
Gulping up of food.
Vomiting, of water; of mucus; of acid; of bile; of blood.
Empty retching.
90. Painful pressure in the pit of the stomach and stomach, especially after eating.
Spasms of the stomach.
Painfully distended abdomen, very sensitive to the touch.
Colic, with restlessness, below the umbilicus, as from clutching and griping with the nails, worse from external pressure.
Flatulent colic, (with protrusion of the transverse colon, like a pad,) ameliorated by bending forwards and by external pressure.
95. Stitches in the left side of the abdomen when coughing, sneezing, and touching it.

Stool and Anus.

Stool in lumps, like chalk.
Frequent small diarrhœic stools of mucus.
Thin, green stools, with frequent micturition and perspiration.
Dysenteric stools.
100. Involuntary evacuations.
Before stool, perspiration.
During stool, shuddering.

Spasmodic stricture of the rectum.
Paralysis of the sphincter ani.
105. Stinging pain in the rectum.

Urine.

Retention of urine.
Difficult discharge of urine, (and then discharge of a few drops of bloody urine only.)
Urine scanty, fiery red, dark, turbid.
Continuous dropping of urine.
110. Paralysis of the sphincter vesicæ.
Strictures of the urethra.

Sexual Organs.

Men. Inflammation of the testicles, great hardness in the drawn-up testicles.
Women. Great pressing in the genital organs, as if every thing would protrude.
Spasmodic contraction of the uterus.
115. Labor-pains too distressing, spasmodic,—too weak, or ceasing.
After-pains.
Congestion and inflammation of the uterus and labia.
Prolapsus and induration of the uterus.
Stitches in the organs.
120. Dryness of the vagina.
Metrorrhagia, blood clotted, with violent pain in the small of the back, and bearing down.
Puerperal fever, nymphomania.
Catamenia too early and too profuse.
Menstrual blood of bright color, or of a bad smell.
125. Lochial discharges in clots, and of bad smell.

Larynx and Trachea.

Larynx very painful, with anxious starts when touching it.
Constriction of the trachea.
Voice rough, with a nasal sound.
Hoarseness, loss of voice.
130. Short, dry cough, from tickling in the larynx, with headache, redness and heat in the face.
Cough, with stitches in the chest, in the lumbar region, in the hip, in the uterus,—pain in the sternum, with tightness of the chest,—with rattling of mucus on the chest.
Dry, spasmodic cough, with vomiturition, especially after midnight.
Barking cough.
Hooping-cough, with crying, or pain in the stomach before the attack, with expectoration of blood, (pale or coagu-

lated,) congestion of blood to the head, sparks before the eyes, spasms in the throat, bleeding from the nose, stitches in the spleen, involuntary stool and urine, oppressed breathing, stiffness of the limbs, shaking of the whole body, and general dry heat.
135. The cough is renewed by the least motion, (especially at night.)

Chest.

Breathing labored, unequal, quick, with moaning.
Vehement expirations.
Feeling of suffocation when swallowing, or when touching and turning the neck.
Oppression of the chest in the morning when rising, cannot breathe in the room, better in the open air.
140. Congestion to the chest.
Stitches in the chest, especially when coughing or yawning.
Violent palpitation of the heart, reverberating in the head.
Mammæ swelled, inflamed or indurated.
Flow of milk.

Back.

145. Stiffness of the neck.
Painful swelling of the glands of the neck.
Intense cramp—pain in the small of the back and the os coccyx; he can only sit for a short time.

Extremities.

Upper. Arms heavy, as if paralyzed.
Scarlet redness and swelling of the arms and hands.
150. Painful twitchings, spasms and convulsions in the arms and hands.
Lower. Coxalgia, with stinging pain or burning in the hip-joint; worse at night; aggravated by the least contact.
Involuntary limping.
Heaviness and paralysis of the legs and feet.
Tottering walk—when rising from bed in the morning, the legs refuse their service.
155. *Phlegmasia alba dolens.*

Generalities.

Over-excitability of all the senses.
Spasms in single limbs, or of the whole body, in children, during dentition.
St. Vitus's dance.
Epileptic spasms.
160. Renewal of the spasms by the least contact, or from the glare of light.
Hydrophobia.

Full habit (plethora.)
Congestions (head, lungs.)
Apoplexia.
165. Burning in the inner parts.
Rheumatic pains (in the joints) flying from one place to another.

Sleep.

Sleeplessness, with drowsiness.
Somnolence—stupor—lethargy (with snoring.)
Fearful visions, when closing the eyes to sleep.
170. Starting, when closing the eyes, or during sleep, as in a fright.
Dreams anxious—night-mare.
Sleep, with moaning and tossing about.

Fever.

Pulse. Pulse accelerated, often full and hard, tense, occasionally soft and small; if slow, the pulse is full.
Chilliness in the evening, especially on the extremities (arms) with heat of the head.
175. Cold limbs, with hot head.
Chilliness not relieved by the heat of the stove.
Chilliness as soon as he moves under the cover.
Internal and external burning heat, with restlessness.
Continuous dry, burning heat, with perspiration only on the head.
180. Internal heat, with restlessness; hot forehead and cold cheeks.
Dry heat, with thirst, and perspiration only on the head and neck (sour smelling.)
Perspiration exclusively on the covered parts, during sleep, ascending from the feet to the head.

Skin.

Dry, burning-hot skin.
Smooth, even, shining (not circumscribed) redness, of the skin, with bloatedness, dryness, heat, burning, itching and swelling of the parts (especially face, neck, chest, abdomen and hands.)
185. Erysipelatous inflammations.
Scarlet-red rash (over the whole body.)
Miliary eruptions.
Vesicular eruptions, with scabs, white edges and œdematous swellings.
Boils (returning every spring.)
190. Glands swelled, inflamed, painful, stinging.
Bleeding soreness of the bends of the joints.
Ulcers, with burning pain when touching them.

Conditions.

Indurations, after inflammation.
Liability to take cold, with great sensitiveness to draft of air, especially when uncovering the head.
195. Bad effects from valerian, mercury, china and opium.
Aggravation, in the afternoon, and after midnight; on moving; from touching the parts even softly; on walking in the wind; from a draft of air; on looking at shining or glistening objects; while drinking.
Amelioration, on bending the affected part backwards or inwards; from leaning the head against something; while standing.

BENZOIC ACID.

Mind and Disposition.

Inclination to dwell on unpleasant subjects.
While writing, he often omits words.

Head.

Giddiness, especially in the afternoon, as if he would fall on his side.
Pressure on the vertex, extending to the spine,—without pain, but with anxiety.
5. Rheumatic pains in the head.
Headache from a draft of air; from uncovering the head; in the morning, when awaking; worse when at rest, returning periodically, and accompanied by pain in the stomach, nausea, and cold hands.
Cold perspiration on the head.

Face.

Burning heat of one side of the face.
Circumscribed redness on the cheeks.
10. Copper-colored spots on the face.
Cold perspiration of the face.

Tongue.

The tongue is spongy on the surface, with deep cracks, and with spreading ulcers.

Throat.

Sensation, as of a lump in the pit of the throat, as if some food had lodged there.
Sensation of swelling or constriction in the throat.
15. The throat symptoms are relieved by eating.

Stool and Anus.

Watery, light-colored, very offensive stools, (in children,) with unusually strong-smelling urine.

Urinary Organs.

Soreness, or hot, burning pain in the (left) kidney.
Frequent desire to urinate.
Urine contains mucus and pus, (with enlargement of prostate gland.)
20. Urine of dark color, with unusually strong smell; heavy, hot.

Chest.

Long-continued, dry cough, after suppressed gonorrhœa.
Pains in the region of the heart.
Awakens every morning at 2 o'clock, with violent internal heat, and hard, beating pulse, compelling him to lie on the back, because the beating of the temporal arteries causes a humming in the ears, and prevents him from going to sleep.
Awakens after midnight with violent palpitation of the heart, and hard beating of the temporal arteries.

Extremities.

25. Tearing and stitches, especially in the right big toe, (gout.

Generalities.

Great weakness, perspiration, and comatose condition.
Trembling, with palpitation of the heart.

Sleep.

Awakens with oppression of breathing, with palpitation of the heart, (after midnight,) with heat and hard pulse.

Fever.

Chilliness before the stool.
30. Great internal heat when awaking.
Perspiration while eating.

Conditions.

The pains suddenly change their locality, but are mostly felt in the region of the heart.
When moving, cracking of the joints.
Aggravation of the headache, when at rest; of the toothache, when lying; of the eye and ear symptoms in the open

air; of the head symptoms, when uncovering one's self, and when in a draft of air.
35. Amelioration of the face symptoms by heat.
The most of the symptoms appear first on the left, and then on the right side.

BERBERIS VULGARIS.

Mind and Disposition.
Indifference, apathy.
Melancholy, inclination to weep.

Head.
Darting and shooting pains in the head, often changing their locality.
Heat in the head after dinner, or in the afternoon.
5. Headache aggravated by movement, relieved in the open air.

Eyes.
Dryness of, or biting,—burning, or itching sensation in the eyes.
Itching in the canthi, eyebrows, and eyelids.

Ears.
Stitches in the ear.

Nose.
Dryness in the nose.

Face.
10. Pale face, with a dingy-grayish tinge, sunken cheeks, and deep-seated eyes, surrounded with bluish and blackish-gray border.

Mouth.
The mouth feels dry and sticky.
Painful white blisters on the tip of the tongue.

Throat.
Inflammation of the tonsils and pharynx, with swelling and fiery redness, and a sensation as if a lump were lodged in the side of the throat; expectoration of a quantity of thick, yellow, jelly-like mucus,—white, sticky tongue, viscid saliva resembling soap-suds.

Appetite and Taste.
Thirst and dryness of the mouth.
15. Taste bitter.

Abdomen.
Pressure in the region of the liver.
Burning under the skin, in the left side of the abdomen.

Stool and Anus.
Hard, scanty stool, (like sheep's dung.)
Watery evacuations.
20. Burning, stinging pain in the anus, before, during, and after stool.
Hemorrhoidal tumors, with burning pain after stool.
Painful pressure in the perinæum; stitches in the perinæum, extending deep into the (left side) pelvis (fistula in ano.)

Urine.
Lancinating or tearing pulsative pains in the region of the kidneys; worse when stooping and rising again, sitting or lying; better when standing.
Violent sticking pains in the bladder, extending from the kidneys into the urethra, with urging to urinate.
25. Frequently recurring, crampy, contractive pain, or aching pain, in the bladder, when the bladder is full or empty.
Stitches in the urethra, extending into the bladder.
Stitches and burning in the urethra.
Frequent urging to urinate.
Urine dark yellow, red, becoming turbid, copious; mucous sediment, or transparent, jelly-like or reddish, bran-like sediment.
30. Greenish urine, depositing mucus.
Blood-red urine, depositing a copious, slimy, bright-red, bran-like sediment.
During urination, burning in the urethra, with pressure on the bladder.
After urination, burning in the urethra, or bladder, pressure in the bladder, cutting, burning, and stitches in the urethra.
Movement brings on or increases the urinary difficulties.
35. With the symptoms in the urinary organs, pain in the loins and hips.

Sexual Organs.
Men. Dragging or lancinating pains in the spermatic cord, extending into the testicles.
Cold feeling in the prepuce and scrotum.
Women. Catamenia too scanty, painful (pain in the small of the back.)

BERBERIS VULGARIS.

Menses, consisting of gray mucus or brown blood.
40. Suppressed menstruation.

Chest.
Stitches in the chest (left side.)

Back.
Stitches in the spine.
Numbness in the small of the back.
Pain in the small of the back; worse when sitting and lying in the morning, when awaking (during menstruation.)

Generalities.
45. Great weakness, like fainting, after a walk, with perspiration and heat on the upper part of the body; cold, pale, sunken face and oppression of breathing.

Sleep.
Great sleepiness during the day and after dinner.
Sleep unrefreshing.

Fever.
Pulse slow and weak, or full, hard and rapid.
Chilliness, with hot face, followed by heat, with perspiration, or burning heat in the afternoon, increasing during the night.
50. Perspires easily from the least exertion.

Conditions.
Rheumatic and gouty complaints, with diseases of the urinary organs.
Movement increases or causes the complaints.

BISMUTHUM.

Mind and Disposition.
Apathy and continual complaints, with peevish dissatisfaction.
Solitude is intolerable to him.

Head.
Sensation of weight in the forehead, temples and occiput.

Face.
Earthy paleness of face, with distorted features, and blue borders around the eyes.

Mouth.
5. White-coated tongue in the evening.
Sensation of soreness in the mouth.

Appetite and Taste.
Great thirst in the evening for cold drinks (without heat.)

Stomach.
Nausea after every meal.
Vomiting (of bile) with oppressive anxiety, small pulse, vertigo and prostration.
10. Vomiting and diarrhœa.
Vomiting of all fluids (children.)
Pressure in the stomach, especially after a meal.
Burning in the stomach. (Inflammation of the stomach.)

Stool and Anus.
Urging to stool in the evening, without any evacuations.

Urinary Organs.
15. Frequent and copious micturition; the urine is watery.

Sexual Organs.
Pressing, aching in the (right) testicle.

Generalities.
Sensation of heaviness in the inner parts.
Screwing pains.
Pressing pains (eyes, head, abdomen, testicles.)
20. Pressing-tearing (bones of the hands and of the feet.)

Fever.
Flushes of heat, especially on head and chest.

Conditions.
Most symptoms disappear during motion.

BORAX.

Mind and Disposition.

Easily frightened, and starting from the least noise.
Anxiety, with sleepiness, increased towards evening.
The child feels an anguish when rocked in a cradle, has an anxious countenance during the downward motion, (when carried down stairs.)
Parts, which are usually red, turn white.

Head.

5. Vertigo in the morning, in bed.
Headache in the forenoon, (10, A. M.,) with nausea and trembling of the body.
Hot head (hot mouth and hands) of the infant.

Eyes.

The eyelashes turn inward into the eye, inflaming it, especially in the external canthus, where the borders of the lids are quite sore.
Itching in the external canthus of the eye.

Ears.

10. Discharge of pus from the ears, with hardness of hearing; with roaring in the (left) ear.

Nose.

Dry scabs in the nose.

Face.

Tetter around the mouth.
Burning heat and redness of the left cheek.

Mouth and Throat.

Aphthæ in the mouth, and on the tongue, bleeding when eating.
15. Tenacious, whitish phlegm in the throat, which can only be loosened with great exertion.

Stomach and Abdomen.

Distention from flatulence after every meal.
Hiccough after dinner.

Stool and Anus.

Frequent soft, light-yellow, slimy stools.
Diarrhœa after breakfast.
20. Stitches in the rectum.

Urinary Organs.

Frequent micturition, (acrid-smelling urine.)
Hot urine in infants.

Sexual Organs.

Men. During cöition, the semen escapes either too early or too late.
Women. Catamenia too early, and too profuse.
25. During the catamenia, spasmodic pressure and stitches in the groin.
Sterility, or easy conception.
Fluor albus, like the white of an egg, or acrid.
Stitches in the region of the uterus.
Sensation of contraction in the left mamma, while the child nurses from the right.
30. Aphthæ on the nipples, they bleed.

Chest.

Stitches in the chest, whenever he coughs, or takes a deep inspiration.

Extremities.

Lower. Stitches in the soles of the feet.
Suppuration of a spot in the heel, where the rubbing of the shoe had occasioned a wound.
Frequent stitches in the corns.
35. Great weakness and debility of the lower extremities.

Generalities.

Restlessness and ebullitions, especially after talking, with nausea.

Sleep.

Sleepiness during the day, and sleeplessness at night.
The child starts from his sleep, and cries.

Fever.

Chilliness, especially during sleep.
40. Flushes of heat, (morning and evening.)
Perspiration during the morning sleep.

Skin.

Unwholesome skin, small wounds suppurate and ulcerate.
Erysipelatous inflammation on the lower leg, with chilliness, followed by heaviness and pulsation in the head; later, bleeding of the nose.

Conditions.

Consequences from getting cold when the weather is wet and cold.
Bad effects from riding; from eating fruit, (apples, pears.)
Aggravation after menstruation.

BOVISTA.

Mind and Disposition.
Sad, depressed, and desponding.
Awkwardness; she lets every thing drop out of her hand.
Weak memory.

Head.
Headache deep in the brain, sensation as if the head were enlarged.
5. Sensation as if bruised in the head.

Eyes.
Dim eyes, without lustre.
Objects seem to be too near the eye.

Ears.
Itching in the ears.
Discharge of fetid pus from the ears.
10. Ulcer in the (right) ear.

Nose.
Scurfs and crusts about the nostrils.
Stoppage of the nose with fluent coryza.
Bleeding of the nose early in the morning, (during sleep.)

Face.
Chapped lips.
15. Eruptions in the corners of the mouth.
Swelling of the upper lip (and cheek, after toothache) in scrofulous subjects.

Teeth.
Bleeding of the gums, (when sucking them.)

Stomach and Abdomen.
Bloatedness of the abdomen; with softness, flatulency, or rumbling, with constipation.

Stool and Anus.
Ineffectual urging to stool.

20. Stool hard and difficult.
    After stool, tenesmus and burning at the anus.
    In the rectum, itching, as from worms.
    Darting from the perinæum to the rectum and the genital organs.

Urinary Organs.

Frequent desire to urinate, even immediately after urination. (Diabetes mellitus.)
25. In the urethra, stinging, itching, burning; the orifice is inflamed, and feels as if glued up.

Sexual Organs.

Catamenia too early and too profuse, or too late, too scanty, too short; 'flowing only at night.
Before the catamenia, diarrhœa.
Leucorrhœa thick, slimy, tenacious, acrid, corrosive.

Extremities.

Perspiration in the arm-pits, smelling like onions.
30. Sensation in the wrist-joint, as if sprained.
Weakness of the hands; they let the least thing drop.
Tremor of the hands, with palpitation of the heart and oppressive anxiety.
Blunt instruments (scissors) make deep impressions in the skin of the fingers.

Generalities.

Ebullitions, with much thirst.
35. Great weakness of the joints.

Sleep.

Sleepiness after dinner, and early in the evening.

Fever.

Chilliness and heat, with thirst.
Morning sweat, especially on the chest.

Skin.

Moist tetters
40. Blunt instruments make deep impressions.

BUFO.

Mind and Disposition.
Inclination to be angry—to bite.
Stupor.

Head.
Giddiness, with heaviness of the head.
Headache in the forehead and on the vertex; the parts are tender to the touch, especially in the evening.
5. One-sided headache (right side) relieved by bleeding of the nose.
Headache, after breakfast.
Headache, aggravated by light and noise; accompanied by cold feet and palpitation of the heart.
Profuse perspiration on the head.

Eyes.
Eyes red, injected—itching, swollen.
10. Appearance of objects as if there were a veil before the eyes.

Nose.
Sneezing in the evening when going to bed.
Bleeding of the nose relieving the headache.

Face.
Pimples on the upper lip, with coryza.
Momentary hot flushes of the face.
15. Erysipelas.

Mouth and Tongue.
Stuttering.
Black tongue.
Fetid odor from the mouth.

Throat.
20. Mucus descends from the nose into the posterior nares.
Dryness in the throat, impeding deglutition (morning.)

Appetite and Taste.
Desire for sugar-water.
Sensation, as if he would faint from emptiness in the stomach.

Stomach and Abdomen.

Eructations, as from rotten eggs.
Vomiting, after drinking.
25. After eating, irresistible sleepiness.
Colic pain after drinking milk, and after smoking tobacco.

Stool and Anus.

Stools white.
Constipation, with coldness of the body and hot head.
Hemorrhoidal tumors, with discharge of bright-red blood.

Urinary Organs.

30. Frequent discharge of pale urine.
Urine brown; of offensive odor.
Burning pain in the kidneys, with oppressed breathing and faintiness.

Sexual Organs.

Men. Inclination to touch the genitals.
Women. Menstruation too early—with headache.

Larynx and Chest.

35. Cough, from stitches in the larynx.
Sensation, as if the chest and the heart were constricted.
Stitches in the chest (right side.)
Palpitation of the heart, after a meal, with nausea.

Extremities.

Upper. The arms go to sleep easily.
40. Large blisters in the palms of the hands and soles of the feet.
Panaritium, swelling blue-black around the nail (thumb,) followed by suppuration.
After a slight contusion of the (little) finger, tearing pain, with redness along the whole arm, following the lymphatic vessels into the arm-pit; causing there painful glandular swellings.
Lower. Cramps in the legs, awaking him from his sleep.
Great weakness of the legs.

Generalities.

45. Great weakness—fainting.
Swelling of the whole body.
Twitching of the muscles.
Convulsions. Epilepsy (after fright.)

Sleep.

Sleepiness, after meals.
50. Inclined to lie on the left side.
Sleepiness when he smokes tobacco in the forenoon.

Fever.
Heat, with apathy or delirium, and cold feet.
Skin.
Yellow color of the skin.
Small wounds suppurate much.
55. Carbuncles.
Ulcers, with burning pains.
Conditions.
Aggravation, morning or evening.
The warm room is unpleasant.

BROMINE.

Mind and Disposition.
Cheerful mind; desire for mental labor.
Low-spirited, and out of humor.
Crying and lamentation, with hoarse voice.
Head.
Headache after drinking milk.
5. Pain over the left eye.
Scald-head.
Eyes.
Lachrymation (right eye) with swelling of the tear-gland.
Darting through the eyes, (left.)
Dilatation of the pupils.
10. Flashes before the eyes.
Protruded eyes.
Ears.
Swelling and hardness of the (left) parotid gland.
Nose.
Soreness in the nose, with scurfs.
Bleeding of the nose, relieving the chest.
15. Coryza, with sneezing; the margins of the nose, and the parts under the nose, are corroded, with stoppage of the nose.
Face.
Paleness of the face.
Heat in the cheek; first in the right, later in the left.

Mouth and Throat.

Ptyalism; much frothy mucus in the mouth.
Inflammation of the throat, with net-like redness and corroded places.
20. Burning from the mouth to the stomach.
Stinging in the tip of the tongue.
Heat in the mouth and œsophagus.

Appetite and Taste.

Desire for acids; and diarrhœa from taking them.
Water tastes saltish.

Stomach and Abdomen.

25. Vomiting of bloody mucus.
Nausea and retching; better after eating.
Feeling of emptiness in the stomach; better after eating.
Feeling of heaviness in the stomach, (inflammation of the stomach.)
Enlargement and induration of the spleen.

Stool and Anus.

30. Diarrhœa; stools yellow, green, black.

Sexual Organs.

Men. Swelling and induration of the (left) testicle, with sore pain, or sensation of coldness.
Swelling of the scrotum, (with chronic gonorrhœa.)
Women. Loud emissions of flatulency from the vagina.
During the menses, pain in the abdomen and in the small of the back.

Larynx and Throat.

35. Hoarseness, aphonia; worse in the evening.
Soreness and roughness in the throat.
Tickling in the trachea during an inspiration.
Dry, spasmodic, wheezing cough, with rattling breathing.
Cough rough, barking, from tickling in the throat.
40. Violent oppression of the chest, as from the vapors of sulphur.
Sensation of weakness in the chest.
Tightness of the chest, (asthma.)
Stitches in the chest, (inflammation of the lungs, right side.)
Violent palpitation of the heart; she cannot lie on the left side.

Neck and Back.

45. Goitre.
Two encysted tumors on both sides of the neck.
The left side of the neck is stiff and painful.

Generalities.
Excessive languor and debility, (worse after breakfast.)
Tremulousness all over.
Sleep.
50. Irresistible drowsiness while reading.
Fever.
Pulse much accelerated.
Chill on alternate days, with cold feet.
Internal burning heat.
Perspiration from the least exertion.
Skin.
55. Swelling and induration of the glands, (thyroid, testes, submaxillary, parotid.)
Boils.
Conditions.
Aggravation in the evening till midnight; in the warm room; and when at rest.
Amelioration from motion, riding on horseback.
More suitable for persons with light hair and blue eyes.

BRYONIA ALBA.

Mind and Disposition.
Exceedingly irritable and inclined to be angry.
Restlessness, with fear of the future; fear of death, which he thinks is near.
Despair of recovery.
Delirium at night of the business of the day.
5. Unconsciousness.
After having been angry he is chilly; has a red face and heat in the head.
Head.
Giddiness, with sensation of looseness in the brain when stooping, and when raising up the head.
Fulness and heaviness in the forehead, as if the brain were pressed out; with bleeding of the nose; 'red, bloated face; worse when opening or moving the eyes; when

stooping; in the evening; from motion; better from closing the eyes; from external pressure.

Tearing in one (right) side of the head, extending into the cheek and jaw-bones; worse from motion, touch and heat; better during rest and from external pressure.

10. Heat of the head, with dark-red face; with coldness of the rest of the body; with much thirst and pain in the limbs when moving them; worse in the evening.

Oily, greasy, sour-smelling perspiration on the head (and the whole body) during sleep; at night, especially towards morning.

Greasiness of the hair of the head.

Eyes.

Stitches in the eyes.
Burning in the eyes and edges of the eyelids.
15. Inflammation of the eyes, aggravated by heat.
Inflammation of the eyes, especially in gouty subjects.
The eyes feel as if pressed out of the head.
The eyes feel very sore to touch, and when moving them.
Swollen eyelids, especially the upper lids.

Nose.

20. Swelling of the nose, with very sore pain when touched.
Bleeding of the nose, especially in the morning—with suppressed menstruation.

Face.

Yellow paleness of the face.
Hot. bloated red face.
Nodosities and indurations on the face.
25. Lips dry, swollen; cracked.

Teeth.

Toothache; shooting from one tooth to another, or into the head and cheeks; from an exposed nerve (sensitiveness of the decayed teeth to contact of the air;) pain worse from smoking or chewing tobacco; from introducing any thing warm into the mouth; relieved, momentarily, by cold water, and when lying on the painful side.

Mouth.

Dryness of the mouth, tongue and throat.
Tongue coated white or yellow, especially in the middle.

Throat.

Great dryness in the throat.
30. Stitches in the throat when swallowing.
Sensation of swelling and constriction in the œsophagus.

Appetite and Taste.
Abnormal hunger; he must often eat something.
Does not drink often, but much at a time.
Taste bitter, even of food.

Stomach.
35. Vomiting of solids, and not of fluids.
Bitter vomiting, when drinking immediately after a meal.
Vomiting, first of bile, then of fluids.
Pressure in the stomach after eating, especially after eating bread.
Stitches in the stomach.
40. Burning in the stomach and pit of the stomach, especially when moving.
Inflammation of the stomach.
Sensitiveness of the pit of the stomach to touch and pressure.

Abdomen.
Bloated abdomen (dropsy.)
Stitches in the liver, when touching it; when coughing and breathing. (Inflammation of the liver.)

Stool and Anus.
45. Constipation.
Stools too large in size; too hard and dry.
Diarrhœa, preceded by pain in the abdomen; during stool burning at the anus.
Diarrhœa putrid; smelling like old cheese; worse (or only) in the morning; during hot weather.
Involuntary stools while asleep.

Urinary Organs.
50. Diminished secretion of hot, red urine.
White, turbid urine.
Burning in the urethra, (when not urinating.)
Cutting in the urethra, or sensation of constriction while urinating.

Sexual Organs.
Men. Stitches in the testicles while sitting.
55. *Women.* Menstruation too early and too profuse, with dark, red blood.
Suppressed menstruation, with bleeding of the nose.
During pregnancy, pain in the abdomen and burning in the uterus.
Swelling and inflammation of the (left) labia majora.
Lumps, indurations and inflammations of the mammæ, with diminished or retarded secretion of milk. (Puerperal fever.)

Respiratory Organs.

60. Hoarseness and roughness of the voice (acute bronchitis.)
Deep, slow breathing.
Difficult breathing, only possible with the assistance of the abdominal muscles.
Frequent sighing, breathing.
Continued inclination to draw a long breath.
65. Breathing quick, difficult and anxious; caused by stitches, principally in the chest, compelling him to sit up.
Cough, from tickling in the throat and pit of the stomach; in the evening and at night without expectoration; during the day the expectoration is yellow, or consists of coagulated brown blood, or of cold mucus of a disagreeable flat taste.
Cough and stitches in the head and chest; or pain, as if the head and chest would burst.
Stitches in the chest, when breathing or coughing.
Heat in the chest (pleurisy, pneumonia.)
70. Palpitation of the heart, with oppression of the chest (carditis.)
Dry, spasmodic cough, after eating and drinking, with vomiting of food.
Cough, with involuntary secretion of urine; hoarseness; thirst; sneezing; stitches in the chest and small of the back; red face; aggravated by motion, talking, laughing, eating and drinking.

Back.

Stitches in the back and small of the back.
Painful stiffness in the small of the back, compelling him to walk and sit crookedly.
75. Painful stiffness of the neck.

Upper Extremities.

Swelling of the elbow and hand joints, and upper parts of the hands.
The wrist feels as if dislocated, when moving it.
Rheumatic swelling of the right shoulder and upper arm, with stitches.
Swollen hands.

Lower Extremities.

80. Cracking and dislocation of the hip-joint, when walking.
Stitches in the hip-joint, extending to the knee.
Painful stiffness of the knees, with stitches, especially when moving them.
The ankle feels as if dislocated, especially when walking.

BRYONIA ALBA.

Swelling of the lower extremities.
85. Hot, inflammatory swelling of the feet, with redness.
Stitches in the feet (soles of the feet, big toe.)
Putrid ulcers on the lower extremities.

Generalities.

Over-sensitiveness of the senses to external impressions.
Rheumatic and gouty pains in the limbs, with tension; worse from motion and contact.
90. Paralysis of the limbs.
Stiffness and stitches in the joints.
Swelling (pale or red) of the affected parts, with inability to move them.

Sleep.

Sleeplessness before midnight, with thirst, heat and ebullitions.
Drowsiness, with half-closed eyes.
95. Yawning and sleepiness in the day-time.
Delirium, as soon as he awakes.

Fever.

Pulse full and hard, tense and quick; seldom intermitting.
Chilliness predominating, frequently with heat of the head, red cheeks and thirst.
Chill, with external coldness of the body.
100. Coldness and chilliness, mostly in the evening, and often only on one (right) side.
More chilliness in the room than in the open air.
Heat. Fever, with bitter taste and thirst.
Dry, burning heat, mostly internal, as if the blood were burning in the veins.
Perspiration, profuse and easily excited when walking slowly in the open, cold air.
105. Profuse night and morning perspiration.
Perspiration sour, or oily.

Skin.

Yellowness.
Burning itching eruptions.
Rash, especially of children, and during child-bed.
110. Petechiæ.
Erysipelatous inflammations, especially of the joints.
Hard knots and blotches.
Putrid ulcers, feeling cold.

Conditions.

Aggravation, in the evening (9, P. M.;)
115. From motion, exertion of the body, on ascending; worse

on sitting up in bed; the patient is made sick at the stomach by sitting up; can't sit up a moment; *gets faint, or sick*, or both, on *sitting up;*
From heat and warm food;
While coughing, after eating, while swallowing;
After the suppression of cutaneous eruptions.
Amelioration, while making an expiration;
120. On descending;
While lying, especially on the painful side;
While sitting;
From eating cold things;
On getting warm in bed.

CACTUS GRANDIFLORUS.

Mind and Disposition.
Sadness and bad humor; taciturnity, melancholy, hypochondriasis.

Head.
Vertigo, from sanguineous congestions to the head.
Pulsating pain, with the sensation of weight in the right side of the head.
Heavy pain, like a weight on the vertex; worse from sounds, even talking.

Eyes.
5. Dimness of sight; cannot see at a distance; objects appear to be obscured.

Ears.
Hearing diminished by the buzzing in the ears.
Pulsations in the ears (otitis.)

Nose.
Profuse bleeding of the nose.

Face.
Face bloated and red, with pulsation in the head.

Throat.
10. Constriction of the œsophagus, which prevents swallowing; which excites the frequent swallowing of saliva.

Stomach and Abdomen.

Nausea in the morning, lasting all day.
Acrid acid in the stomach, which rises in the throat and mouth.
Burning pulsation or heaviness in the stomach.
Constriction or pulsation in the scrobiculus.
15. Pulsation in the cœliac artery (after dinner.)
Copious vomiting of blood.

Stool and Anus.

Constipation; stool hard and black.
Diarrhœa, watery, mucous, bilious (in the forenoon.).
Sensation of great weight in the anus.
20. Swollen, painful varices at the anus.
Copious hemorrhage from the anus.
Itching in the anus.

Urinary Organs.

Constriction of the neck of the bladder.
Irritation in the urethra, as if he would pass water constantly.
25. Urine passes by drops, with much burning.
Profuse urine, of a straw color.
Urine, on cooling, deposits a red sand.
Hæmaturia.

Sexual Organs.

Women. Pulsating pain in the uterus and ovaries.
30. Sensation of constriction in the uterine region.
Very painful menstruation.
Labor suppressed.

Chest.

Feeling of constriction in the chest, as if bound; hindering respiration.
Sensation of constriction in the heart, as if an iron hand prevented its normal movement.
35. Acute pains and stitches in the heart.
Difficulty of breathing; attacks of suffocation, with fainting, cold perspiration on the face, and loss of pulse.
Palpitation of the heart; worse when walking, and at night when lying on the left side.
Chronic bronchitis, with rattling of mucus.
Hæmoptysis, with convulsive cough.
40. Spasmodic cough and copious mucous expectoration.
Pricking pains in the chest, with oppressed respiration, intense cough, sanguinolent sputa. (Pneumonia.)

Extremities.

Formication and weight in the arms.
Œdema of the hands; worse in the left.
Œdema of the feet, extending to the knee; the skin is shining; pressure with the fingers leaves an indentation.

Generalities.

45. General weakness and prostration of strength.
Sensation of constriction in the throat; chest; heart; bladder; rectum.
Hemorrhages, nose; lungs; rectum; stomach.

Sleep.

Sleeplessness without cause; or from arterial pulsations in the scrobiculus, and in the right ear.
Delirium at night, on waking up.

Fever.

50. Slight chilliness towards 10 A. M.
Chilliness, with chattering of the teeth.
Burning heat, with shortness of breath.
Scorching heat at night, with headache, following a chill and terminating in perspiration.
Intermittent fever (quotidian) recurring every day at the same hour. One o'clock in the afternoon slight chill, then burning heat, with dyspnœa, pulsating pain in the uterine region, terminating in slight perspiration:—(quotidian) 11 A. M., great coldness for two hours; then burning heat, with great dyspnœa, violent pain in the head, coma, stupefaction, insensibility till midnight, then unquenchable thirst and perspiration.

Skin.

55. Dry, scaly herpes on the outside of the elbow, and on the right internal malleolus.

Conditions.

The intermittent fever attacks recur at the same hour.
Aggravation in the forenoon (diarrhœa.)
At night (palpitation of the heart; headache.)
When lying on the left side (palpitation of the heart.)
60. After eating (weight in the stomach.)
From noise and light (headache.)

CADMIUM SULPHURICUM.

Mind and Disposition.
Great irritability.
Aversion to be alone, or at work.

Head.
Sensation of constriction in the head.
Stitches and pulsations in the temples.
5. Headache, with restlessness, icy coldness of the body, bleeding of the nose, constriction in the throat, thirst, nausea, and vomiting; mostly present when awaking, in the open air, from a draft of air, in the sun.

Eyes.
Cannot read small print.
Night-blindness.
Dimness of, or spots on the cornea.
Hot tears.

Stomach.
10. Vomiting of acid or yellow substances, with cold perspiration in the face, and cutting pain in the abdomen.
Burning and cutting pain in the stomach.

Chest.
Oppression; sensation as if the lungs were in a state of adhesion.

Extremities.
Upper. Perspiration in the palms of the hands.

Generalities.
Cutting pains in the limbs.

Conditions.
15. Aggravation, in the morning, forenoon; after grief; after intoxication; when sitting or lying.
Amelioration, from eating.

CALADIUM SEGUINUM.

Mind and Disposition.
Low spirits and gloomy thoughts, (with impotence.)
Forgetfulness.

Mouth.
Swelling of the tongue with excessive ptyalism; the saliva resembling the white of an egg; the eyes are violently inflamed, the chest is oppressed, pulse small and accelerated, cold perspiration all over.

Throat.
Dryness in the fauces and pharynx, with aversion to cold water.

Stomach and Abdomen.
5. Frequent rising of air, as if the stomach were filled with dry food, (with asthma.)
Burning in the stomach, not relieved by drinking.

Stool and Anus.
Discharge of thin, red blood after the stool.
Discharge of mucus from the rectum after stool.

Urinary Organs.
The bladder feels full, without desire to urinate.
10. Fetid urine, (with impotence and secondary gonorrhœa.)

Sexual Organs.
Men. The sexual organs are bloated, relaxed, and sweaty.
Swelling of the prepuce, (border,) with smarting during micturition.
After coition, the prepuce remains behind the glans; it is painful and swollen.
Glans red, dry, dotted with fine points, which are still redder.
15. Painful erections without sexual desire, alternating with sexual desire with relaxed penis.
Imperfect erections, and premature ejaculation of the semen.
Impotence; the penis remains relaxed, even when excited.
Feeling of coldness, and cold perspiration of the sexual organs.

Larynx and Trachea.
Sensation of constriction in the larynx and trachea.

Generalities.

20. Attacks like fainting after writing and thinking, when lying down, or when rising.

Disinclination to move, and desire to lie still.

Sleep.

Sleepiness in the day-time, but cannot go to sleep on account of vertigo.

At night, cramps in the soles of the feet.

Fever.

Chilliness in the evening, without thirst.

25. Internal heat, going off from sleep.

Heat with thirst, pain in the ears, swelling of the submaxillary glands, and retention of stool.

Sweat towards evening, with prostration, yawning and drowsiness.

The perspiration (after the heat) attracts the flies.

Skin.

Itching, burning rash, (forearm and chest,) alternating with asthma.

Conditions.

30. All the symptoms are ameliorated by perspiration, and after sleeping in the day-time.

CALCAREA CARBONICA.

Mind and Disposition.

Easily frightened, or offended.
Inclination to weep.
Children are self-willed.
Apprehensive anxiety about his health, or of some future misfortune.

5. Anguish, with palpitation of the heart.

She fears she will lose her understanding, or that people will observe her confusion of mind.

Despairing mood, with fear of disease and misery.
Thinking is difficult.

Head.

Vertigo, when ascending a height, walking in the open air, or turning the head quickly, or looking upwards (in the morning.)
10. *Mania a potu,* with delirious talk about fire, rats, mice and murder.
Congestion of blood to the head, with heat and stupefying headache; with redness of the face and bloatedness; worse in the morning when awaking, and from spirituous drinks.
Headache, from overlifting.
Fulness and heaviness in the head.
Pulsations in the occiput.
15. Heat in the vertex.
Headache, with empty eructations and nausea, vertigo; aggravated from mental exertions, stooping, or walking in the open air; ameliorated by closing the eyes, and by lying down.
Internal and external sensation of coldness of one (right) side of the head, as if a piece of ice were lying there; with pale, puffed face.
Enlargement of the head, with open fontanelles.
Profuse perspiration, mostly on the back part of the head and on the neck (in the evening.)
20. Tumors and suppurating boils on the head.
Itching of the hairy scalp—scabs on the head.
Falling off of the hair (sides of the head—temples.)

Eyes.

Pressure, itching, burning and stinging in the eyes.
Cutting in the eyes and lids; worse when reading by candle-light.
25. Inflammation of the eyes, from foreign bodies coming into them; in infants, or scrofulous subjects.
Ulcers, and specks on the cornea.
Dimness of the cornea.
Oozing of blood from the eyes.
Watering of the eyes in the morning, or in the open air.
30. Fungus medullaris.
Fistula lachrymalis.
Pupils dilated.
Dimness of sight (mist before the eyes when looking sharp.)
Bright light dazzles the eyes.

Ears.

35. Stitches, or pulsations in the ear.
Inflammation of the external and internal ear.
Discharge of pus from the ears.

Tingling in the ears.
Polypus of the ear.
40. Hardness of hearing, especially after the suppression of intermittent fever by quinine.
Inflammatory swelling of the parotid gland.

Nose.

Inflamed, swollen, red.
Dryness of the nose.
Nostrils ulcerated and scabby.
45. Bleeding of the nose (in the morning.)
Polypus of the nose.
Stench before the nose (as from manure, gunpowder or putrid eggs.)
Stench from the nose.
Smell diminished.

Face.

50. Pale bloatedness of the face.
Yellow color of the face.
Moist, itching, scurfy eruption on the cheeks and forehead (with burning pain.)
Eruptions on the lips; around the mouth; in the corners of the mouth.
Ulcerated corners of the mouth.
55. Itching of the face and under the whiskers.
Swelling of the upper lip (in the morning.)
Painful, hard swelling of the submaxillary glands.

Teeth.

Difficult dentition.
Gums swollen and bleeding.
60. Toothache, drawing, stinging, from a draft of air; aggravated by noise, from drinking any thing cold, during and after the catamenia, during pregnancy.
Fistula dentalis.

Mouth.

Dryness of the tongue at night, and when awaking.
Ranula.
Accumulation of mucus in the mouth.

Throat.

65. Spasmodic contraction of the œsophagus.
Inflammatory swelling of the palate, with blisters on it.
Stinging in the throat when swallowing.
Swelling of the tonsils.

Appetite and Taste.

Continued violent thirst for cold drinks (at night.)
70. Canine hunger (in the morning.)
Desire for wine, salt or sweet things.
After drinking milk, nausea and sour eructations.
After eating, heat, or bloatedness, with nausea.
Sour taste of the food, or by itself.

Stomach and Abdomen.

75. Eructations tasting like the ingesta.
After eating, heartburn, and continued loud belching of wind.
Morning nausea.
Sour vomiting, especially in children, and during dentition.
Vomiting of the ingesta (tasting sour.)
80. Pit of the stomach swollen and painful to pressure.
Pressure and cramp-like pain in the stomach, especially when fasting, or after meats, with vomiting of the ingesta.
Stinging pain in the liver, (during or after stooping.)
Cutting in the upper part of the abdomen.
Sensation of coldness in the abdomen.
85. Enlargement of the abdomen, with swelling of the mesenteric glands.
Incarcerated flatulence.
Inguinal glands swollen and painful.

Stool and Anus.

Constipation; stools hard and undigested.
White stools.
90. Diarrhœa, of sour smell; putrid; during dentition.
Involuntary stool, (as if fermented.)
Tapeworm, and ascarides, with the stool.
Discharge of blood from the rectum.
Prolapsus ani.
95. Itching of the anus.
Varices, swollen, protruding, burning.

Urinary Organs.

Frequent micturition, also at night.
Urine dark, brown; with white sediment; of putrid smell.
Bloody urine.
100. During micturition, burning in the urethra.
Polypus in the bladder.

Sexual Organs.

Men. Inflammation of the prepuce, with redness and burning pain.
Frequent nocturnal, involuntary emissions.
During coition, erections of too short duration.

105. Burning and stinging while the semen is discharged during coition.
Women. Catamenia too early, and too profuse.
Suppressed menstruation, with full habit.
During menstruation, cutting in the abdomen; griping in the back; heat and congestion to the head.
Stitches in the os uteri.
110. Itching or pressing in the vagina.
Varices on the labiæ.
Prolapsus uteri, with sensation of pressing on it.
Sterility, with catamenia too early, and too profuse.
Fluor albus, like milk; burning; itching; in starts; during micturition; before the catamenia.

Larynx and Trachea.

115. Hoarseness, (painless.) Sensation, as if something were torn loose in the trachea.
Tickling cough, caused by a sensation of dust in the larynx.
Ulceration of the larynx.
Cough in the evening in bed, at night; while sleeping; with expectoration through the day, but not at night.
Expectoration of thick mucus; gray, yellow, of putrid smell; bloody; purulent; tasting sour.
120. Hæmoptysis.
Ulceration of the lungs.

Chest.

Tightness of the chest, as if too full, (filled with blood.)
Arrest of breath, when walking against the wind, or when stooping.
Burning in the chest.
125. Inclination to draw a deep breath.
Sensitiveness and sensation of soreness in the chest, when drawing a deep breath, and when touching it.
Stitches in the chest, and sides of the chest when moving; when taking a deep inspiration; when leaning against the painful side.
Palpitation of the heart at night; after eating; with anguish.
Trembling pulsation of the heart.
130. Hot swelling of the mammæ.
Secretion of milk too abundant, (galactorrhœa,) or suppressed.

Back and Neck.

Pain in the small of the back, or in the neck from over-lifting.
Pain in the small of the back, (as if sprained;) he can scarcely rise from his seat, after being seated.
Pressing pain between the shoulder-blades, impeding breathing, when moving.

135. Curvature of the dorsal vertebræ.
Painful swelling of the cervical glands.
Thick, struma-like swelling of the thyroid gland.

Extremities.

Upper. Suppuration of the axillary glands.
Weakness and lameness of the arms, (left.)
140. Pain as if sprained in the wrist-joint, (right.)
Arthritic nodosities on the hand and finger-joints.
Deadness of the fingers.
Trembling of the hands.
Lower. Coxalgia, with drawing stitches, or tearing, cutting.
145. The child is late learning to walk.
Heaviness and stiffness of the legs.
Swelling of the knee.
Tearing and stinging in the knee.
Cramp in the bend of the knee, in the calves of the leg; soles of the feet; toes; especially when extending the leg, (pulling on the boots.)
150. Erysipelas, (lower leg, with swelling.)
Phlegmasia alba dolens.
Itching on the lower limb and foot-joint.
Burning of the soles of the feet.
Perspiration on the feet, (foot-sweat.)
155. Perspiration of the palms of the hands.
Coldness and deadness of the feet, especially at night, in bed.
Corns, sore, with burning pain.

Generalities.

Great weakness and debility, from a short walk; from talking.
Cramps in single parts, which draw the limbs crooked, especially the toes and fingers.
160. Epileptic attacks, at night; during the full moon; with hallooing and shouting.
St. Vitus' dance.
Fainting, with loss of sight and coldness.
Full habit and ebullitions.
Tendency in children and young persons to grow very fat.
165. Bloatedness of body and face, with swelled abdomen, in children.
Great emaciation, with swelled abdomen and good appetite.
Visible quivering of the skin, from the feet to the head, with which he becomes dizzy.
Trembling of inner parts.
170. Bleeding from inner parts.
Pulsating pains.
Sensation of dryness of inner parts.

Sensation of coldness in inner parts.
Stinging and cutting in outer and inner parts.
175. Arthritic tearing in the muscles.
Arthritic nodosities.

Sleep.

Sleeplessness, from many thoughts crowding his mind.
When closing his eyes, he has many horrid visions.
He falls asleep late.
180. Awakens early in the night.
Fearful of fantastic dreams during sleep.
At night, oppression of the chest, with heat and restlessness, thirst.
Sleepy the whole day, and early in the evening.

Fever.

Pulse full, accelerated or tremulous.
185. Chilliness, when rising in the morning.
Chilliness, mostly in the evening; internal with external heat.
Frequent flushes of heat, with anxiety and palpitation of the heart.
Heat, with thirst, followed by chilliness.
Heat, after eating.
190. Perspiration from the least exertion, even in the open, cold air.
Perspiration, in the first sleep.
Night sweat, especially on head, neck and chest.
Night sweat, sticky only on the legs.

Skin.

Flaccidity of the skin.
195. Bloatedness.
Nettle rash, mostly disappearing in the cold air.
Eruptions moist, scurfy. (Milk crust.)
Herpes, burning; chapped; furfuraceous.
Rhagades, especially in those who work in water.
200. Unwholesome, readily ulcerating skin; even small wounds suppurate and do not heal.
Polypus (nose, ear, uterus.)
Ulcers, deep; fistulous; carious.
Steatoma, reappearing and suppurating every four weeks.
Warts, inflamed; stinging; suppurating.
205. Painful swelling of the glands.
Varices.
Bones, swelling; softening; curvature of; stinging in; caries.

Conditions.

Easy straining, from which he gets sore throat, stiff-neck, backache, or headache.
Sprains, from overlifting.
210. Liability to take cold, and great sensitiveness to moist, cold air.
Aversion to the open air.
Full habit and ebullitions.
Puffiness. (Chlorosis.)
Desire to be magnetised.
215. *Aggravation.* Morning; evening, or after midnight.
In the cold air, and in wet weather.
After washing, and by cold water.
On awaking.
After eating (smoked meat, milk.)
220. From exertion of the mind (after writing.)
From pressure of the clothes.
From sexual excess.
From suppressed perspiration.
Amelioration. After breakfast; on rising; from drawing up the limbs; from loosening the garments.

CALENDULA OFFICINALIS.

External wounds and lacerations, with (or without) loss of substance.
The wound is raw and inflamed; is painful, as if beaten; the parts around the wound become red, with stinging in the wound during the febrile heat.

CAMPHOR.

Mind and Disposition.

Great anguish and discouragement.
Mania to dispute.
Confusion of ideas; delirium.

Head.

Giddiness, with heaviness of the head and vanishing of the senses.

5. Sensation of constriction in the brain, especially in the cerebellum; the pain ceases when he thinks of it.
Inflammation of the brain, (after sun-stroke,) with pulsation and sensation of constriction in the brain, spasmodically turned head, (to the side or backward,) worse from movement, or in the cold air; better when lying down, or when thinking of it.

Eyes.
Staring, wild look.
Eyes sunken.
Contraction of the pupils.
10. Aversion to light; the objects appear too bright and shining.

Ears.
Lobules red, hot.
Ulcer in the (left) meatus auditorius, (with stinging pain.)

Nose.
Dry coryza.

Face.
Death-like paleness of the face, alternating with redness.
15. Icy-cold, purple, pale face.
Distorted countenance.
Lock-jaw.
Foam at the mouth.

Throat.
Burning in the mouth and throat, extending to the stoma h.
20. Dry, scraping sensation of the palate.

Appetite and Taste.
Thirstlessness, or violent thirst.
Food tastes bitter.
The taste is more acute.

Stomach and Abdomen.
Burning in the stomach.
25. The pit of the stomach is very sensitive to the touch.
Burning heat in the abdomen.

Stool and Anus.
Constipation, from want of peristaltic motion of the intestines.
The rectum feels narrow and swollen; is painful during the emission of flatulence.
Involuntary diarrhœa; stools blackish.

Urinary Organs.
30. Strangury, with tenesmus of the neck of the bladder.

Burning of the urine during emission.
The stream is thin, as if the urethra were contracted.
The urine is yellowish-green.

Sexual Organs.
Sexual desire wanting; impotence.
35. Sensation of contraction in the testes.

Chest.
Violent oppression of breathing, with constriction of the throat, as if produced by the vapor of sulphur.
Accumulation of mucus in the air-passages, with danger of suffocation.
Audible palpitation of the heart, (after eating.)
Trembling of the heart.

Extremities.
40. *Upper.* Hands icy cold.
Convulsive rotation of the arms.
Lower. Great weakness of the legs.
Cramps in the calf of the leg and feet.

Generalities.
Epileptic and convulsive attacks; he falls down insensible.
45. Diminished circulation of the blood to the parts most distant from the heart.
Icy coldness of the whole body, with paleness of the face.
Sudden and great sinking of strength.

Sleep.
Torpor, with delirium or snoring.
Sleeplessness from nervous over-excitability.
50. During sleep, the inspirations are shorter than the expirations.

Fever.
Pulse small, weak, and slow.
The blood does not circulate to the parts distant from the heart.
Chilliness, and sensitiveness to cold air.
Coldness, with chilliness and shaking.
55. Icy coldness of the whole body, with congestion to the head and chest.
Heat, with distended veins, aggravated from every movement.
Cold perspiration, often clammy, and always very debilitating.

Skin.
Dryness of the skin.
Erysipelatous inflammation.

Conditions.

Most pains are felt during a half-conscious condition, and disappear when thinking of them.
Great sensitiveness to cold and cold air; the pains are aggravated by it.

CANNABIS SATIVA.

Mind and Disposition.

The mind is too active; crowded with ideas.
The ideas seem to stand still; he unconsciously stares, as if hurried in thoughts.

Head.

Sensation as if intoxicated.
Congestion of blood to the head, with pulsation, and not unpleasant warmth in it.
5. Sensation of a heavy weight on the vertex.
Sensation as if drops of cold water were falling on the head.

Eyes.

The cornea becomes opaque.
Specks and pellicle on the cornea.
Weakness of the eyes, and diminished vision.
10. Cataract.

Ears and Nose.

Throbbing, pushing pain in the ear, disappearing when stooping, and re-appearing when raising the head again.
Pulsation in the ears.
Dryness of the nose, with heat.
Stupefying pressure on the root of the nose.
15. Swelling and copper-redness of the nose.
Bleeding at the (dry) nose, even to fainting.

Face.

Pale face.
Hot face, with red cheeks.

Mouth and Throat.

Dryness of the mouth; viscid saliva, without thirst.
20. Eruption in the vermilion border of the lips.
Difficult speech.
Burning in the throat.

Stomach and Abdomen.

Rising of air.
Gulping up of a bitter-sour, acrid fluid.
25. Vomiting of green bile.
Sensation of soreness of the stomach when touching it, relieved by eating.
Cramp in the stomach, with perspiration of the pale face.
Sensation of soreness in the abdomen, (dropsy.)
Shuddering in the abdomen, as if cold water were running through it.

Stool and Anus.

30. Constipation; stool hard.
Diarrhœa after colic.
Sensation in the anus, as if something were dropping out of it.

Urinary Organs.

Sensation of soreness and inflammation of the kidneys.
Strangury; painful urging to urinate; he discharges only a few drops of bloody, burning urine.
35. During micturition, burning, smarting, or stinging pain in the urethra.
Burning, during and after micturition, (forepart of the urethra.)
Spreading stream.
The urethra feels inflamed.
Discharge of watery mucus from the urethra, (gonorrhœa.)
40. Painless discharge of mucus from the urethra.

Genital Organs.

Men. Inflammatory swelling of the prepuce, with dark redness.
The penis feels sore and burnt when walking.
Painful erections.
Sexual desire increased.
45. Swelling of the prostate gland.
Women. Profuse menstruation.

Chest.

Asthmatic attacks; he can only breathe when standing up.
Oppressed breathing, as from a weight on the chest, with wheezing, rattling breathing.
Difficult respiration when lying down.
50. Loss of voice.
Cough dry, or with green, viscid expectoration.
Inflammation of the lungs, with stitches low downward, or with inflammation of the heart, or with vomiting of bile.

Violent palpitation of the heart.
Shocks and beats in the region of the heart.
55. Sensation as if drops were falling from the heart.
Inflammation of the heart.

Back.
Pain in the back, arresting the breathing.

Extremities.
Upper. Cramp-like contraction of the metacarpal bones, of the (right) hand.
Lower. Pain in the legs, as from great fatigue.
60. Heaviness of the legs; he walks in a stagger—and painful weariness of the knees, as from over-exertion.
The patella starts out of its normal position, when going up stairs.

Generalities.
Great debility after dinner, and from exertion.
Exhaustion from talking and writing.
Tetanic spasms of the upper limbs and the trunk.
65. Sensation, as if drops of cold water were falling, (on the head, from the anus, from the heart.)

Sleep.
Great sleepiness in the day-time.
Sleeplessness at night from heat; he feels as if hot water were poured over him.

Fever.
Pulse weak, slow, almost imperceptible.
Chilliness, with thirst.
70. External coldness of the body, with the exception of the face.
Heat only in the face.
Burning heat at night.

Skin.
Rheumatic tearing, as it were in the periosteum, during motion.

Conditions.
Fatigue after great bodily exertion, or from over-exertion; fatigue after a very long foot journey.
The weariness is worse after a meal; from talking; or writing; from a little exercise.

CANTHARIDES.

Mind and Disposition.

Anxious restlessness, ending in rage.
Paroxysms of rage, with crying, barking and beating; they are renewed by the sight of dazzling, bright objects; when touching the larynx; when trying to drink water.
Amorous frenzy, with shameless, unchaste gesticulations.
Delirium. Hydrophobia.

Head.

5. Soreness and burning in the brain.
Burning in the sides of the head, ascending from the neck, with soreness and giddiness; worse in the morning and afternoon; when standing or sitting; better when walking or lying down.

Eyes.

Eyes protruding; fiery, sparkling, staring look.
Involuntary spasmodic movement of the eyes.
The eyes look yellow.
10. Burning and soreness in the eyes.
Things look yellow.

Nose.

Erysipelatous inflammation of the dorsum of the nose, extending to the cheeks (right side) with hardness and subsequent desquamation.

Face.

Death-like appearance; expression of terror and despair.
Sunken, hippocratic countenance.
15. Yellow complexion.
Hot, red, swollen face.

Mouth and Throat.

Suppuration of the gums.
Fistula dentalis (suppurating) (upper incisors.)
Burning in the mouth, extending down the pharynx, œsophagus and stomach; worse from drinking cold water.
20. Inflammation of the mouth and pharynx.
Inflammation and suppuration of the tonsils, with inability to swallow.

Painless inability to swallow.
Expectoration of frothy saliva, streaked with blood.
Feeble voice, from debility of the organs.
25. Inflammation and suppuration of the tongue.

Appetite and Taste.
Thirst, with aversion to all fluids.

Stomach and Abdomen.
Violent burning pain (inflammation) in the stomach.
Sensitiveness of the stomach; also externally.
Inflammation of the liver.

Stool and Anus.
30. Diarrhœa of mucus, followed by pain in the abdomen, or bloody discharges.
Dysentery; discharges of blood-streaked mucus, or white mucus, looking like the scraping from the intestines.
During stool, burning in the anus; prolapsus ani.
After stool, chilliness and tenesmus.

Urinary Organs.
Burning, stinging and tearing in the kidneys. (Inflammation of the kidneys.)
35. Pressing pain in the kidneys, extending to the bladder; along the ureters; relieved by pressing upon the glans.
Desire to urinate constant, with inability to urinate, or with difficult emission of a few drops only.
Discharge of blood by drops; hemorrhage from the urethra.
Spasmodic pain in the bladder, with suppression of urine.
Discharge of bloody mucus from the bladder. (Inflammation of the bladder.)
40. During micturition, burning or cutting pain in the urethra. (Inflammation of the urethra.)

Sexual Organs.
Men. Inflammation of the genitals.
Painful erection (with gonorrhœa) with strong sexual desire (priapism.)
Women. Catamenia too early and too profuse (blood black.)
Inflammation of the ovaries.
45. Swelling of the neck of the uterus.

Chest.
Sensation of weakness in the respiratory organs.
Oppression of breathing, with sensation of constriction of the pharynx.
Stitches in the chest, during an inspiration. (Inflammation of the lungs.)

Burning and stinging in the larynx, especially when attempting to hawk up tough mucus.
50. Hoarseness; weak, indistinct voice.

Back.

Tearing in the back (after rising from a seat.)
Stiffness in the nape of the neck, with tension when bending it over.
Opisthotonos.

Extremities.

Lower. Coxalgia, with spasmodic pains in the bladder, and strangury.
55. Soles of the feet sore (ulcerating pain.)

Generalities.

Over-sensitiveness of all parts.
Burning, with soreness, especially in the cavities of the body.
Tearing (rheumatism) in the limbs; relieved by rubbing.

Fever.

Pulse hard, full and rapid.
60. Pulsation through the trembling limbs.
Chilliness, principally in the evening; not relieved by heat.
Burning heat, with anxiety and thirst.
Perspiration; cold, especially on the hands and feet; on the genitals.
Perspiration smells like urine.

Skin.

65. Erysipelatous inflammation; burning; raising blisters.
Itching pustules, burning when touched.
Itching and tearing in the ulcers.
Blisters, from burns.

Conditions.

The conditions return every seven days.
70. The right side is mostly affected.
Aggravation from coffee (and oil.)
Amelioration, from lying down.

CAPSICUM ANNUUM.

Mind and Disposition.
Peevish, easily offended.
Home-sickness, with redness of the cheeks and sleeplessness.

Head.
Vertigo and giddiness, especially during the cold stage of the intermittent fever.
Pressing headache, as if the head would burst, with fulness, nausea, and vomiting; worse in the evening,—from moving the head,—when walking in the cold air; better when lying with the head high, and from heat.
5. One-sided headache, pressing, with nausea and vomiting; worse from moving the head and eyes.
Darting pain through the head; worse during rest; better from moving about.

Eyes.
Burning in the eyes, (in the morning,) with redness and lachrymation.
Objects appear black when brought before the eyes, (incipient amaurosis.)

Ears.
Swelling behind the ears, painful to the touch.
10. Hardness of hearing after previous burning and stinging in the ear.

Nose.
Bleeding from the nose, in the morning in bed.

Face.
Redness of the cheeks, (without heat,) often changing to paleness.
Dull, pressing pain in the cheek bone, excited by touching the parts.
Swollen, cracked lips.
15. Lips peel off; burning of the lips.

Mouth and Throat.
Burning blisters in the mouth.
Stomacace. Fetid odor from the mouth.

Spasmodic contraction of the throat.
Inflammation, with dark redness and burning of the throat.
The pain in the throat is worse between the acts of deglutition.
Appetite and Taste.
20. Unnaturally increased appetite, alternated with aversion to food.
Taste sour.
Thirstlessness.
Stomach and Abdomen.
Burning in the stomach, (after eating.)
Distention of the abdomen, with suffocative arrest of breathing.
25. Colic from flatulence.
Painless rumbling in the abdomen.
Stool and Anus.
Dysentery; stools of bloody mucus with tenesmus, and strangury.
Diarrhœa at night, with burning at the anus.
Hæmorrhoidal tumors, with burning, (bleeding.)
Urinary Organs.
30. Strangury, with tenesmus of the bladder.
Spasmodic contraction of the neck of the bladder.
Burning while urinating.
Discharge of blood from the urethra, which is painful to the touch.
Sexual Organs.
Men. Impotence, with coldness of the scrotum.
35. Purulent discharge from the urethra.
Dwindling of the testes.
Chest.
Oppressed breathing appearing to come from the abdomen, or from fulness of the chest.
Asthma with redness of the face, eructation and sensation as if the chest were extended.
Deep breathing, almost like a sigh.
40. Dry, hard cough in the evening and at night, with pain in distant parts, (stitches in the bladder, pain in the knees or legs, ears, throat.)
When coughing, he exhales fetid smelling air.
Generalities.
Aversion to exercise.
Phlegmatic temperament, and relaxed fibres.

CARBO ANIMALIS.

Fever.
Pulse irregular, and often intermitting.
45. Chill almost always with violent thirst; worse after drinking.
Heat, with perspiration, and no thirst.
Perspiration after the chill, without previous heat.
On the upper part of the legs cold perspiration.

Skin.
Sensation over the whole body, as if the parts would go to sleep.

Conditions.
50. Stiffness and painfulness of all the joints when beginning to move.
Cracking of all the joints, (finger joints, knee.)
Most complaints are aggravated from eating and drinking; are most severe on beginning to exercise; and are relieved or ameliorated by continued exercise.

CARBO ANIMALIS.

Mind and Disposition.
Alternate cheerfulness and melancholy.
Fright in the dark.

Head.
Heaviness in the cerebellum; worse in the forenoon,—in the cold air,—relieved after dinner.
Pain in the vertex, as if the skull were open.
5. Tightness and tension of the skin of the forehead and vertex.
Heat in the head in the evening in bed, better after rising.

Eyes.
Sensation as if the eyes were lying loose in their sockets.

Ears.
Hardness of hearing; the sounds appear confused, does not know from what direction they come.
Discharge of pus from the ears.
10. Swelling of the parotid gland.

Nose.
The tip of the nose is red, chapped, burning, the skin feels tight.

Face.
Erysipelas of the face.
Red, smooth, elevated blotches in the face.
Vesicles and cracks on the lips.
15. Heat of the face and head in the afternoon.
Swelled, burning lips.

Mouth and Throat.
Burning blisters in the mouth and on the tongue.
Gums red, swollen, painful.
Looseness of the teeth.
20. Dryness of the mouth and tongue.

Appetite and Taste.
Ravenous hunger.
Repugnance to greasy food.
Bitter taste in the morning.

Stomach and Abdomen.
Weak digestion; almost all food causes distress.
25. Pressure in the stomach, even in the morning and in the evening, in bed.
Spasmodic cramp in the stomach.
Considerable inflation after a meal.
Audible rumbling in the abdomen.

Stool and Anus.
Constipation; unsuccessful desire for stool; he passes only very offensive flatus.
30. Stools hard, knotty.
During stool, pain in the small of the back, with inflation of the abdomen.
Varices, burning; stinging.
A viscid, indorous humor oozes out of the rectum, and from the perinæum.

Urinary Organs.
Frequent desire to urinate, with increased secretion of urine.
35. Burning soreness in the urethra when urinating.
Involuntary discharge of fetid-smelling urine.

Sexual System.
Women. Menses too early.
Fluor albus, leaving yellow stains on the linen.
Mammæ swollen, inflamed (erysipelatous) during confinement.
Hard, painful nodosities in the mammæ.

Chest.

40. Hoarseness and roughness in the throat in the morning, after rising.
Loss of voice (during the night.)
Breathing, panting and rattling.
Oppression of breathing in the morning, and after eating.
Soreness in the chest.
45. Burning in (right side of) the chest.
Sensation of coldness in the chest.
Cough, with discharge of greenish pus (suppuration of the lungs.)

Neck and Back.

Painful swelling and induration of the glands of the neck, and of the parotid glands.
Stitches in the small of the back when drawing a long breath.

Extremities.

50. *Upper.* Swelling and induration of the axillary glands.
Oozing of moisture from the arm-pits.
Gouty stiffness of the joints of the fingers.
Pain in the wrist-joint, as if sprained.
The hands go to sleep.
55. *Lower.* Stitches in the left hip when sitting.
Drawing and sensation of contraction under the knee.
The ankle-joint and toes bend easily when walking.
Frost-bitten feet and toes, inflamed; burning.

Generalities.

Numbness of all the limbs.
60. Burning pains.

Sleep.

Cannot go to sleep in the evening, from restlessness, anxiety, and frightful visions.
During sleep, groaning, talking and shedding of tears.

Fever.

Pulse accelerated, especially in the evening.
Chill, especially in the afternoon, in the evening, and after eating.
65. Chill in the evening, followed by perspiration.
Heat after a chill, mostly at night, in bed.
Perspiration after the heat, especially towards morning.
Perspiration of bad odor; debilitating; coloring the linen yellow; more on the upper legs.

Skin.

Erysipelatous swellings, with burning pain.

70. Inflammation, swelling and induration of the glands.
Itching over the whole body in the evening, in bed.

Conditions.

Easy straining; great debility and spraining of the joints.
Aversion to the open, cold, dry air.

CARBO VEGETABILIS.

Mind and Disposition.

Restlessness and anxiety (in the evening, 4–6, P. M.)
Periodical weakness of the memory.
Sensitiveness and irritability.

Head.

Giddiness when moving the head.
Congestions to the head.
5. Pressing headache, with tears in the eyes; they are painful when moving them; the hairy scalp is painful to the touch; worse in the afternoon and evening, and after eating.
Spasmodic tension in the brain.
The external head is painfully sensitive to pressure, especially the pressure of the hat; worse from taking cold, or when getting warm in bed.
Falling off of the hair, with itching of the scalp in the evening, when getting warm in bed.

Eyes.

10. Weakness of the eyes from using them too much, and from fine work.
Hemorrhage from the eyes, with congestion to the head.
Nightly agglutination of the eyes.
Burning and pressing in the eyes.
Itching of the margins of the eyelids.
15. Black, flying spots before the eyes.

Ears.

Every evening heat and redness of (the right) the external ear.

Deficiency of wax.
Suppuration (fetid) of the inner ear.
Pulsations in the ears.
20. Swelling of the parotid gland.

Nose.
Frequent and continuous bleeding from the nose, especially in the morning, or after straining to stool, with paleness of the face before and afterwards.
The tip of the nose is red and scabby.
Itching around the nostrils; coryza, with hoarseness.

Face.
Greenish color of the face.
25. Great paleness of the face.
Swollen face and lips.
Lips swelled, chapped.

Teeth.
Looseness of the teeth.
30. Tearing toothache from salt food.
The gums recede from the teeth, (incisors.)
The gums bleed easily and often.

Mouth and Throat.
Dryness of the mouth, without thirst.
Tongue coated white or yellow-brown.
35. Stomacace.
Sensation of constriction in the throat.
Feeling of coldness of the throat.
Burning; roughness; rawness in the throat.
The throat is full of mucus, which can be hawked up easily.
40. Swelling and inflammation of the uvula, with stitches in the throat.

Appetite and Taste.
Excessive hunger or thirst.
Great desire for coffee.
Aversion to meat and fat things.
Bitter or salty taste.
45. The food tastes too salt.
Acidity in the mouth after eating.
Weakness of digestion: the plainest food inconveniences him.

Stomach and Abdomen.
Nausea in the morning.
Eructations of the (fat) food.
50. Bloated abdomen after eating and drinking.
Vomiting of blood; of the food in the evening.

Colic, with the sensation of a burning pressure; much flatulence and sensitiveness of the pit of the stomach.
Pain in the stomach after loss of fluids, (while nursing.)
Stitches under the ribs, especially in the region of the liver.
55. Pain in the liver, as if bruised.
Distention of the abdomen from flatulency, with heat, and frequent discharge of very fetid flatus.
Pain in the abdomen from riding in a carriage.
He cannot bear any tight clothing around his waist and abdomen.

Stool and Anus.

Constipation; hard, tough, scanty stool.
60. Diarrhœa; thin, pale, mucous.
The stool, even if it be soft, is passed with difficulty.
Discharge of blood from the rectum.
Burning varices.
Burning at the anus, (after stool.)
65. Soreness of, and oozing of moisture from the perinæum.

Urinary Organs.

Frequent and anxious urging to pass urine.
Copious emission of light-yellow urine, (diabetes.)
Wetting of the bed at night.
Constriction of the urethra every morning.
70. Red, dark urine, as if mixed with blood.

Sexual Organs.

Men. Frequent, involuntary seminal emissions.
Rapid discharge of semen during cóition, followed by roaring in the head.
Women. Itching, burning and soreness of the parts.
Aphthæ and itching at the pudendum.
75. Menses too early and too profuse, (blood pale.)
Menstrual blood thick; corrosive; of an acrid smell.
Thick, yellowish white leucorrhœa.
Varices on the parts, (pudendum.)
Disposition to miscarriages.

Larynx and Trachea.

80. Hoarseness aggravated by talking; worse in the evening.
Roughness of the throat, causing cough.
Soreness and ulcerative pain in the larynx and pharynx.
Loss of voice at night, or when talking.

Chest and Lungs.

Oppression of breathing.
85. Sensation of rawness and soreness in the chest.

Burning, pressing, and stinging in the chest, (hydrothorax.)
Wheezing and rattling of mucus in the chest.
When breathing, painful throbbing in the head and teeth.
Spasmödic, hollow cough, (hooping-cough;) four to five attacks every day, caused by a tingling irritation in the larynx; expectoration only in the morning, yellow, like pus,—brownish,—bloody,—tasting putrid, sour, salt, and of offensive smell.
90. Cough, with spitting of blood and burning pain in the chest.
Cough, with expectoration of pus.
The cough is worse in the evening; till midnight; from movement; when walking in the open air; from cold, wet weather; from going from a warm to a cold place; after lying down; after eating and drinking, especially cold things; from talking.
Brown-yellow blotches on the chest.
Palpitation of the heart, especially when sitting.
Erysipelatous inflammation of the mammæ.

Back.

95. Stitches in the back.
Rheumatic tearing in the back.
Painful stiffness of the back in the morning, when rising.
Swelling of the cervical glands.

Extremities.

Upper. Pain, as from contusion in the elbow joints.
100. Tearing in the wrists.
Paralytic weakness of the fingers when seizing any thing.
Heat in the hands; burning in the hands.
Icy cold hands. The tips of the fingers are covered with cold sweat.
Lower. Heaviness in the lower extremities.
105. The legs go to sleep.
Cramps in the legs, and especially the soles of the feet.
Perspiration of the feet.
Toes red, swollen, stinging, as if they had been frozen.
Ulcerated tips of the toes.

Generalities.

110. Numbness of the limbs.
Burning pains (limbs, bones, ulcers.)
The limbs go to sleep easily.
Great debility and weakness as soon as he makes the least exertion.

Sleep.

Sleepiness in day-time (forenoon) with sleeplessness at night, on account of great restlessness.

115. No sleep, with inability to open the eyes.

Fever.

Pulse small, weak, imperceptible; uneven; intermitting.
Chilliness and chill, especially in the evening, with thirst—sometimes on one side only; with great debility and icy coldness of the body. (Intermittent fever, with thirst only during the chill.)
Heat after the chill, or by itself, in the evening and at night, in bed; flushes of heat; burning heat, generally without thirst.
Perspiration smelling putrid, or sour; easily excited, even when eating; cold.
120. Night-sweat. Morning sweat smelling sour.

Skin.

General itching all over in the evening, when getting warm, in bed.
Burning on different parts of the skin.
Ulcers; bleeding readily; putrid; with burning pain; with acrid, corroding pus.
Lymphatic swelling, with suppuration and burning pain.
Glands swollen, indurated.

Conditions.

Evil effects from the loss of fluids.
The rheumatic pains in the limbs are often accompanied by flatulency.
The great debility is worse at noon.
Bad effects from over-lifting, and from getting cold in cold, wet weather.
The soreness in the limbs is worse in the morning, on riding.
Bad effects from the abuse of china, or chinium sulphuricum.
It follows well after veratrum, especially in hooping-cough.
China follows well after carbo vegetabilis.

CASCARILLA.

Ears.

Burning heat of the inner and outer ear.

Stool and Anus.

Constipation; stool hard; in pieces, covered with mucus.

Frequent and excessive discharges of light-colored blood from the rectum, during and after hard, brown stool in large lumps; and without stool.

CASTOR EQUORUM.

Excessively sore nipples, bleeding, suppurating, and only hanging on strings.

CAUSTICUM.

Mind and Disposition.
Melancholy, peevish.
Low-spirited, with fearful anxiety, day and night.
Attacks of anger, with scolding.
Afraid at night (in the dark room; the child does not want to go to bed alone.)

Head.
5. Giddiness, with sensation of weakness in the head.
Stitches in the temples.
Tension and tightness in the head, and of the scalp (forehead and temples.)
Congestion to the head, with roaring in the head and ears.
Involuntary nodding of the head while writing.

Eyes.
10. Pressure in the eyes, as if sand were in them.
Agglutination of the eyes (in the morning.)
Inflammation of the eyes, with burning and itching of the eyes and eyelids.
Old warts; on the eye-brows; on the upper eye-lid (nose.)
Movements before the eyes, as of a swarm of insects.
15. Dim-sightedness, as if a thick fog were before the eyes.

Ears.

Buzzing and roaring in the ear and head.
Spasmodic pain in the ear, as if the inner parts were pressed out.
Stitches in the (right) ear.
Painful swelling of the external ear.
20. Feeling of obstruction in the ears.
Words spoken and steps re-echo in the ear.

Nose.

Pimples on the tip of the nose.
Old warts on the nose (orbits, upper eyelids.)
Itching in the nose, and of the nostrils.
25. Coryza, with hoarseness, preventing loud speech.
Continuous dry coryza, with obstruction of both nostrils.

Face.

Yellowness of the face, (temples.)
Spasmodic sensation of the lips.
Sensation of tightness and pain in the jaws, rendering it very difficult to open the mouth, or to eat.
30. Arthritic pains in the lower jaw.
Semi-lateral paralysis of the face.
Itching eruption on the face.

Teeth.

Painfully elongated teeth, (incisors.)
Stitches in the teeth.
35. Gums suppurating, (fistula dentalis.)

Mouth and Throat.

Swelling of the inner side of the cheek; he bites it when chewing.
Dry mouth and tongue.
Accumulation of much mucus in the mouth and throat.
Speechlessness from paralysis of the tongue.
40. Distortion of the tongue and mouth when talking.
Stuttering, difficult, indistinct speech.
Dryness in the throat, without thirst.
Constant disposition to swallow, (pain as if a tumor were in the throat.)
Audible cracking in the throat.
45. Sensation as if something cold were rising in the throat.

Appetite and Taste.

Aversion to sweet things.
Greasy taste in the mouth.
Violent thirst, (cold drinks.)
Fresh meat causes nausea; smoked meat agrees.

CAUSTICUM. 125

Stomach and Abdomen.

50. Violent distention of the abdomen after a meal, (breakfast.)
Sour vomiting, often followed by sour eructation.
Colic, with heat in the head, chilliness over the whole body; better when lying down.
Swelled abdomen in children.
Painful swelling of the navel.
55. The clothes press the hypochondria painfully.
Stitches in the liver.

Stool and Anus.

Constipation; painful, fruitless urging to stool, with anxiety and redness of the face.
The hard, tough stool, is covered with mucus, and shines as if greased.
The stool is too small-shaped.
60. Diarrhœa, with tenesmus and burning in the rectum.
Bloody stool, with soreness and burning of the rectum.
Itching at the anus, (after dinner.)
Varices of the rectum, hindering stool; large; painful; stinging; burning when touched; increased by walking, and when thinking of them.
Pulsation in the perinæum. (Fistula in ano.)
65. Soreness of, and oozing of moisture from the rectum.

Urinary Organs.

Frequent and urgent desire to urinate, with thirst and scanty emission.
Involuntary emission of urine by day and night; at night, when asleep; when coughing, sneezing, and walking.
Burning in the urethra when urinating.
Itching of the orifice of the urethra.

Sexual Organs.

70. *Men.* Increase of smegma about the glans.
Aching in the testes.
Itching of the scrotum.
Women. Menses too late, but profuse; blood clotted.
Difficult first menstruation.
75. During the menses, no blood is passed at night.
Pain in the back, (during the menses;) yellowness of the face; vertigo.
Aversion to coition.
Leucorrhœa at night.
Sore, cracked nipples, surrounded with herpes.
80. Deficiency of milk.

Larynx and Trachea.

Burning and roughness.
Hoarseness and roughness, (early in the morning.)
Aphonia, (in the morning,) or from weakness of the organs.
Sensation of soreness of the larynx.
85. Hawking up of mucus early in the morning.

Chest.

Asthma, especially when sitting or lying down.
Stitches in the sternum, or deep in the chest, during a long inspiration.
Rattling in the chest.
Burning, stitches, and soreness in the chest.
90. Palpitation of the heart, with languor.
Stitches about the heart.
Tight dressing about the chest oppresses the breathing.
Short, dry cough.
Dry, hollow cough, with soreness in the chest, caused by tickling and mucus in the throat, with expectoration only at night, of acrid-tasting mucus, which he cannot raise, but has to swallow it again.
95. Cough, with pain in the hip, with involuntary passage of some drops of urine.
Cough is worse in the evening till midnight, from exhaling; drinking coffee; cold air; draft of air; when awaking from sleep.
Cough is relieved by a swallow of cold water.

Back and Neck.

Stiffness and tension in the neck.
Swelling, like goitre, on the throat.
100. Painful stiffness between the scapulæ, and of the back, especially when rising from a seat.
Itching and humid tetter in the nape of the neck.
Pain, as from a bruise in the nape of the neck.

Extremities.

Upper. Dull tearing in the arms and hands.
Great heaviness and weakness in the arms.
105. Trembling of the hands.
Great heaviness in the right hand.
Paralytic feeling in the right hand.
Sensation of fulness in the interior of the hand when grasping any thing.
Tension of the posterior joints of the fingers when bending them.
110. Numbness, insensibility and tightness of the fingers.

Tearing in the right wrist-joint.
Lower. Sensation of dislocation of the hip-joint when walking.
Tension in the knee and ankle-joints.
Contraction and tension in the heel and tendo Achillis.
115. Marbled skin of the legs.
Swelling of the feet.
Cold feet; cramp in the feet.
Unsteady walk of children; they fall easily.

Generalities.

Paralytic, trembling weakness of the limbs, paralysis (one-sided.)
120. Epileptic spasms (at night during sleep.)
St. Vitus' dance.
Tension and shortening of the muscles, contracting the joints and bending the limbs; they become paralyzed.
Rheumatism in the limbs.

Sleep.

He starts from the sleep.
125. Sleeplessness at night, with anxiety and heat.
Great sleepiness during the day.

Fever.

Pulse only accelerated towards evening.
Chilliness predominating, frequently with coldness of the left side.
Internal chilliness, followed by perspiration, without previous heat.
130. Heat in the evening, from 6 to 8, P. M.
Flushes of heat, followed by chilliness.
Perspiration when walking in the open air.
Morning sweat (smelling sour.)

Skin.

Itching of the whole body at night. (Itch.)
135. Injuries of the skin, which had been healed, become sore again.
Humid tetters.
Painful varices.
Soreness of children.

Conditions.

In the evening, great restlessness of the body (legs.)
140. Aggravation in the evening; in the open air; from colic.
Amelioration, especially of the rheumatic pains in the limbs, in bed, and from heat.

CHAMOMILLA VULGARIS.

Mind and Disposition.

Anger, with rage, violence and heat.
Great anguish and restlessness.
Crying and howling.
Weeping uneasiness; the child wants different things, and repels them when given to him.
5. The child cries and wants to be carried on the arm.
Seeks a cause for quarrel.
Peevishness and ill humor; taciturn; absence o mind.

Head.

Vertigo, when rising from bed; from drinking coffee.
Pulsating headache, generally in one side of the head, with one red cheek; worse at night; in the open air; in the wind; better from warm coverings and when walking about.
10. Lancinating pain in one side of the head, with thirst; better from walking about.
Headache, which is felt even during sleep.
Hot, clammy perspiration on the scalp and forehead.

Eyes.

Burning heat in the eyes.
Inflammation of the eyes, especially the edges of the lower eyelids, which are swollen.
15. Distortion of the eyes.
Yellowness of the whites.
Hemorrhage from the eyes.
Spasmodically closed eyelids.
Twitching of the eyelids.
20. Aversion to bright light.

Ears.

Otalgia, with stitches and tearing.
Discharge of thin pus from the ears.
Inflammatory swelling of the paratid gland.
Sensitive hearing.

Nose.

25. Wrinkled skin of the nose.
Ulcerated nostrils.
Sensitive smell.

Face.

Bloatedness of the face.
Redness and burning heat, particularly of the cheeks; sometimes of *one* cheek only, with paleness and coldness of the other.
30. Swelling, with hardness and blueness of one cheek.
Red rash on the cheeks.
Convulsive movements and twitchings of the facial muscles and lips.
Rhagades in the middle of the lower lip.
Heat of the face, while the rest of the body is cold.
35. Wrinkles on the forehead.

Mouth and Throat.

Putrid smell from the mouth.
Dry mouth and tongue, with thirst.
Red tongue, cracked.
Tongue coated thick, yellow or white.
40. Convulsive movements of the tongue.
Inflammation of the soft palate and the tonsils, with dark redness.
Sensation of a plug in the throat.
Inability to swallow while lying.
Inability to swallow solid food.
45. Sore throat, with swelling of the parotid or submaxillary glands.

Teeth.

Insupportable (drawing) toothache (at night) with swelling of the hot, red cheek, and thirst.
The toothache recommences when entering the warm room.
Toothache, aggravated from drinking any thing warm, especially coffee.
Toothache, after a cold and suppressed perspiration.
50. Toothache, with redness and swelling of the gums
Dentition, with convulsions.

Appetite and Taste.

Aversion to food; loathing of food.
Great thirst; longing for cold water.
Bitter taste in the mouth early in the morning.
55. Desire for coffee.

Stomach and Abdomen.

Sour eructations (the existing pain is aggravated by eructations.)
Vomiting, of food; sour; of bile.

9

After eating or drinking, heat and perspiration of the face.
Distention of the abdomen after a meal.
60. Painful bloatedness of the epigastrium (in the morning.)
Nausea (after drinking coffee.)
Colic, after anger.
Oppression of the stomach, as if a stone were pressing downwards.
Burning in the pit of the stomach.
65. Pressing towards the abdominal ring, as if hernia would protrude.

Stool and Anus.

Nightly diarrhœa, with frequent small discharges and colic.
Hot, diarrhœic stools, smelling like rotten eggs.
Stools green, chopped.
Stools consisting of white mucus, with colic.
70. Diarrhœa during dentition (green mucus.)
Diarrhœa from cold, from anger, from chagrin.
Stools corroding the anus.

Urinary Organs.

Ineffectual urging, with anguish during micturition.
The urine is hot, with flocculent sediment; turbid.
75. Smarting pain in the urethra during micturition.

Genital Organs.

Men. Itching, stinging pain in the margin of the prepuce.
Soreness of the border of the prepuce. (Sycosis.)
Excited sexual desire.
Women. Pressure towards the uterus, like labor-pain.
80. Metrorrhagia; the blood is passed in clots, and smells putrid.
Discharge of blood between the regular catamenia.
Abdominal spasms, before the catamenia; of pregnant women; or while nursing.
The labor-pains are not sufficient, but cause great restlessness and anguish (over-sensitive to the pains.)
Violent after-pains.
85. Suppression of milk (milk is cheesy, or mixed with pus; (milk fever.)
Puerperal fever.
Erysipelas of the mammæ and soreness of the nipples.
Induration and swelling of the mammæ; they are painful to the touch.

Larynx and Trachea.

Wheezing and rattling in the trachea.
90. Hoarseness, from tenacious mucus in the trachea.
Catarrhal hoarseness.

Stitches and burning in the larynx, with hoarseness.
Hoarseness and cough, from rattling mucus in the trachea.

Chest.

Burning of the chest.
95. Oppression of the chest, as from flatulence.
Constriction of the upper part of the chest.
Sudden stoppage of the chest, in children.
Stitches in the sides of the chest.
Burning pain under the sternum.
100. Rattling of mucus in the chest.
Cough, from irritation in the chest; from tickling in the pharynx and larynx, during the day, with expectoration of small quantities of tough mucus, tasting bitter or putrid.
Dry nightly cough of children, from tickling in the throat-pit.
Nightly dry cough during sleep.
Cough worse at night; aggravated from crying; from cold air; dry winds; open air; during sleep.
105. Amelioration of the cough when getting warm in bed.

Back.

Pain in the small of the back, especially at night.
Stinging pain in the back.

Extremities.

Upper. The arms go to sleep, especially when taking hold of any thing.
Convulsions of the arms, with clasping in of the thumb.
110. Convulsive twitchings of the fingers.
Cold hands, with cold perspiration in the palms of the hands.
Swelling of the palms of the hands.
Lower. Cracking of the knee during motion.
Burning of the soles of the feet, (at night, he puts his feet out of bed.)
115. Sensation of numbness in the toes.

Generalities.

Over-sensitiveness of the nerves; (pain is insupportable, and drives to despair.)
Over-sensitiveness of the senses, (especially from coffee and narcotics.)
Great, prostrating debility as soon as the pain begins.
Convulsive twitchings in the limbs. Convulsions, (during dentition.)
120. Sensation of numbness, (extremities.)

Sleep.

Yawning and stretching.
Drowsiness, with short breathing; groaning; starts.
Nightly sleeplessness from anxiety and visions.
Restless sleep, with weeping and howling, groaning and tossing about.
125. Snoring breathing when asleep.
Sleep full of vivid, fanciful dreams.

Fever.

Pulse small, tense, and accelerated.
Chilliness; frequently on some parts, while others are hot.
Chilliness, with internal heat.
130. Chill and coldness of the whole body, with burning hot face and hot breath.
Chilliness and coldness of the fore part of the body, while the back part is hot, or vice versa.
Chilliness from exposure to the air, (undressing,) or in the cold air.
Heat, with occasional chills, and one hot, red cheek, while the other is pale.
Heat, with anxiety and perspiration of the face and scalp.
135. Continuous burning heat, with violent thirst, and starts during sleep, and furious delirium.
Perspiration during sleep, mostly on the head, smelling sour, and with biting sensation of the skin.
Suppressed perspiration.

Skin.

Yellow skin, (over the whole body.)
The skin becomes unhealthy, and every injury ulcerates.
140. Rash of infants, and during nursing.
Red rash on the cheeks, on the forehead.
Ulcers, with darting and lancinating pain in the night, and excessive sensitiveness to the touch.
Itching pimples form around the ulcer, covered with scurf, and suppurating.
145. Inflammatory swelling of the glands.

Conditions.

Extreme sensitiveness to pain, with great irritability.
Over-sensitiveness to the open air, and aversion to being in the wind.
At night, tearing (rheumatic) pains in the limbs, with sensation of numbness.
The pains are worse at night, and are accompanied by thirst and heat.

150. Aggravation at night; from anger, (colic;) after taking cold; while lying down; during perspiration; during sleep. Amelioration while fasting; from bending the head backward; after perspiration; on rising.

CHELIDONIUM MAJUS.

Mind and Disposition.
Low-spirited and desponding, with inclination to weep.

Head.
Sensation of coldness in the occiput, ascending from the nape of the neck; worse when moving, better at rest.
Stitches in the vertex, particularly when walking fast.
Tingling in and on the head.
5. Scald-head.

Eyes.
Contraction of the pupils.
Painful pressure on the upper eye-lid.
Inflammation and nightly agglutination, with dimness in the morning.
Fistula lachrymalis.

Ears.
10. Sensation in both ears, as if wind were rushing out.
Whizzing before the ears, like wind.
Loss of hearing during cough.

Nose.
Dry coryza, with partial (one-sided) stoppage.

Face.
Redness of the face, without heat.
15. Tension and drawing in the (left) malar bone.
Itching in the face, and on the forehead.
Herpes in the face, especially the chin.

Throat.
Sensation as if the larynx were pressed on the œsophagus, impeding deglutition.
Sensation of choking in the throat, as if too large a morsel had been swallowed.

Appetite and Taste.
20. Longing for milk, which agrees well with him.
Bitter taste in the mouth.
Stomach and Abdomen.
Hiccough.
Frequent rising of air.
Eructation, tasting like juniper berries.
25. Nausea, with sensation of heat in the stomach.
Gnawing sensation in the stomach, relieved by eating.
Burning in the stomach.
Feeling of coldness in the stomach.
Cutting pain in the stomach when yawning; soon after eating.
30. Colic; the navel is drawn in; nausea.
Stool and Anus.
Constipation, stool hard in hard lumps.
Mucous diarrhœa at night.
Urinary Organs.
Pressure in the bladder, with scanty emission.
Urine pale.
35. Burning, darting and cutting in the urethra.
Sexual Organs.
Women. Menstruation too late; too profuse, and of too long duration.
Vanishing of milk.
Chest.
Oppression of the chest and respiration.
Stitches in the left chest during an inspiration.
Back.
40. Pain (pinching) under the right scapula (hindering the motion of the arm.)
When bending forwards or backwards, tearing pressing pain in the back, as if the vertebræ were being broken assunder.
Extremities.
Upper. Paralytic pressure in the upper-arm.
Stiffness of the wrist.
The anterior joints of the fingers (of the right hand) became yellow, cold and dead; the nails were blue.
45. Fine tearing in the tips of the fingers of the (right) hand.
Lower. Paralytic weakness of the (left) thigh and knee, when stepping.
Stiffness of the ankles.
The toes are without sensation, and feel dead.

Generalities.
The limbs feel paralyzed.
50. Stiffness in the joints (wrist, ankle.)

Sleep.
Goes to sleep late.
Sleeplessness, with sleepiness.
Perspiration during the morning sleep.

Fever.
Pulse small and rapid; full, hard, but not very much accelerated, towards evening.
55. Chill, internally, when walking in the open air; better in the room.
Chilliness and coldness of the whole body, mostly on the hands and feet.
Internal heat in the evening, after lying down, without thirst.
Perspiration during sleep, after midnight; in the morning hours; ceasing soon after awaking.

Skin.
Old, putrid, spreading ulcers.

Conditions.
60. Great debility and lassitude after eating; after awaking in the morning.
Desire to lie down after a meal.
Aversion to move; he feels tired from the least exertion.
Aggravation in the morning.

CHENOPODIUM.

Head.
Dulness in the head, as if from coryza, with flushes of heat in the face; violent pressing in the forehead or the cerebellum, aggravated by motion, with sensation as if the brain were balancing to and fro; drawing-tearing in the scalp.

Eyes.
Burning of the eyelids in the evening.

Ears.
Tearing in the ears, now in one, then in the other.
Nose.
Sensation of soreness of the nostrils.
5. Violent sneezing, with soreness of the larynx.
Coryza, with burning and biting on the margins of the nostrils, particularly of the septum.
Fluent coryza, with secretion of thin mucus; with accelerated pulse; with coldness of the feet up to the knees, and a chill over the back.
Face.
Pale or yellowish color of the face.
Flushes of heat in the face, with dulness of the head (evening.)
10. Dryness of the lips, especially in the morning.
Mouth and Throat.
Painful vesicle on the tip of the tongue.
Dryness of the mouth and throat, sometimes with increased secretion of mucus.
Much mucus in the mouth and throat, tasting flat, with continual disposition to hawk or spit.
Secretion of frothy mucus from the mouth and throat.
15. Scraping and burning in the throat.
Appetite and Taste.
Increased thirst, from dryness in the throat.
Stomach.
Frequent cutting pain in the abdomen, especially at night, or during the day, with urging to stool, emission of large quantities of flatulence.
Frequent rumbling of flatulence in the bowels.
Congestion of blood to the organs in the pelvis.
Stool and Anus.
20. Ineffectual urging, with pressure on the bladder and rectum.
Evacuations liquid, papescent, with burning in the anus and renewed urging, or with pinching in the abdomen before and after the stool.
Urinary Organs.
Pressure on the bladder, especially with ineffectual desire to stool.
Irritation in the urethra, as from acridity, compelling him to urinate frequently.
During micturition, burning in the urethra, especially at the orifice.

25. Frequent and copious emission of saturated, yellow, foaming urine, attended with an acrid sensation in the urethra, brownish red, depositing a thick, yellowish sediment during the night.

Larynx and Trachea.

Frequent roughness and huskiness of the voice; going off by hawking.

Burning scraping in the larynx, as from acridity; titillating burning or stinging, particularly in the open air during wet and cold weather, with constant irritation in the larynx, obliging him to cough or to hawk, with constant expectoration of mucus.

Back.

Pain below the left shoulder-blade.

Extremities.

Upper. Pain, as if bruised in the arms, with rheumatic pains in the shoulders and upper arms.

30. *Lower.* Rheumatic pains, especially on the tibia and soles of the feet.

Sensation of weariness in the legs.

Tearing-drawing above the knee, especially in the morning.

Cold feet up to the knees.

Stinging burning in the corns.

Generalities.

35. The limbs feel bruised.

Rheumatic drawing pains in temples, ears, decayed teeth, shoulders, upper arms, soles of the feet, above the knees, and on the tibia.

Fever.

Pulse accelerated, especially in the evening.

Chills, especially over the back.

Burning in the palms of the hands.

40. Perspiration in the palms of the hands, especially in the forenoon.

CHINA.

Mind and Disposition.

Indifference and apathy.

Disposition to be alone.

Ill-humor, with disposition to hurt other people's feelings.

Nervous irritation, with slowness of ideas.
5. Full of projects and ideas, especially in the evening and at night.

Head.

Congestion of blood to the head, with twitching in the temples.
Headache, from suppressed coryza.
Sensation, as if the whole head were bruised; worse from exertion of the mind.
Sensation, as if the head should burst, with sleeplessness at night; aggravated from touch, motion and stepping hard, ameliorated in the room, and when opening the eyes.
10. Stitches in the head, with pulsation in the temples, which can be felt by the finger; ameliorated by hard pressure, but aggravated by the movement of the head.
Sensitiveness of the scalp, especially the root of the hair, to the least touch; worse when walking in the open air and from a draft of air; ameliorated by strong external pressure and when scratching the head.
The headache is aggravated by a draft of air, in the open air, from the slightest contact, and relieved by hard pressure.

Eyes.

Pressure in the eyes, as from drowsiness.
Pressure, as from sand in the eyes, when moving the lids, with inflammation of the eyes, and worse in the evening.
15. Redness of the eyes, with heat in them.
Yellow color of the eyes.
Sensitiveness of the eyes to the bright sun-light.
Dimness and weakness of sight.
When reading, the letters look pale, confluent, and surrounded with a white border.
20. Incipient amaurosis after loss of animal fluids, (in drunkards.)

Ears.

Humming in the ears. (Hardness of hearing.)
Stitches in the ears.
Heat of the outer ear.

Nose.

Redness and heat of the nose.
25. Tearing in the dorsum of the nose.
Frequent bleeding from the nose. (Hemorrhage from the nose and mouth.)
Bleeding of the nose, after blowing it.
Dry coryza, with toothache and lachrymation.
Suppressed coryza, (headache from it.)

Face.

30. Face pale, sunken, (hippocratic,) pointed nose, sunken eyes, surrounded by blue margins.
    Pale, sickly appearance, as after excesses.
    Complexion gray-yellow, or black.
    Bloated, red face.
    Hot face, especially when entering a warm room, when coming from the cold air.
35. Face-ache, (neuralgia,) irritated from the slightest touch.
    Lips dry, coated black, wrinkled and chapped.
    Swelling of the lips.
    Swelling of the submaxillary glands, with pain in the glands during deglutition.

Teeth, Mouth and Throat.

Twitching tearing in the upper molar teeth, from taking cold in a draft of air.
40. Painful numbness in decayed teeth.
    Throbbing toothache.
    Looseness of the teeth.
    The toothache is caused by a draft of air, aggravated by smoking, the slightest contact, and relieved by pressing the teeth firmly together.
    Black coating of the teeth.
45. Swelling of the gums.
    Putrid taste in the mouth in the morning.
    Accumulation of mucus in the mouth.
    Ptyalism, (with nausea,) (from the abuse of mercury.)
    Tongue coated white or yellow.
50. Thick, dirty coating of the tongue.
    Blackish, parched tongue.
    Burning biting, as from pepper, on the tip of the tongue, succeeded by ptyalism.
    Voice husky or weak.
    When he talks or sings, the voice is too deep.

Appetite and Taste.

55. No desire for eating and drinking.
    Desire for various things, without knowing which.
    Longing, for acid fruit, wine.
    Bitter taste of the food, (bread, beer, tobacco.)
    The food tastes too salt.
60. Canine hunger, especially during the night.
    Violent thirst, for cold water, (drinks but little at a time, but often.)
    Shuddering and chilliness, with goose-flesh after every swallow he takes.

Weakness of digestion; the food is not digested, if taken too late in the day.
After a meal, distention of the abdomen, oppression of the stomach, general languor, and disposition to lie down.
65. Sour eructations after swallowing milk.
The thirst in intermittent fever only between the cold and hot stages, or during the perspiration.

Stomach and Abdomen.

Colic, from weakness and loss of animal fluids.
Milk deranges the stomach easily.
Pulsations in the pit of the stomach.
70. Eructations, tasting of the ingesta.
Bitter eructations, (after a meal.)
Vomiting; sour, mucus, water, and food, blood, bile.
Distention of the abdomen, (meteorism,) (dropsy.)
Accumulation of flatulence.
75. Incarceration of flatulence.
Rumbling, especially in the epigastrium.
Fermentation after eating fruit.
Emission of a quantity of flatulence, frequently very fetid.
Liver swollen, and very painful when slightly touched.
80. Swelling, inflammation, induration of the spleen.
Stitches in the spleen, (when walking slowly.)

Stool and Anus.

Difficult passage of the fæces, even when soft, (papescent,) as from inactivity of the bowels.
Painless, very debilitating diarrhœa.
Stools loose, watery, yellow mucus, blackish, bilious, white.—undigested food.
85. Diarrhœa from eating fruit.
Diarrhœa, particularly after meals, at night, involuntary.
In the rectum, stitches, also during stool.
Tingling in the anus, as from ascarides. (Ascarides.)
Discharge of mucus from the rectum.
90. Bleeding hæmorrhoids.

Urinary Organs.

Urine dark, turbid, scanty.
Scanty urine, greenish-yellow, with brick-dust sediment.
Frequent micturition.
Burning at the orifice of the urethra, especially painful if the clothes rub against the parts.
95. Stitches in the urethra.

Sexual Organs.

Men. Sexual desire excited, with lascivious fancies.
Impotence, with excited lascivious fancy.

Nocturnal emissions, after onanism; very debilitating.
Women. Congestion to the uterus, with feeling of fulness and painful pressing to and sense of heaviness of the genital organs, particularly when walking.
100. Profuse menses (black clots.)
During the menses, spasms in the chest and abdomen; congestion of blood to the head.
Metrorrhagia, with discharge of black blood; with fainting and convulsions.
Discharge of bloody serum from the vagina, alternating with discharge of pus.
Painful induration in the vagina.

Larynx, Trachea, Chest.

105. Hoarseness, from mucus in the larynx.
Sensation of soreness in the larynx and trachea.
Deep, husky voice when talking or singing.
Breathing, wheezing, crowing, rattling, tight, oppressed and painful.
Difficult inspiration and quick expiration.
110. Suffocative fits, as from mucus in the larynx.
Oppression of the chest, in the evening (at night, while lying.)
Inclination to take a deep breath.
Oppression of the chest, as from fulness in the stomach, and caused by continued talking.
Stitches in the chest; diaphragm.
115. Congestion of blood to the chest, with violent palpitation of the heart.
Suppuration of the lungs, after hæmoptysis (frequent venesections) with stitches in the chest, which are aggravated by pressure.
Nightly suffocative cough, with stitches in the chest.
Hæmoptysis, (clotted blood mixed with pus.)
The cough is aggravated in the evening, or after midnight; from laughing; from continued talking; from lying with the head low; from slightly touching the larynx; from draft of air, after awaking; from loss of fluids.
120. Cough, with pain in the larynx and sternum.

Back.

Pressure as from a stone between the shoulder blades.
Pain in the small of the back at night when lying on it.
Insupportable pain in the small of the back, like a cramp, aggravated by the least movement.
Perspiration in the back and neck on the least motion.
125. Stitches in the spine and shoulders.

Extremities.

Upper. Trembling hands, (when writing.)
Icy coldness of one hand, while the other is warm.
Swelling of the dorsum of the left hand.
Blue nails.
130. Lower. Hot swelling of the right knee, painful to the touch.
Weakness in the knees.
Uneasiness in the legs, obliging him to curve them and draw them up.
Swelling of the feet.
Rheumatic pains in the metatarsal bones and the phalanges of the toes, worse from contact, not from motion.
135. Soft swelling of the soles.

Generalities.

Over-sensitiveness of the nerves, (from loss of fluids.)
Numbness of the parts on which one lies.
Congestions. Veins are much enlarged.
Emaciation.

Sleep.

140. Sleeplessness from crowding of ideas and making of plans.
Irresistible sleepiness during the day and after eating.
As soon as he goes to sleep, confused, absurd dreams.
While asleep, snoring, and blowing expiration.

Fever.

Pulse small, hard and rapid, less frequent after eating; irregular.
145. Chilliness over the whole body, aggravated by drinking, with thirst before and after, not during the chill.
Internal violent chill with icy cold hands and feet, and congestion to the head.
Chilliness and heat alternating in the afternoon.
In the evening, in bed, he cannot get warm.
Heat over the whole body with enlarged veins.
150. During the heat, thirstlessness, or only desire for cold drink.
After the heat, violent thirst.
Long continued heat, often coming late after the chill.
During the heat, desire to be uncovered; delirium.
Perspiration very profuse, and very debilitating.
155. Profuse perspiration during sleep, and from exercise in the open air.
Very debilitating morning and night sweats.
During the perspiration, increased thirst.
Perspiration on the side on which he lies.
Suppressed perspiration.

Skin.

160. Yellowness of the skin. (Jaundice.)
Skin flaccid and dry.
Swelling of the limbs.
Rheumatic, hard, red swellings.
Humid gangrene (of external parts.)

Conditions.

165. Paroxysms of pain caused by the slightest contact, and then gradually increasing to a great height.
The least draft of air causes suffering.
Bad effects from the loss of animal fluids. (Masturbation.)
Aggravation at night after drinking, after the chills, from milk, from touching the parts softly.

CICUTA VIROSA.

Mind and Disposition.

Moaning and howling.
Insanity, she does all sorts of absurd and foolish things, with heat of the body and longing for wine.
He confounds the present with the past.
He thinks himself a young child.
5. Excited and apprehensive about the future.
Anxiety, sadly affected by sad tales.
Want of confidence in and dread of man, retires into solitude.

Head.

Giddiness, with falling forwards.
Vertigo, reeling, as if all the objects turned around him.
10. Affections of the brain, from concussion of the brain.
Semi-lateral headache, as from congestion to the head; relieved when sitting erect.
Compression from both sides of the head.
Feeling of looseness of the brain, as if it were shaken in walking; early in the morning; disappearing when thinking of the pain intensely.
The head is bent backward.
15. The headache is relieved by sitting erect, or by emission of flatulence.
Burning, suppurating eruptions on the hairy scalp.

Eyes.

Contraction of the pupils.
Staring at one and the same object, which she is not able to distinguish correctly.
The objects appear double and black.
20. Staring at an object, the head inclines forward; is frequently bent back again, with twitching, trembling and tension in the neck while moving it.
When reading, the letters turn, and are surrounded with a colored areola, the same as the light.
Twitching of the orbicularis muscle.

Ears.

Sore pain behind the ear, as after a blow.
Hemorrhage from the ears.
25. Detonation in the right ear when swallowing.
Hardness of hearing.
Burning, suppurating eruption on and around the ears.

Nose.

Yellow discharge from the nose.
Scurfs in the nostrils.
30. Frequent sneezing, without coryza.

Face, Mouth and Throat.

Deadly paleness of the face, with coldness of the face and hands.
Red face.
Burning, suppurating, confluent eruptions on the face.
Thick, honey-colored scurf on the chin, upper lip, and lower portion of the cheeks, (milk crust,) burning, soreness and oozing, accompanied with swelling of the submaxillary glands, and insatiable appetite.
35. Painful, burning, ulcerated lips.
Grinding of the teeth.
Lock-jaw, the teeth pressing firmly against one another.
Foam in and at the mouth.
Swelling of the tongue; white, painful, burning ulcers on the edges of the tongue.
40. Speech difficult; when talking, he feels a jerk in the head from before backwards, as if he had to swallow the word, as in hiccough.
Inability to swallow; the throat appears to be closed, and feels bruised when touched externally, (with eructations.)

Stomach and Abdomen.

Great desire for coal.

Continual hunger and appetite, even shortly after a meal.
Violent thirst (during the spasms).
45. Nausea in the morning and when eating.
Hiccough.
Vomiting of blood.
Vomiting, alternating with tonic spasms in the pectoral muscles and distortion of the eyes; (the vomiting does not relieve the lock-jaw.)
Burning pressure at the stomach and abdomen.
50. Swelling, and throbbing in the pit of the stomach.
Colic, with convulsions (in children from worms).
Distention and painfulness of the abdomen.

Stool and Anus.
Frequent liquid stools.
Itching in the rectum, with burning pain after friction.

Urinary Organs.
55. Frequent micturition; the urine is propelled with great force.
Involuntary emission of urine.

Genital Organs.
Men. Sore, drawing pain under the penis as far as the glans, obliging one to urinate.
Women. Menses delayed.
Spasms during parturition.

Chest.
60. Want of breath, caused by tonic spasms of the pectoral muscles.
Tightness in the chest; she is scarcely able to breathe all day.
Burning in the chest.
Sensation of soreness (as if bruised) at the lower end of the sternum (when walking).

Back.
Tension in the muscles of the neck; if he turns the head, he cannot easily turn it back again.
65. Tonic spasms in the neck.
Tonic spasms of the cervical muscles.

Extremities.
Upper. Deadness of the fingers.
The veins on the hands are enlarged.
Jerking in the left arm all day.
70. Frequent involuntary jerking and twitching in the arms and fingers.

Lower. Painful feeling of stiffness and rigidity in the muscles of the lower limbs.
Violent trembling of the left leg.
The feet turn inwards when walking.
Spasms in the muscles, especially of the neck and chest.
75. Twitchings of the extremities.
Tonic spasms.
Epileptic convulsions and epilepsy.
Sensation on many parts of the body, as from a bruise.

Sleep.

Vivid dreams, which cannot be recollected.
80. Frequent waking with profuse general perspiration, which relieves very much.

Fever.

Pulse weak, slow, trembling.
Chill and chilliness, with desire to go to the warm stove.
The chilliness begins in the chest and extends down the legs and into the arms, with staring.
Heat only internally.
85. Perspiration at night (in the morning hours), principally on the abdomen.

Skin.

Burning, itching.
Suppurating eruptions, with yellow scurf and burning pain.
Swelling of the neck, arising from wounding the œsophagus with a splinter (bone) or similar sharp body.

Conditions.

Worm complaints in children, with convulsions.
90. Aggravations from concussions (brain).

CIMEX LECTULARIUS.

Head.

Violent headache, which almost deprives him of the power of thinking during the chill; worse when he drinks.

Nose.

Dryness of the nostrils.
Constant sneezing in the forenoon.
Fluent coryza, with pressure in the frontal sinuses

Mouth and Throat.

5. Tongue coated white.
   Swollen feeling of the tongue.
   Feeling as if burnt on the tongue, in the region of the palate and the upper anterior gums.
   Dryness of the throat, causing him to drink all day.

Stomach and Abdomen.

Sour eructations.
10. Pain in the liver, as if it had been strained by bending the right side inward; the spot is painful when touching it and when coughing.
    Colic, followed by emissions of flatulence or liquid stools.

Stool and Anus.

Stools hard, in small balls.
After the discharge of a small piece of white stool the rectum closes firmly.
Stools with hæmorrhoidal sufferings.

Urinary Organs.

15. Urine brown, with a deposit of sediment (during the fever, when he drinks)

Respiratory Organs.

Dry cough, with gagging, as if he would vomit, with perspiration.

Back.

Pain in the small of the back, extending over the abdomen, with distention of the abdomen.
Pain in the small of the back; worse when sitting.

Extremities.

Upper. Pain in the right shoulder and the anterior muscles of the chest, extending through the whole arm down t the nails; the fingers feel as if they had gone to sleep.

Fever.

20. Pulse feeble; intermitting.
    Before the cold stage, thirst; heaviness in the lower extremities.
    At the beginning of the chill, clenching of the hands and violent rage.
    Chilliness over the whole body, followed by dry heat which is succeeded by some moisture over the skin.

During the chill painfulness in all the joints; sensation as if the tendons were too short; the knee joints are most contracted; the legs cannot be extended; the chest feels oppressed, obliging one to take a long breath frequently; irresistible sleepiness.

25. At the end of the chill the legs feel tired; the position of the legs has to be changed constantly; this ceases during the hot stage.

After the chill thirst, and when he drinks he is attacked with violent headache, which almost deprives him of the power of thinking; tickling in the larynx, causing a continuous dry cough; oppression of breathing; heaviness in the middle of the chest; anxiety. Amelioration if he does not drink.

During the hot stage gagging in the œsophagus, which impedes inspiration; thirstlessness; the water drank to allay the gagging goes down at intervals only; the œsophagus feels constricted.

If he drinks during the fever he passes soon after very hot brown urine, depositing a good deal of sediment.

The perspiration, after the hot stage, is accompanied by hunger.

30. Perspiration mostly on the head and chest.

During the intermittent fever, constipation; stools dry.

Sleep.

Great drowsiness; falls asleep when sitting, in the morning.

CINA.

Mind and Disposition.

Piteous complaints and weeping.

Ill-humor; the child is averse to being caressed and rejects every thing which is offered.

The child will not be touched.

Disposition to be offended by trifling jests.

Head.

5. The head falls to the side and is jerked backwards, with twitches in the limbs and cold perspiration of the face.

Headache, before and after the epileptic attacks; after attacks of intermittent fever.

CINA.

The headache is aggravated by walking in the open air and from exertions of the mind.
Cold perspiration on the head (forehead) and on the pale, cold, bloated face, with blueness around the mouth; twitching of the limbs and sleepiness, worse at night (after attacks of hooping-cough and epilepsy).

Eyes.

Pain in the eyes when using them at night by the candle-light.
10. Dilatation of the pupils.
When looking at a thing steadily (reading) he sees it as through a gauze, which is relieved by wiping the eyes.
Weakness of sight (from onanism).
Aversion to light.

Nose.

Bleeding of the nose and from the mouth, with burning in the nose.
15. Disposition to bore in the nose.
The child rubs the nose constantly, and bores with the fingers in the nose until blood comes out.
Sneezing, violent, with stitches in the temples.
Stoppage of the nose in the evening; fluent coryza at noon; the nose burns.

Face.

Paleness of the face, with sickly appearance around the eyes.
20. Bloated, pale face, with blueness around the mouth.
Pale, cold face, with cold perspiration.
Pain (tearing) in the zygomata, aggravated or renewed by contact and pressure.

Teeth.

Grinding of the teeth.
Sensitiveness of the teeth to cold air and cold water.
25. The teeth feel sore.

Mouth and Tongue.

Sensation of dryness and roughness of the mouth, especially of the palate.
Inability to swallow, especially fluids.

Appetite and Taste.

Canine hunger; he is hungry soon after a full meal.
The child refuses to take the mother's milk.
30. Increased thirst.

Gastric Symptoms.

Vomiting (and diarrhœa) after drinking.
Vomiting of lumbrici (and ascarides); of food and mucus.
Vomiting during the fever, with clean tongue.
Vomiting of the food and of bile.
35. Frequent hiccough.

Stomach and Abdomen.

Cutting and pinching pain in the abdomen from worms.
Pain in the pericardial region, oppressing the breathing.
Painful twisting around the navel.
Unpleasant sensation of warmth in the abdomen.
40. Bloated abdomen, especially in children.
Feeling of emptiness in the abdomen.
Audible gurgling from the throat into the stomach when drinking.

Stool and Anus.

Involuntary diarrhœic, white stools.
Discharges of lumbrici and of ascarides.
45. Itching of the anus.

Urinary Organs.

Involuntary emission of urine (at night).
Turbid urine.

Sexual Organs.

Women. Menstruation too early and too profuse.
Hemorrhage from the uterus.
50. Labor-like pains in the abdomen, frequently recurring, as if the menses would appear.

Respiratory Organs.

Oppression of the chest, as from a cramp-like, contracted sensation in the chest.
Short, interrupted breathing.
Respiration wheezing and panting.
Suffocative attacks.
55. Hoarseness, with much mucus in the larynx and trachea.
Dry, spasmodic cough, preceded by rigidity of the body and unconsciousness.
Hooping-cough, in violent periodically returning attacks, from a titilating sensation in the throat, as of a feather, and much tough mucus—in the morning without expectoration, in the evening with difficult expectoration of white, occasionally blood-streaked, mucus, which is

tasteless; worse in the morning and in the evening; better during the night; aggravated by drinking, walking in the open air, pressing on the larynx, when lying on the right side, in the cold air, and when awaking from sleep.
Burning, stitches, and soreness in the chest.

Back.

Pain in the small of the back, as if bruised.

Extremities.

60. *Upper.* Twitching of the fingers.
Spasmodic contraction of the hand.
Weakness of the hand; he can hold nothing with it.
Cramp-like drawing pains in the arms and hands.
Sprained feeling in the wrist-joint.
65. *Lower.* Rigidity of the lower limbs; spasmodic stretching and twitching of the feet.

Generalities.

Epileptic attacks, especially at night, with or without consciousness, lying on the back; violent screams and violent jerks of the hands and feet.
The body is stretched out and becomes rigid.
Dull stitches in different parts of the body.
Twitching and distortions of the limbs.

Sleep.

70. Sleeplessness, with restlessness, crying and lamentations.
At night, restless, tossing about, and crying (children).
Wakes in the morning, restless and lamenting, in a start.

Fever.

Pulse small, hard, and rapid.
Chilliness, with shaking or trembling, ascending from the upper part of the body to the head.
75. Chill, with coldness of the pale face and heat of the hands.
Chill, not relieved by external heat, with great paleness of the face, and mostly in the evening.
Heat, mostly in the face and head, often with paleness of the face.
Heat at night, with thirst.
Perspiration, generally cold, on the forehead, around the nose, and on the hands.
80. After the perspiration (sometimes before the chill) vomiting of food; at the same time canine hunger.

Conditions.

Suitable for children, especially when they suffer from worms.
When touched, or when moving, the body feels sore.
External pressure renews or aggravates the suffering.
Bad effects from onanism (eyes).
85. Aggravation at night; on looking fixedly at an object; from external pressure.

CINNABARIS

Mind and Disposition.

Indisposition for mental labor.
Sensation of fulness of the head from mental application.
Forgetfulness (forgets things he has to do).
Fretful, easily provoked.
5. Desire to be alone.

Head.

Giddiness in the morning after rising, when stooping, with nausea.
Fulness in the head; the eyes are reddened.
Congested sensation over the whole head, principally the forehead.
Congestion of blood to the head, particularly to the vertex; worse after eating.
10. Intense headache; he cannot raise his head from the pillow; relieved by external pressure.
Dull pain in the forehead, which is cold; relieved by heat.
Sensation as if touched by a cold metallic body, on a small space over the root of the nose.
In the morning, after waking, pain in the forehead and top of the head; worse when lying on the left side and back; better and going off, when turning on the right side, and after rising.
Shooting pain in the left side of the head, with increase of saliva and great flow of urine.
15. Sensitiveness of the head to the touch—even the hairs are sore.

Eyes.

Shooting pains in the inner canthus of the right eye, with burning and itching.
Inflammation of the right eye; itching, pressing and pricking at the inner angle and lower lid; constant lachrymation on looking steadily, with profuse discharge of mucus from the nose.
Flow of tears.
Sticking pain about the punctum lachrymale of the upper eyelid.
20. Redness of the whole eye, with swelling of the face.

Ears.

Roaring in the ears, with swelling of the face (after eating).
Scurfy eruption in the right external ear.
Itching in the right ear.

Nose.

Itching of the nose, with bleeding (very dark blood) after blowing it.
25. Coryza, with lameness of the thighs and aching pain in the small of the back; lumps of dirty yellow mucus are discharged from the posterior nares.

Face.

Heat of the face, which is much swollen, mostly about the eyes.

Mouth and Throat.

Both corners of the mouth are chapped.
Tongue coated white in the morning.
A small ulcer on the roof of the mouth, on the right side of the tip of the tongue; on the tip of the tongue.
30. Soreness in the roof of the mouth.
Dryness in the mouth and throat at night, which causes him to drink often.
Inflammation, with great dryness of the throat and mouth; worse at night.
Dryness and irritation of the throat (posterior nares, tonsils, fauces) at night, with soreness during the day; in the morning, secretion of tenacious mucus also, in lumps, from the posterior nares.
Contracting pain in the throat during empty deglutition.
35. Fulness in the throat, causing a constant desire for swallowing.
Taste bitter (in the morning).
Increased flow of saliva (and of urine).

Salivation.
Scanty, tenacious, frothy saliva in the mouth, without thirst; better after drinking.
40. Dryness and putrid taste in the mouth.

Stomach and Abdomen.

Appetite increased.
Soreness in the stomach, with dizziness and lightness in the head and tightness in the temples.
Nausea, alleviated by eructations.
Nausea, with water-brash (in the evening).
45. Flashes of heat confined to the abdomen, with great flatulence (worse in the forenoon).

Stool and Anus.

Soft, scanty stools twice a day, preceded by pinching; less afterwards.
Bloody dysentery.
Sensation of formication in the anus, as if from a large worm.
Little pimples around the anus, with burning and itching; thin stools and tenesmus.

Urinary Organs.

50. Frequent and increased emission of watery urine; also during the night.
Pain, as if from a sore in the urethra when urinating; this pain wakes him up at night.

Genital Organs.

Men. Swelling of the penis.
Redness and swelling of the prepuce, with painful itching.
Violent itching of the corona glandis, with profuse secretion of pus.
55. Small, shining red points on the glans penis.
Blennorrhœa of the glans penis.
Sycotic excrescences.
Violent erections in the evening.
Women. Leucorrhœa, causing, during its discharge, a pressing in the vagina.

Respiratory Organs.

60. Hoarseness in the evening.
Chest oppressed, feels contracted; relieved by stretching himself.
Dyspnœa, with heat.
Pain running over the ensiform cartilage, from the seventh rib on the right side diagonally through the chest.
Cough from tickling in the throat.

Back.

65. The muscles of the back part of the neck seem as if contracted.
Aching in the small of the back, as if bruised.
Pain all over the back down to the loins, aggravated on drawing a long breath.

Extremities.

Upper. Pain in the left shoulder, between the clavicle and scapula, interiorly.
Pain in the middle of the upper part of the right arm, as though it would break.
70. Periodical shooting pains in the arms.
Sensation of lameness in the right arm.
Numbness of the left arm, from the elbow to the end of the little finger.
It feels as if the "crazy-bone" was struck.
The joints of the fingers and knuckles are red (and hot).
75. *Lower.* Shooting, drawing and aching pains in the thighs, from the hip-joints nearly down to the condyles; worse at night.
Violent itching on the inside of the thighs, knees and legs; worse on the knees, especially at night.
Profuse perspiration between the thighs (when walking).
Rheumatic pain in the right knee-joint; worse when walking (ascending), better at rest.
Pain in the tendo Achilles and os calcis after walking.
80. Coldness in the joints.
Coldness of the feet, day and night.

Generalities.

Sensation of lameness in all the limbs.
Weariness, languor, tired and prostrated; worse before eating, better when riding in the open air.
General nervous, uneasy sensation.

Sleep.

85. Sleepiness in the day-time and sleeplessness at night; unconquerable desire to sleep after dinner, early in the evening (during the day).
Restlessness and sleeplessness at night, from a constant flow of ideas changing from one thing to another.
Restless sleep, with vivid dreams and much talking.

Fever.

Pulse slower in the forepart of the day, accelerated in the evening.
Coldness and chilliness in the warm room.
90. Internal and external heat of the body during the whole night.
Profuse perspiration between the thighs.
Perspiration most at noon.

Skin.

Itching of the nose (bleeding after blowing it), of the eyelids, canthi (outer), ears, face (left side), palms of the hands (right), thighs (inside), knees, legs, at the anus (at night), on the shoulders (evening).
Sensation as if pimples were coming out over the body.
95. Red papulous eruption, without itching, on both elbows.
Redness of the skin.

Conditions.

The pains intermit in severity.
Aggravations in the evening and at night, except of the perspiration, which is worse at midday; after sleeping (headache).
Amelioration in the open air, and after dinner.

CISTUS CANADENSIS.

Mind and Disposition.

Bad effects from vexation.
Mental excitement increases the suffering (stitches in the throat, producing cough).

Head.

Pressure above the eyes, in the forehead.
Headache, worse towards evening, lasting all night.
5. Head drawn to one side by swelling on the neck.

Eyes.

Feeling of weight above the eyes.
Stitches in the left eye.
Feeling as if something were passing around in the eye, with stitches (scrofulous inflammation of the eyes).

Ears.

Discharge from the ears (of water and bad-smelling pus).
10. Inner swelling of the ears (with discharge).
Tetters on and around the ear, extending to the external meatus.
Swelling of the parotid glands.

Nose.

Frequent and violent sneezing (evenings and mornings).
Cold feeling in the nose.
15. Inflammation and swelling of the left side of the nose (burning).
The tip of the nose is painful.

Face.

Flushes of heat in the face.
Heat and burning in the facial bones.
Vesicular erysipelas in the face.
20. Caries of the lower jaw.
Lupus extends to the mouth and nose.

Mouth and Teeth.

Scorbutic gums, swollen, separating from the teeth, easily bleeding, putrid.
Dryness of the tongue and roof of the mouth.
Sore tongue, as if raw, on the surface.
25. Sensation of coldness of the tongue, larynx, and trachea: the saliva is cool; the breath feels cold.
Impure breath.

Throat.

Dryness and heat in the throat; he must constantly swallow saliva to relieve it (drinking water and eating relieve it).
Periodical itching in the throat.
Fauces inflamed and dry without feeling dry; hawking up of tough, gum-like, thick, tasteless phlegm (in the morning).
30. Hawking of (bitter) mucus, relieving the throat.
Sore pain in the throat and dryness of the tongue in the morning.
Stitches in the throat, causing cough, whenever mentally agitated.

Stomach and Abdomen.

Cool eructations.
Cold feeling in the stomach before and after eating.
35. Pain in the stomach immediately after eating.
Cold feeling in the whole abdomen.

Stool and Anus.

Diarrhœa, after eating fruit, after drinking coffee.
Thin hot stools, of grayish yellow color, from midnight till noon.

Genital Organs.

Male. Itching on the scrotum.

Respiratory Organs.

40. Cool feeling in the larynx and trachea.
Feeling as if the trachea were not wide enough (asthma).
Pain in the trachea.
Feeling of rawness, extending from the upper part of the chest into the throat.
Fulness of and pressure on the chest.
45. Cough, from stitches or painful tearings in the throat.
Cough; the neck is thickly studded with tumors.
Bleeding at the lungs.

Back and Neck.

Glands on the neck and throat swollen.
Scrofulous swelling and suppuration of the glands of the throat.
50. Itching on the back.
A burning, bruised pain in the os coccygis, preventing sitting; aggravated by contact.

Extremities.

Upper. Sprained pain in the wrists.
Pain in the fingers (right hand) while writing.
Tearing in the finger-joints.
55. The tips of the fingers are very sensitive to the cold.
Tetter on the hands.
Lower. Pains in the knee and right thigh when walking or sitting.
Tearing in the knees (evening).
Piercing pain in the right great toe (evening).
60. Cold feet.

Generalities.

Trembling (with the fever).
Sensation as if ants were running through the whole body (in the evening, with anxious, difficult breathing).

Fever.

Chilliness.
Cold feeling in the abdomen, larynx.

65. Chill, followed by fever, with trembling, accompanied by a quick swelling and great redness of the glands below the ear and in the throat.
Heat, with thirst (drinks frequently).

Sleep.

Very restless at night.
Sleeplessness because of the dryness of the throat.
Night sweats.

Skin.

70. Itching all over the body without eruption (abdomen, navel scrotum).
Vesicular erysipelas on the face.
Tetter (ears, hands).
Lupus on the face.
Hard swelling around the mercurial, syphilitic ulcers on the lower limbs.

Conditions.

75. *Aggravation.* Evening; during the night; in the morning.
Cold air (sore throat).
When lying down (difficulty of breathing).
From drinking coffee (diarrhœa).
From motion.
80. *Amelioration.* Fresh air (difficult breathing).

CLEMATIS ERECTA.

Mind and Disposition.

Low-spirited and fear of approaching misfortunes.
Aversion to talk.
Fear of being alone, but disinclined to meet otherwise agreeable company.
Memory impaired.

Head.

5. Giddiness, if he lift his head up, or when moving the head.
Boring pains in the temple.
Head feels full and heavy, hanging down.
Heaviness in the forehead.
Headache, aggravated by bending the head backwards.

10. Eruptions on the back part of the head and neck; moist, sore, tingling and stinging itching; often drying up in scales; when getting warm in bed, violently itching; only temporarily relieved by scratching; with soreness and rawness.

Itching on the hairy scalp.

Eyes.

Itching in the canthi.
Burning of the eyelids.
Burning and heat in the eyes, with dryness, as if fire were streaming from the eyes.

15. Redness, biting and lachrymation from the eyes.
Inflammation of the iris.
The white of the eyes has a yellow tint.
The closed eye is very sensitive to the air (cold air), and when it is opened very sensitive to light.
While writing, the letters momentarily run one into another; at times, double vision, with flickering before the eyes.

Ears.

20. Ringing, as from bells in the ear.
The external ear is hot and burns.

Nose.

Dryness of the nose, with heat.
Violent coryza, with sneezing; the secretion is streaked with blood.

Face.

Sickly paleness of the face.

25. Cheeks red and hot (momentary flushes).
White blisters on the nose and face, as if burned by the sun.
Moist eruption on the face, preceded by stinging pain.
Cancer of the lips.

Mouth and Throat.

Pricking or drawing toothache; worse, and becoming insupportable at night, in a horizontal position.

30. Toothache in a decayed molar tooth, much aggravated from a crumb of bread coming into it; relieved by cold water.
Sensation as if the decayed tooth were too long; the least contact is exceedingly painful, with an excessive flow of saliva.
Aggravation of the toothache by smoking tobacco.
Increased secretion of saliva.
Small blisters on the tongue and in the throat, which soon become ulcers.

CLEMATIS ERECTA.

35. Heat and burning in the mouth and throat.
Sensation of roughness in the throat.

Appetite and Taste.

Aversion to beer.
Increased thirst, with desire for ice.
After eating, nausea and sleepiness.

Stomach and Abdomen.

40. Nausea after smoking tobacco.
Disagreeable sensation of coldness in the stomach.
Tension of the stomach.
Pain in the liver, aggravated by pressure.
Stitches in the liver.
45. Sensation of constriction in the lower abdomen, which is hard.
Swelling, induration and twitching pains in the inguinal glands.

Stool and Anus.

Hard stool, difficult to discharge (in the evening).
Loose stools, with burning at the anus.
Burning heat, and itching at the anus (in the evening); better after an evacuation.
50. Hæmorrhoids, itching, discharging some mucus.

Urinary Organs.

Increased secretion of urine.
Urine turbid, milky, dark, with flakes of mucus and frothy.
Secretion diminished; the last drops cause violent burning.
Secretion slow and in a small stream.
55. During micturition, burning in the urethra; stitches in the urethra; stitches from the abdomen into the chest.
After micturition, itching, tingling in the urethra, lasting half an hour; burning in the urethra; involuntary dripping of urine.
The urethra is painful to pressure.
Spasmodic stricture of the urethra.
Discharge from the urethra, thick, pus.

Genitals.

60. *Men.* Itching at the genitals.
Drawing pain from the testicles into the spermatic cords upwards; the right testicle is drawn up.
Sensation of soreness of the testes.

CLEMATIS ERECTA.

Violent, long-continuing erections, with stitches in the urethra.
Painful swelling and induration of the testes (right).
65. Scrotum swelled, indurated.
Women. Swelling and induration of the mammary glands; cancer of the breast.

Respiratory Organs.

Violent cough, with irregular respiration, at times too slow, at times too rapid; barking cough, with burning pain in the sternum and stitches in both sides of the lungs.
Sharp stitch in the heart, from within to without.

Back and Neck.

Moist eruption in the neck, extending into the head.
70. Pain in the small of the back, as if broken, with tension; worse when stooping.

Extremities.

Upper. Swelling and induration of the axillary glands.
The hands feel as if they were too large; they are dry and hot.
Spreading blisters on the swollen hands and fingers, aggravated by cold water.
Arthritic nodosities in the finger joints.
75. *Lower.* Dry, scaly tetter on the legs.
Itching of the toes and perspiration between them.

Generalities.

Great emaciation.
Twitching of the muscles.
Great debility and weakness, (3—5 P. M.)

Sleep.

80. Sleepiness during the day (morning).
Restless sleep, with tossing about and vivid, lascivious dreams; profuse perspiration after midnight.

Fever.

Pulse accelerated.
Chilliness with shuddering, followed by perspiration.
Chilliness from being uncovered.
85. Dry heat, with sensation of general heat (at night).
Profuse perspiration at night, towards morning, with disinclination to be uncovered.

Skin.

Painful swelling and induration of the glands.

Ulcers, with tingling, pulsation, burning; stitches in the edges when touching them.
Itching over the whole body.
90. Skin inflamed, red, burning; eruption of blisters, which burst and form ulcers.
Moist tetter, itching in the heat of the bed, and after washing.
Painful (not itching) tetter over the whole body; red and moist during the increasing moon, pale and dry during the decreasing moon.
Scaly tetter, with thick crusts.
Itching and moist eruptions, with ichorous discharges excoriating the surrounding parts, with redness, heat and swelling of the skin.
95. Aggravation of all skin symptoms by the heat of the bed and from washing.

COCCIONELLA SEPTEM PUNCTATA.

Mind and Disposition.
Ill-humored, irritable.

Head.
Giddiness; the head feels dull, as if he had drank too much, with a white-coated tongue.
Congestion of blood to the head when entering a warm room; better in the open air.

Eyes.
Sensation as if a foreign body were lodged between the eyelid and the eye.
5. Sensation as if the edges of the eyelids were swollen.

Ears.
Sudden violent stitch in the left internal ear, extending to the left side of the neck and into the sternum.
Intolerable itching in the left ear.

Nose.
Dryness of the nose, with inclination to sneeze.
Swelling of the nose, with itching, violent sneezing and increased secretion of mucus.
10. Redness of the edges of the nostrils.
Crusts on the edges of the nostrils.

Mouth and Throat.

Sensation as if cold air were blown on the teeth.
Great soreness of the teeth to contact.
Scraping and dryness in the throat.
15. Sweetish, metallic taste in the mouth.
Dry, brown-coated tongue.
Stitches and burning in the throat and on the tongue.
Swelling and redness of the right tonsil.
Sensation as if the palate were elongated, with continuous hawking.
20. Swelling of the tonsils, with continuous desire to swallow, and sensation as if a plug were lodged in the throat.

Appetite and Taste.

Desire to eat often and much at a time.
Sensation of hunger, with colic.
Canine hunger.
After dinner much thirst, and when he drinks water then chill.

Stomach and Abdomen.

25. Spasmodic empty eructations.
Heartburn.
Sensation as if something indigestible were lying in the stomach.
Nausea and vomiting; vomiting of mucus.
Stitches in the pit of the stomach when inhaling.
30. Fulness in the abdomen, as if he had eaten too much, with swelling and tenderness of the pit of the stomach.

Stool and Anus.

During stool, burning in the rectum; stitches in the rectum.
Itching at the anus, with tenesmus, from slight exertion.
Stitch from the anus, extending into the urethra.

Urinary Organs.

Stitches extending from the kidneys through the urethra into the bladder.
35. Spasmodic pain in the bladder, with alternate coldness and heat.
Itching at the end of the urethra.
Great desire to urinate in the morning (with erection).
Frequent micturition.
The discharge of urine is slow, in small quantities, with violent burning pain.
40. Red sediment like brick-dust.

Genitals.

Men. Genitals hot, red, swollen.
Sexual desire increased.
Women. Catamenia too early and too profuse.

Respiratory Organs.

Hoarse voice, with roughness and scraping sensation in the throat.
45. Hawking and coughing, with increased thirst.
Cough, in a warm room; better, in a cold room.
Periodical attacks of cough, with expectoration of mucus.
Hooping-cough; nightly, periodical attacks of cough from tickling in the larynx, ending with expectoration of a large quantity of viscid, stringy mucus.
Morning cough; first barking, dry cough, followed by expectoration of viscid mucus; the difficult expectoration causes vomiturition and vomiting.
50. Cough, with expectoration of viscid, stringy, yellow, sour-tasting or reddish mucus.
The bronchial tubes are loaded with mucus.
Burning under the sternum.
In the chest sensation of heat, of soreness.
Sensation as if every thing were pressed towards the heart.
55. Heavy pressure in the region of the heart.

Extremities.

Upper. Sensation as if a fine glass splinter were sticking in the tips of the fingers, under the nails.
Lower. Violent stitches in the right hip-joint.
Hot swelling of the knees.
Pain in the right patella when walking.

Sleep.

60. Frequent awaking during the night, with excitement, as if he had taken too much coffee.
Great sleepiness (after dinner).
Vivid dreams.

Fever.

Chilliness all day; cold feet in the morning, with perspiration of the whole body.
Chill in the evening, with heat in the head, followed by general heat, and then perspiration all night, which relieves.
65. Perspiration, when walking, on the lower extremities, in the morning.

Conditions.

Especially affects the mucous membranes.
Aggravation from motion and heat (headache).

COCCULUS.

Mind and Disposition.

He sits as if wrapped up in deep, sad thoughts, and does not take notice of any thing; anxiety.
The time passes too quickly.

Head.

Giddiness, with nausea, when raising himself up in bed.
Vertigo, as from intoxication.
5. Stupid feeling in the head (cold perspiration on forehead and hands).
Cloudiness in the head, increased by eating and drinking.
Sensation of emptiness in the head.
Headache, with nausea.
The headache is aggravated after sleeping, eating or drinking (coffee), in the open air, while riding in a carriage; and is relieved in a warm room, or when becoming warm in bed.
10. Spasmodic trembling of the head, caused by weakness of the muscles of the neck; worse after sleeping and in the open air, from coffee and tobacco; better in the warm room.

Eyes.

Pain in the eyes, as if they were torn out of the head (with headache).
At night the eyes cannot be opened; they are aching.
Dim-sightedness (after reading a short time the print is all blurred).
Black spots before the eyes.
15. Dryness of the eyelids.

Ears.

Hardness of hearing, with noise, as from rushing water.
The right ear feels closed.

Nose.
Very acute sense of smell.
Swelling of the right half of the nose.

Face.
20. Heat in the face and redness of the cheeks.
Flushes of heat in the face after drinking.
Swelling and induration of the submaxillary glands.

Mouth and Throat.
Dryness of the mouth (in the night, without thirst).
Dryness of the œsophagus, with feeling of heat.
25. Inability to swallow; the œsophagus feels paralyzed.
Difficulty of speech, as from paralysis of the tongue.
Foamy phlegm before the mouth.
Taste in the mouth coppery, metallic, sour (after eating and coughing).

Stomach and Abdomen.
Aversion to food, drinking, tobacco and acids.
30. Intense thirst, especially while eating.
Frequent empty eructations, leaving a bitter taste in the mouth and throat.
Eructations, with nausea and sticking pains in the pit of the stomach.
Paroxysms of nausea, with tendency to faint.
Excessive nausea and vomiting when riding in a carriage, or from becoming cold.
35. Nausea, with headache and pains in the intestines, as if bruised.
Spasm of the stomach (cramp) during and after a meal, with griping tearing.
Fulness and pinching in the stomach, with oppressed breathing.
Constrictive pain in the stomach, preventing sleep.
Sensation of emptiness in the abdomen.
40. Hysterical spasms in the abdomen, in women.
Distention of the abdomen.
Flatulent colic, at night, aggravated when coughing.

Stool and Anus.
Constipation; the hard stool is expelled with difficulty.
After the evacuation, violent tenesmus.
45. Ineffectual desire for stool, with constipation.
Contractive pain in the rectum, preventing sitting (in the afternoon).
Diarrhœa, with emission of flatulency before the stool.

Urinary Organs.

Frequent desire to urinate, with small discharges.
Watery (pale) urine.

Sexual Organs.

50. *Men.* Increased excitability of the sexual organs.
The testicles feel bruised, especially when touched.
Women. Menstruation too early, blood coagulated, or suppressed, with violent uterine spasms or abdominal colic.
Discharge of bloody mucus during pregnancy.

Respiratory Organs.

Oppressed breathing, from contractive sensation in the trachea, as if irritated by smoke, causing constant coughing.
55. Oppression of the chest, caused by cough.
Tightness and constriction of the right side of the chest.
Stitches in the chest (sternum) when walking.
Burning in the chest, extending into the throat.
Sensation of emptiness of the chest.
60. Hysterical spasms in the chest, with sighing and moaning.
Palpitation of the heart, nervous, with anxiety.

Back and Neck.

The muscles of the neck are weak; they do not support the head.
Cracking of the cervical vertebræ.
Tremor in the back.
65. Paralytic pain and paralysis of the back and small of the back.

Extremities.

Upper. Pain, as if bruised, in the shoulder and bones of the arms, when lifting them up, and when touching them.
Lameness of the arm (cannot write).
The arms go to sleep, are insensible.
Hot swelling of the hands.
70. The hands are alternately hot and cold.
Lower. Cracking in the left hip-joint.
Paralytic immobility of the lower limbs.
Paralysis of the lower limbs, from the small of the back downwards.
The thighs feel paralyzed and bruised.

75. Cracking of the knee during motion.
Inflammation and swelling of the knee, with stitches.
Hot swelling of the feet (evening, the left foot).
Burning of the feet.
Cold perspiration of the feet.
80. Pain in the heel (os calcis), as if bruised.

Generalities.

Paralysis, one sided, with numbness of the limbs.
Paralytic immobility of the limbs, with drawing pains in the bones.
Sensation of emptiness, or of constriction in internal parts.
Disposition to tremble (trembling of all the limbs).
85. Hysterical spasms, with anguish.
Great debility from slight exertion and inclination to faint.
Attacks of gout, with swelling of the affected parts.

Sleep.

Constant drowsiness.
Sleeplessness on account of anxiety and bodily restlessness.
90. Vivid dreams, exciting fear.

Fever.

Pulse small and spasmodic; sometimes it cannot be felt.
Chilliness alternating with heat.
Chill in the afternoon and evening, principally on the legs and in the back; not relieved by heat.
Continuous chilliness, with hot skin.
95. Dry heat during the night.
Flushes of heat, with burning heat of the cheeks and cold feet.
Perspiration during the night, which is only cold on the face.
Morning sweat, especially on the chest.
Slight perspiration over the whole body, from the least exertion.
100. Perspiration of the affected parts.
Intermittent fever, with colic and lameness of the small of the back.

Skin.

Induration; cold swelling of the glands, with stinging pains.
Pale (chlorotic) skin.
Ulcers very sensitive to contact.

Conditions.

105. Great sensitiveness to the open (cold and warm) air.
Aggravation from eating, drinking, riding in a carriage, talking and sleeping.

COCHLEARIA ARMORACIA.

Mind and Disposition.

Difficult thinking in the evening.

Head.

Headache, now in one, then in another side of the head; worse when opening the eyes widely.

Urinary Organs.

Frequent desire to urinate; the urine is discharged with difficulty, causing burning, tenderness and inflammation of the urethra, as in the first (inflammatory) stages of gonorrhœa.

Generalities.

Pain in every joint, during rest; going off during motion.

COFFEA CRUDA.

Mind and Disposition.

Over-sensitiveness; weeping mood.
Great anguish; cannot be composed; is not able to hold the pen; trembles.
Sentimental ecstasy; excited imagination; increased power to think.
Excessive weeping and lamentations over trifles.
5. The pains seem insupportable, driving to despair.
Fright from sudden pleasant surprises.

Head.

Congestion of blood to the head, especially after a pleasant surprise.
Headache, as if the brain were torn or dashed to pieces.
In the vertex he feels and hears a cracking, when sitting quietly.
10. One-sided headache, as from a nail driven into the head; worse when walking in the open air.

Eyes.

Eyes look reddish; the power of vision is increased; can read small writing more distinctly.

Ears.

Music has a shrill sound to the ears.
Sense of hearing more acute.

Nose.

The sense of smell is more acute.
15. Bleeding from the nose.

Face.

Dry heat in the face, with red cheeks.

Mouth and Teeth.

Toothache, with restlessness, anguish and weeping mood, especially at night and after a meal.
Toothache, relieved by cold water.
Swelling and painfulness of the throat; worse when swallowing.

Appetite and Taste.

20. Increased hunger, with rapid, hurried eating.
Nightly thirst, which wakens him.
Taste more acute.
Sweetish taste in the mouth.

Stomach and Abdomen.

Colic, as if the stomach had been overloaded, as if the abdomen would burst; cannot suffer the clothes to be tight on the abdomen.
25. Pressure in the abdomen as from incarcerated flatulence.

Stool and Anus.

Diarrhœa, during dentition.

Urinary Organs.

Emission of large quantity of urine (midnight).

Sexual Organs.

Men. The sexual organs are very much excited without emission of semen, and with dry heat of the body.
Women. Labor and after-pains insupportably painful.

Respiratory Organs.

30. Oppression of the chest; obliged to take short inspirations; the breathing heaves the chest visibly.
Short, dry cough, as from constriction of the larynx.
Night cough (cough with measles).

Generalities.

The pains are felt intensely, driving to despair, and inclination to weep.
He feels unusually well.
35. Twitching of the limbs.
Great movability of all the muscles.

Sleep.

Sleeplessness, from over-excitability of mind and body (sleeplessness of lying-in women).

Fever.

Chilliness, increased by every movement.
Internal chilliness, with external heat of the face and body.
40. Chills running down the back.
Dry heat in the evening after going to bed, with chilliness in the back.
Nightly, dry heat, with delirium.
Perspiration on the face, with internal chilliness.

Skin.

Eruptions (measles), with over-excitability and weeping.

Conditions.

45. Bad effects from sudden, pleasurable surprise.
Aversion to the open air, which aggravates the symptoms.
Bad effects from wine-drinking, taking cold, and excessive exaltation.
Amelioration by cold water (odontalgia).

COLCHICUM.

Mind and Disposition.

Peevish; dissatisfied with every thing.
His sufferings seem intolerable to him.
Slight causes, external impressions (bright light, strong smells, contact, bad manners) disturb his temper at once.
Great desire for rest and disinclination to every mental exertion; forgetfulness; absence of mind.

Head.
5. Giddiness when sitting down after walking.
Sensation of constriction over the eyes.
Pulsations in the head.
Pressing pain in the occiput, from mental exertion.
The headache is relieved, after supper, from warmth and lying quiet in bed.

Eyes.
10. Watering of the eyes in the open air.
Ulceration of the meibomian glands (left lower lid), with swelling of the eyelids.
Burning and redness of the edges of the eyelids.

Ears.
Discharge from the ears, with tearing in the ears (after measles).
Stitches in the ears (evening).
15. Dryness of the ears.

Nose.
Fluent coryza, with thin, tenacious discharge from the nose.
Tingling in the nose.
The sense of smell is painfully acute.
Bleeding of the nose in the evenings.

Face.
20. Piteous, sad features, as if he were ill.
Very great paleness of the face.
Cheeks red and hot (afternoon).
Œdematous swelling of the face.

Mouth and Throat.
Increased secretion of saliva; profuse ptyalism, with dryness of the throat.
25. Sensation of warmth and dryness in the mouth.
Lips chapped.
The tongue is heavy, stiff, and insensible.
Tongue coated white.
Smarting and sensation of dryness of the tongue and throat.
30. Biting-tingling in the throat and fauces.
Frequent hawking of (greenish) mucus.
Inflammation and redness of the palate, of the fauces.

Appetite and Taste.

Aversion to food, and loathing when merely looking at it, and still more when smelling it; the smell of broth nauseates, and that of fish, eggs, or fat meat almost makes him faint.

Taste bitter; violent thirst.

Stomach and Abdomen.

35. Constant singultus.

Nausea, in an erect position, when moving, at table, with inclination to vomit, with constant flow of saliva.

Vomiting of bile or mucus, of the ingesta, with trembling, violent gagging, colic, succeeded by bitterness in the mouth and throat.

Every motion excites or renews the vomiting.

Sensitiveness of the region of the stomach; it does not bear contact.

40. The stomach feels icy cold.

Burning in the stomach, with heavy pain.

Sensation of gnawing hunger in the stomach.

Abdominal dropsy, with a fold over the pubic region.

Stitches in the pit of the stomach.

45. Pulsation in the abdomen.

Stool and Anus.

Stool scanty, discharged only by hard straining even of the soft stool, with pain in the small of the back.

Extremely painful stools.

Watery discharges, going off without sensation.

Ineffectual pressing to stool; he feels the fæces in the rectum, but cannot expel them.

50. Frequent evacuations of transparent, jelly-like mucus, relieving the colic.

Fall dysentery, with discharges of white mucus and violent tenesmus; bloody stools, mingled with a slimy substance.

During stool sensation as if the sphincter ani were torn to pieces; burning at the anus.

Prolapsus ani; spasms in the sphincter ani.

Urinary Organs.

Frequent micturition.

55. Whitish sediment in the urine.

Burning in the urinary organs, with diminished secretion.

Brown, black urine.

Sexual Organs.

Men. Itching at the prepuce and orifice of the urethra.
Tearing in the glands and left spermatic cord.
60. *Women.* Catamenia too early.

Respiratory Organs.

Hoarseness in the morning, with roughness of the throat.
Nightly cough, with involuntary discharge of urine.
Oppression of the chest, with anxiety; relieved by bending forward.
Frequent pressure in small spots in the chest.
65. Pressure and oppression in the region of the heart, as if an attack of apoplexy threatened; relieved by walking.
Lancinating pain or cutting, as with a knife, in the right side of the chest.
Hydrothorax.

Back and Neck.

Tearing and lancinations in the back.
Soreness in the small of the back when touching it.
70. Drawing in the small of the back; worse during motion.

Extremities.

Upper. Stitches in the right shoulder.
Painful lameness in the arms, which makes it impossible to hold the lightest thing.
Trembling of the right hand, preventing writing.
Bubbling sensation in the left upper arm.
75. Rheumatic pain in the arms, extending into the fingers, especially the joints of the fingers.
Heat of the palms of the hands.
Fingers cold; tingling in the tips of the fingers.
Lower. Rheumatic pains in the legs, extending to the toes.
Œdematous swelling of the legs and feet.
80. The feet feel heavy.
Tingling in the tips of the toes.

Generalities.

Great weakness, with sensation of lameness through all the limbs.
Tearing twitches, like electric shocks, through one side of the body, with sensation of lameness.
Frequent starting.
85. Tingling in many parts of the body, as if frost-bitten, when the weather changes.

Sleep.

Irresistible sleepiness, drowsiness.
Sleeplessness, without entire consciousness.
Sleeplessness because he cannot lie on the left side, on which he is accustomed to go to sleep.

Fever.

Pulse hard, full, and accelerated.
90. Coldness and chilliness, running through all the limbs.
Frequent shiverings down the back.
External dry heat of the skin.
At night dry, external heat, with excessive thirst.
Perspiration wanting or suppressed.

Skin.

95. Œdematous swelling and anasarca.
Suppressed perspiration.

Conditions.

Rheumatic pains in the limbs during warm weather; stitches in the limbs during cold weather.
The pains increase towards evening, and do not diminish before daybreak.
Sensitiveness of the body, especially of the affected parts, to motion and contact.
100. Aggravation while walking.
Amelioration while reposing, sitting (when stooping).

COLOCYNTHIS.

Mind and Disposition.

Aversion to talk; disinclined to answer questions.
Inclined to be angry and indignant.
Delirium, with eyes open and desire to flee.
Disinclined to occupy oneself, even averse to visit his otherwise well-liked friends.

Head.

5. Easy intoxication (from drinking beer).
One-sided headache, with nausea and vomiting, (5 P. M.)

COLOCYNTHIS. 177

Pressing and heaviness in the forehead; aggravated when stooping and lying on the back.
Pressing pain in the forehead and root of the nose, as if a coryza would appear.
Profuse perspiration on the head, itching, smelling like urine (also on the hands, thighs and feet); worse at night, in bed; relieved after rising and walking in the warm room.
10. Biting, burning pain in the scalp.

Eyes.

Sensitive pressure in the eyes, especially when stooping.
Burning and cutting in the eyes.
Secretion of acrid tears from the eyes.
Stitches in the eyes (and forehead).
15. Obscuration of the sight.

Ears.

Pulsation and rushing in the ears.

Nose.

Coryza, fluent; worse in the open air; better in the room.

Face.

Face pale and relaxed, with sunken eyes.
Dark redness of the face.
20. Prosopalgia, left side; tearing or burning and stinging pain, extending to the ear and head.
Cramp-like sensation in the left malar bone, extending into the left eye.
Swelling of the face, with redness and heat of one cheek.

Mouth and Throat.

Burning at the tip of the tongue.
Sensation as if the tongue had been scalded by some hot fluid.
25. Tongue coated white or yellow.
Burning of the under lip.
Feeling of constriction in the throat, with empty eructations and palpitation of the heart.

Stomach and Abdomen.

Bitter taste of all the food and drink.
Vomiting of food; greenish vomiting.
30. Pressure in the stomach, with sensation of hunger.
Canine hunger; intense thirst, without hunger.
After taking the least nourishment, diarrhœa and vomiting.

12

Pain in the abdomen when walking (navel).
Bruised feeling in the abdomen.
35. Feeling in the whole abdomen as if the intestines were being squeezed between stones; tympanitis.
The (colic) *pains in the abdomen compel one to bend double—worse in any other position.*
Colic, with great sensitiveness of the abdomen, after anger, with cramps in the calves of the legs.
Pain in the abdomen, cutting as.with knives.
Sensation of increasing constriction in the intestines.
40. Rumbling in the bowels.
The colic and abdominal pains are relieved by bending double, by violent exercise, by coffee and tobacco; every other food or drink causes an aggravation.

Stool and Anus.

Constipation, and evacuations retarded (during pregnancy).
Diarrhœa; stools frothy, smelling acid and putrid.
Dysentery; discharges of mucus and blood, with tenesmus.
45. Constriction of the rectum during stool.
Discharge of blood from the rectum, with stinging, burning pain in the small of the back and anus (daily).

Urinary Organs.

Frequent tenesmus vesicæ, with but small discharges.
Urine fœtid; it soon thickens; is viscid and like jelly.
Abundant micturition.
50. Urine (like that in dropsy after scarlet fever) of a faint flesh color, with a white-brown, flocculent, transparent sediment, depositing on the chamber small, red, hard, solid crystals, which adhere firmly to the vessel.
Itching at the orifice of the urethra, with desire to urinate.
Burning in the urethra after micturition.

Sexual Organs.

Men. Retraction of the prepuce behind the glans, during sleep.
Impotence.
55. *Women.* Stitches in the ovaries.
Lochia suppressed; puerperal fever after vexation.

Respiratory Organs.

Constriction in the larynx, which induces frequent deglutition, with oppression of breathing; better in the open air.
Nightly attacks of oppression, as if the chest were constricted.
Cough caused by smoking tobacco.
60. Dry cough from tickling in the throat.

Back.

Pain in the shoulder-blades and back, extending into the neck, with tension.

Great weakness in the back, especially the small of the back, with pressing headache (morning).

Extremities.

Upper. Swelling and suppuration of the axillary glands; subsultus of muscles.

Pain in the palms of the hands, as if the muscles were contracted and the hand and fingers could not be opened; worse when at rest.

65. Hands feel stiff.

Lower. While in motion, pain in the right thigh, as if the psoas muscle were too short; on stopping it ceased, but began again when he commenced to walk.

Cramp-like pain in the hip, from the kidneys to the thighs, with sensation as if the hip joint were fastened by iron clamps.

Stitches in the knee joints.

The knees feel stiff, preventing one from stooping down.

70. Sensation of coldness in the knees (in the morning).

The feet go to sleep (first the left, then the right foot).

Swelling of the feet.

Generalities.

Tension and constriction in external and internal parts.

Stiffness of the joints.

75. Twitching of the muscles.

General shortening of the tendons.

All the extremities are contracted.

Faintness, with coldness of the extremities.

Stitches extending along the body.

80. Swelling of various parts, with oppression of breathing.

Pulsations through the body.

Burning pains.

Sleep.

Sleep restless, disturbed by dreams.

Sleeplessness after anger.

85. Very wakeful and sleepless.

Fever.

Pulse full, hard and accelerated. Strong pulsation in the arteries.

Coldness and chilliness of the body, frequently with heat of the face.

Coldness of the hands and soles of the feet, while the rest of the body is warm.
External dry heat.
90. Internal heat, with attacks of flushes of heat.
Perspiration at night, smelling like urine, causing itching of the skin.
Perspiration, principally on the head and on the extremities.

Skin.

The skin of the whole body scales off.
Carbuncles, with continuous burning pain.
95. Small ulcers, with itching and burning.

Conditions.

The pains are often accompanied by stiffness and retarded motion of the affected parts; they often affect the hip joints; the pains are generally worse during rest, except those affecting principally the joints; they are also much worse from motion; the painful tearing (rheumatic pain) in the limbs is relieved by discharge of flatus.
Bad effects from anger with indignation and silent grief.

CONIUM MACULATUM.

Mind and Disposition.

Hypochondria and hysteria from suppression of, or from too free an indulgence in, the sexual instinct, with low spiritedness, anxiousness and sadness.
Forgetfulness; excessive difficulty of recollecting things.
Dread of men when they approach him; nevertheless he dreads being alone.
Inclination to start, as with fright.
5. Want of disposition to work.

Head.

Giddiness when looking around.
Intoxication from the smallest quantity of stimulus; even wine and water in small quantities intoxicates him.
Apoplexy with paralysis (in old people).

Stupifying headache, first in the forepart of the head, later in the back part, with coryza; worse in the open air; relieved on stooping and moving the head.
10. Tearing in the temples and sides of the head, with the sensation as if the brain were gone to sleep; worse from contact, motion, and after eating; better in a recumbent position, or while stooping.
Lancinating pain, especially in the vertex.
Sensation of a great lump in the brain.
One-sided headache, with nausea.
Headache caused by too small but frequent stools, with tenesmus.
15. Hydrocephalus; the pains are aggravated when awaking, after eating, in the open air; ameliorated on external pressure, on lying down, and on closing the eyes.

Eyes.

Sensation of coldness or burning of the eyes in the open air.
Aversion to light, without inflammation of the eyes.
Cataract from contusion.
Yellowish color of the eyes.
20. Things look red.
Shortsightedness.

Ears.

Stitches in and around the ears.
Accumulation of ear-wax, looking like decayed paper or blood-red; hardness of hearing, ceasing when the wax is removed and returning with the wax.
Great and painful sensitiveness of hearing.
25. Roaring and humming in both ears.
Induration of the parotid gland.

Nose.

Excessively acute smell.
Purulent discharge from the nose.
Frequent bleeding from the nose (when sneezing).
30. Sickly and pale complexion; pale purple, bloated face.
Heat in the face.
Stinging, tearing faceache (at night).
Moist and spreading herpes in the face.
Cancer of the lips (from the pressure of the pipe).
35. Dry and scaly lips.

Mouth and Throat.

Drawing, extending from the jaws to the ears and head
Gnashing of the teeth.

Toothache in a hollow tooth when eating anything cold.
Gums swollen, blue-red, bleed readily.
40. Stiff, swollen, painful tongue; dry tongue.
Involuntary deglutition, especially when walking in the wind.
Violent ptyalism.
Pressure in the œsophagus, as if a round body (globus hystericus) were ascending from the stomach.
Spasmodic constriction of the throat.

Stomach and Abdomen.

45. Nausea as soon as food is taken.
Nausea and vomiting during pregnancy.
Great desire for coffee, for salt food and acids.
After taking milk sensation of inflation of the abdomen.
Suppressed eructations, with subsequent pain in the stomach.
50. Sensation of soreness and rawness of the stomach and of the abdomen when walking on the stones.
Spasmodic pains in the stomach.
Hardness of the abdomen from swelling of the mesenteric glands.
Lancinations in the abdomen, as if knives were plunged in; stitches in the spleen.
Emission of cold flatulence; rumbling and grumbling in the abdomen.

Stool and Anus.

55. Constipation, with ineffectual desire for stool; constant urging, without stool.
Hard stool, with tenesmus (headache; discharge of prostatic fluid).
During stool burning in the rectum.
After stool tremulous weakness.
Frequent stitches in the anus.
60. Heat in the lower part of the rectum.
Diarrhœa; stools undigested, with colic; very debilitating.
Involuntary discharge of fæces during sleep.

Urinary Organs.

Strangury.
The flow of urine suddenly stops, and continues after a short interruption.
65. Urine thick, white and turbid; bloody.
Diabetes, accompanied by great pain.
While urinating, cutting pain in the urethra.

After urinating, burning in the urethra (in the morning); pressure in the neck of the bladder, with stitches; worse when walking, better when sitting.

Pressure on the bladder.

70. Frequent micturition, during the night; the urine cannot be retained.

Sexual Organs.

Men. Impotence; insufficient erections.

Excessive pollutions.

Discharge of prostatic juice, while expelling the fæces, during every emotion.

Swelling of the testes (after contusion).

75. *Women.* Menstruation too early and too scanty.

Painful abdominal spasms during the menses.

Suppressed menstruation (with barrenness).

Acrid, burning leucorrhœa, preceded by pinching pains in the abdomen.

Inflammation of the mammæ, with stitches; scirrhus of the mamma after contusion.

Respiratory Organs.

80. Shortness of breathing when walking; suffocative attacks; oppressed breathing, in the morning, when waking.

Stitches in the chest (sternum).

Violent spasmodic nightly cough (hooping-cough), caused by itching in the chest and throat, or from a small dry spot in the larynx, without expectoration at night, and difficult, bloody, purulent, offensive expectoration during the day.

Cough during pregnancy.

Aggravation at night, when lying down; from acids and salt food.

85. Cough relieves the tightness of the chest.

Loose cough, with inability to expectorate; he must swallow what he coughs up.

Cough, with pain in the abdomen.

Back and Neck.

Pain, as from a sprain in the left side of the back and neck.

Extremities.

Upper. Humid tetters on the forepart of the arms.

90. The shoulder feels as if bruised and sore.

Cracking in the wrist joint.

Lower. Red spots on the calves, which turn yellow or green, as from contusion, preventing movement.

Cracking of the knee joint.
From a slight exposure of the feet he catches cold.

Generalities.

95. Sensation of debility in the morning, in bed.
Sudden loss of strength while walking.
Hysterical and hypochondriacal attacks.

Sleep.

Sleepiness in the daytime and early in the evening.

Fever.

Pulse irregular; generally slow and full, alternating with small and frequent beats.
100. Coldness and chilliness in the morning and forenoon.
Chilliness, with desire for heat, especially the sunshine.
Heat internally and externally, with great nervousness.
Heat, with profuse perspiration.
Perspiration day and night, as soon as one closes the eyes and goes to sleep.
105. Perspiration at night and in the morning, smelling offensively, and causing biting on the skin.

Skin.

Swelling of the glands, with tingling and stitches after contusions and bruises.
Humid tetters.
Blackish ulcers, with bloody, fœtid, ichorous discharges, especially after contusions.
Petechiæ (in old persons).
110. Urticaria, from violent bodily exercise.

Conditions.

Especially suitable for old men.
Most symptoms appear while at rest, especially at night, and in periodical attacks; some, when walking in the open air.
Bad effects from suppressed sexual desire, or from excessive indulgence.
The glands are much affected by contusions and bruises; hard swelling.
115. *Aggravation*, during eating, while standing, while lying down (cough), while at rest, when lifting the affected part, from masturbation.
Amelioration in the dark; from letting the affected limb hang down, from moving, when walking.

COPAIVÆ BALSAMUM.

Stool and Anus.
White, diarrhœic stools, generally in the morning, with chilliness and colic, obliging one to bend double.
Involuntary stools.
Bloody stools.
Stools, with tenesmus.
5. Intolerable burning at the anus.

Urinary Organs.
Inflammation of the urinary organs; swelling and dilatation of the orifice of the urethra, with pulsative pain throughout the penis.
Constant, ineffectual desire to urinate; contraction of the urethra; emission of urine in drops.
Hæmaturia.
Urine foaming; greenish-turbid, smelling like violets.
10. Itching, biting and burning in the urethra, before and after micturition.
Yellow, purulent gonorrhœa.

Sexual Organs.
Men. Burning and sensation of dryness in the region of the prostate gland; induration of the prostate gland.
Swelling and induration of the testicles.

Respiratory Organs.
Dry, painful cough, with dryness in the larynx.
15. Profuse expectoration of a greenish-gray, purulent mucus, of a disgusting smell.
Spitting of blood.

Extremities.
Lower. Pain and swelling of the knees and malleoli.

Generalities.
Burning pain (skin, abdomen, urethra, prostate gland, chest).
Heaviness and pressure (abdomen, chest, perineum).

Fever.
20. Chilliness and coldness, in the forenoon, with pain in the dorsa of the feet; in the afternoon, heat and thirst for water.
Perspiration profuse, of a pungent smell.

Skin.

Scarlet-red or dark, rose-colored eruption, of an irregular, broad shape.
Dark-colored or bright-red, elevated, intolerable itching, lentil-sized, measle-shaped exanthema, in clusters, flowing one into another.
Nettle-rash, pale-red or bright-red, with violent itching.
25. Jaundice.

Conditions.

Rheumatism after suppressed gonorrhœa.
Increased secretion of mucus from the mucous membranes.

CORALLIUM RUBRUM.

Head.

Sensation of emptiness and hollowness of the head.
Violent headache, with pressure, particularly in the forehead, obliging one to move the head from one place to another; this gives no relief, nor does sitting up ameliorate it—it is only relieved for a short time by uncovering the whole body, which is burning hot.
When moving the head quickly, or rocking it, sensation as if wind were blowing through the skull.
The head feels as if it were too large (three times its size).
5. Pressing headache in the forehead; she cannot keep the eyes open; relieved by walking in the open air.
Congestion of blood to the head on stooping.

Eyes.

Pressure, as from sand, in the reddened eyes (evening).
On closing the eyes they feel hot, as if bathed in tears.
Burning of the eyes from candle-light.

Nose.

10. Painful ulcer on the inside of the right wing, with the sensation as if the nasal bones were pressed asunder.
Bleeding of the nose, from one nostril at a time (at night).
Profuse secretion of mucus through the posterior nares, obliging one to hawk frequently.
Violent coryza; discharge resembles molten tallow.

Face.

Heat in the face on bending the head forward.
15. Pain, as if bruised, in the left malar bone; worse on touching the part.
The lips are chapped and painful.
Painful swelling of the left submaxillary glands; worse when swallowing and on bending the head forward.

Mouth and Throat.

Every tooth on the left side feels as if set on edge; it feels as if the teeth were too close to one another, or as if a tenacious body were lodged between them.
Great dryness of the fauces.
20. Constant hawking, owing to an accumulation of mucus in the posterior nares.

Stomach and Abdomen.

Food tastes insipid.
Beer tastes sweet.
Violent thirst; longing for acids and salt food.
After dinner, hot cheeks and forehead, with cold feet.
25. Nausea, with dryness of the tongue and violent headache; worse when sitting up.

Stool and Anus.

Constipation (for six days), followed by copious papescent stool.

Urinary Organs.

Loam-colored urine, with similar sediment.
Burning urine.

Sexual Organs.

Men. Profuse perspiration of the genitals.
30. Swelling of the prepuce; the margin of the prepuce feels sore when the linen touches it.
The frænum is painful, as if pricked by needles.
The glans is sensitive, red, and swollen, and the inner surface and glans secrete yellow-green, fetid pus.
Red, flat ulcers on the glans and inner surface of the prepuce, with secretion of a quantity of yellow ichor.
Involuntary seminal emissions during sleep (without dreams or erections).

Respiratory Organs.

35. During a deep inspiration a sensation as if the air passing through the air-passages were icy cold, an inclination to cough, with difficult hawking up of bronchial mucus (in the morning).

Back and Neck.

Stiffness of the neck.
Pain, as if the small of the back were broken.

Extremities.

Upper. Pain in the wrists, as if he had been writing much and rapidly.
Lower. Pain in the knees, tibia and tarsal joint, as if he had walked a great deal.

Sleep.

40. Yawning, with pain in the articulation of the jaw.
Great sleepiness; falls asleep while standing.
As soon as she falls asleep she starts up, on account of frightful dreams.
Cannot sleep before midnight—tosses about; if he uncovers himself, he feels too cold, and when covered, he feels too hot.

Fever.

Pulse full and hard.
45. Chill; the skin is of the ordinary temperature, with headache and violent thirst; relieved by external heat.
Dry heat without thirst, and not followed by perspiration.
The hot parts feel cold when uncovered.

Skin.

Smooth spots on the palms of the hands and fingers, first of a coral color, then dark-red, and lastly copper-colored.

Conditions.

After a short walk in the evening, great lassitude in the upper and lower limbs.
Artificial heat relieves the heat and coldness.
50. The pains make him scold and swear.

CREOSOTUM.

Mind and Disposition.

Low-spirited, inclined to weep, longing for death; music and other subduing emotions cause him to weep.
Ill-humor (in the morning), with disposition to weep.

Head.

Weakness of memory.
Painful dulness of the head, as after intoxication.
5. Heaviness in the forehead and sensation as if the brain would fall out.
Pulsation in the forehead, vertex (when awaking in the morning), with heat in the face.
Painfulness of the scalp when combing the hair (the hair falls off).

Eyes.

Itching and biting in the eyes, on the edges of the eyelids; when rubbing them they become red and feel worse.
Burning and heat in the eyes, with tears, especially when looking into a bright light.
10. Discharge of hot, acrid, smarting tears, like salt water; worse when rubbing the eyes, or early in the morning, on waking.
Twitching of the lids (uncontrollable).
Dim-sightedness, as if looking through gauze.
Sensation as if something were floating before the eyes, obliging one to wipe them constantly.

Ears.

Stitches in the ears.
15. Itching in the ears (and soles of the feet).
Humid herpes on the ears, with swelling of the cervical glands and livid, gray complexion.
Inflammation of the (left) outer ear, red, hot, swollen, burning, proceeding from a pimple in the concha, with stiffness and pain in the left side of the neck, shoulder and arm.

Nose.

Bad smell before the nose (on waking).
Bleeding of the nose (in the morning).

Face.

20. Livid complexion, with swelling of the cervical glands.
Great heat and brown redness of the face (during the siesta), with throbbing in the cheeks and forehead, and frequent micturition.
Scaly herpes on the eyelids, cheeks and around the mouth.
Dry lips, with peeling off.

Mouth and Throat.

Toothache, extending to the temples, to the left side of the face.

25. The teeth feel as if they were too long.
    Gums inflamed (left upper side).
    Scraping in the throat, with roughness and dryness.

Appetite and Taste.

Bitter taste of the food when it is swallowed.

Stomach and Abdomen.

Eructations sour or empty, after dinner, followed by expectoration of frothy saliva.
30. Nausea during pregnancy.
    Vomiturition, straining to vomit, in the morning; vomiting in the morning of sweetish water, with dryness in the nose and fullness in the forehead; cold hands and feet, with thirst.
    Tightness of the stomach and pit of the stomach; the tight clothing is insupportable.
    Painful hard place on the left side of the stomach.
    Scirrhus or cancer of the stomach.
35. Stitches in the region of the liver.
    Pressure in the region of the spleen; the spot is painful to external pressure, especially when sitting down soon after rising from the bed in the morning.
    Sensation of contraction in the abdomen, as if a hard-twisted ball were lying in the umbilical region.
    Labor-like pain, with drawing in of the upper part of the abdomen, extending to the small of the back and pressing toward the lumbar vertebræ, with flushes of heat in the face, palpitation of the heart, ineffectual urging to pass urine, which is finally emitted in small quantities and hot; after the paroxysm, chilliness and milky leucorrhœa.
    Sensation of soreness in the abdomen (when taking a deep inspiration).
40. Painful sensation of coldness in the abdomen.
    Distention of the abdomen, as after a copious meal.

Stool and Anus.

Constipation; stool hard, dry, and only expelled with difficulty.
Stitches in the rectum, extending towards the left groin.

Urinary Organs.

Diminished secretion of urine; also, he drinks much, with frequent desire to micturate (at night), passing but little at a time.

45. Frequent and profuse micturition (pale urine).
    Urine has a bad smell; of the color of chestnuts, reddish, with red sediment.
    Before urinating, discharge of mild leucorrhœa.
    During micturition, burning between the labia.

Sexual Organs.

Men. Burning in the genitals and impotence.

50. *Women.* Itching in the vagina, inducing rubbing in the evening, succeeded by smarting, swelling, heat and induration of the external parts, with soreness in the vagina when urinating.
    On the neck of the uterus a hard lump, and ulcerative pain during an embrace; the pain worse in the morning than in the evening.
    Prolapsus uteri.
    During an embrace, burning in the parts, followed next day by menstrual discharge of dark blood.
    Menstruation too early and too profuse.
55. Before and during menstruation, hardness of hearing.
    Leucorrhœa, mild, corrosive, debilitating.
    Appearance of the menses in the third month of pregnancy (blood black, flows in a stream).

Respiratory Organs.

Scraping and roughness in the throat, with hoarseness, relieved by sneezing, in the morning.
Cough (in the evening, in bed), caused by crawling below the larynx, with involuntary micturition.
60. Dry, wheezing, hollow cough, caused by scraping and roughness and crawling in the chest, without expectoration.
    Cough, with expectoration of thick, yellow or white mucus.
    Aggravation of the cough morning and evening, while exhaling, from motion, from music, when awaking, when lying on the side, or when turning in bed.
    Cough, with pain in the chest and sternum, compelling to press the hand on it; stitches and soreness in the chest.
    Pain in the back; great sleepiness and profound sleep.
65. Frequent desire to take a deep breath on account of a sensation of heaviness on the chest.
    Shortness of breath, with sensation of heaviness on the chest.
    The chest feels bruised, especially the sternum.
    Stitches in the chest above the heart, with oppression of breathing; in the right side, extending under the shoulder-blade, arresting the breathing.
    Stitches in the heart.

Back.

70. Pain, as if the small of the back would break; worse at rest; better from motion.

Pain in the small of the back like labor-pains; strong pressure to urinate, and ineffectual desire to go to stool.

Pain in the back at night; worse when lying.

The scapulæ feel as if bruised.

Extremities.

Upper. Pain in the shoulders as if they had been uncovered all night.

75. Stitches in the arm from the shoulder-joint through the fingers; they feel as if gone to sleep, insensible.

Deadness of the fingers, which grow pale and insensible (early in the morning, when rising), (with tingling and going to sleep).

Pain in the left thumb, as if sprained or stiff.

Lower. Humming and buzzing sensation in the lower limbs.

Pain of the soles of the feet, as from subcutaneous ulceration.

80. Œdematous, white swelling of both feet (feel cold and heavy).

Burning itching of the soles.

Sleep.

Great drowsiness, with frequent yawning.

Sleeplessness (before midnight); tosses about all night without any apparent cause.

Generalities.

Faintness (in the morning, when rising too early).

85. Sensation of soreness, as if bruised.

Restlessness in the body while reposing.

Stitches in the joints.

Fever.

Pulse small and weak; when at rest, pulsation in all the arteries.

Chilliness predominating while at rest.

90. Chill, with flushes of the face; red cheeks and icy cold feet.

Chill, with great bodily restlessness.

Heat, mostly in the face.

Flushes of heat, with circumscribed redness of the cheeks.

Perspiration only during the morning, with heat and redness of the cheeks.

Skin.

95. Blotches like nettle-rash.
Large, greasy-looking, pox-shaped pustules over the whole body.
Herpes, furfuraceous and pustulous, dry, humid (on the backs of the hands and fingers, in the palms of the hands, on the ears, elbows, knuckles, and malleoli).
Itching, very violent towards evening.

Conditions.

Aggravation, in the open air; on moving; from eating cold food.
100. *Amelioration*, from warmth.

CROCUS SATIVUS.

Mind and Disposition.

Gaiety; uncommon mirth and cheerfulness; witty; joking loquacious.
Sings involuntarily, and then laughs.
Immoderate, improper laughter; changeable disposition.

Head.

Vertigo when raising the head, with heat of the whole body.
5. Great forgetfulness; loses his ideas when he undertakes to write them down.
Giddiness, as if intoxicated, in the forehead; in the room, but not in the open air.
Giddiness, with fainting.
Pulsating pains in one side of the head (left), extending into the eye.
Pain in the forehead in the evening by candle-light, with burning and pressure in the eyes.
10. Sudden shock in the forehead and temples.
Sensation, when moving the head, as if the brain were loose, and were tottering to and fro.

Eyes.

Twitching of the eyelids; twitching and itching of the upper eyelids.
Nightly spasms of the lids.

13

Inclination to wink and to wipe the eyes, as if a pellicle of gum were drawn over them.
15. When reading (in the evening) sees as through a gauze.
Dilatation of the pupils.
When reading, the white paper is pale-red.
Sudden flashes before the eyes like electric sparks (during the day).
A quantity of tears rush from the dim eyes as soon as he begins to read.
20. Lachrymation in the room; not in the open air.
Heating and lancinating pains in the eyes after surgical operations.

Ears.

Humming and roaring in the ears, with hardness of hearing; worse on stooping.

Nose.

Discharge from the nose (one nostril at a time) of tenacious, thick, dark-black blood, with cold perspiration on the forehead.

Face.

Livid complexion.
25. Circumscribed, burning red spots in the face.
Alternate redness and paleness of the face.
Red, hot face.
Lips cracked.

Mouth and Throat.

White-coated tongue (better after breakfast); the papillæ are very much erect.
30. Unusual warmth in the mouth.
Scraping in the throat in the evening before and after, but not during the time he takes his food.
Sensation in the œsophagus as from a plug.
Sensation as if the uvula had been elongated, during and after deglutition.

Stomach and Abdomen.

Thirst in the evening.
35. Nausea, disappearing in the open air.
Heartburn after eating.
Bloated abdomen.
Sensation as if something living were hopping about in the stomach, abdomen, pit of the stomach (arms and other parts of the body).

Distention of the stomach and abdomen (the stomach feels distended in the morning before eating anything).
40. Sensation of heaviness in the abdomen, with pressing towards the uterus.

Stool and Anus.

Creeping in the anus, as from ascarides.
Stitches and itching at the anus (stitch extending from the anus through the small of the back into the left groin, increasing during an inspiration).

Genitals.

Men. Excitement of the sexual desire.
Women. Menstruation too early and too profuse.
45. Hemorrhage from the uterus (during the least movement); blood viscid, black, smelling badly (miscarriage third month).

Respiratory Organs.

Oppression of the chest, with the desire to draw a long breath; relieved by yawning.
Disagreeably-smelling breath.
Violent, dry cough, from irritation in the pharynx; relieved by pressing with the hand on the pit of the stomach.
Cough, with spitting of blood.
50. Great feeling of emptiness in the pit of the stomach.
Sensation as if something living were hopping in the chest.

Back.

Sensation of coldness in the back.
Swelling of the neck.

Extremities.

Upper. In the shoulder-joint sensation as if the head of the humerus were loose; cracking.
55. Sensation as if the arms and hands were gone to sleep.
The arms (fore-arm) feel heavy, as if bruised.
Burning-tingling and tension in the tips of the fingers.
Chilblains on the hands and fingers.
Lower. Violent cracking of the hip-joint, of the knee-joint (when stooping).
60. Great sensation of weariness in the knee-joints and lower legs.
Chilblains on the toes.
The soles of the feet ache from standing.

Sleep.

Continuous yawning and desire to sleep.
Sleepiness after each meal; somnolency.
65. Sings while sleeping.

Generalities.

Sensation as if something living were hopping and jumping in the body.
Tingling in different parts of the body.
Hemorrhages from various organs (blood black, viscid).
St. Vitus' dance (every seven days, with singing, dancing, laughing and singing).
70. Some limbs go to sleep (at night).

Fever.

Pulse accelerated; feverish.
Chill in the afternoon, growing worse in the evening, with chilliness extending from the back into the legs, with trembling.
During the chill (and heat), thirst.
75. Chilliness, only the back part of the body.
Flushes of internal heat, with pricking and tingling of the skin.
Heat, mostly of the head and face, with paleness of the cheeks and thirst.
Perspiration very little, and only at night; cold and debilitating.
Perspiration only on the lower part of the body.

Skin.

80. Scarlet redness of the whole body.
Painful suppuration of bruised parts (old cicatrized wounds open again, and suppurate).
Chilblains.

Conditions.

Especially suitable for women.
Frequent and great changes in the sensations; the feelings changing suddenly from the greatest hilarity to the deepest despondency.
85. *Aggravation*, in the morning early (while fasting), (lassitude, debility).
Amelioration, in the cool, open air.

CROTON TIGLIUM.

Head.

Vertigo, with dulness of the head, pale complexion, debility and nausea; worse in the open air.
Heaviness of the head.
Sensitiveness of the head to the pressure of the hat.
Headache; worse in the morning.

Eyes.

5. Itching of the eyelids.
Œdematous swelling of the eyelids (eyelids look puffed).
Twitching of the eyelids.
Stinging in the eyeball.
Burning pain in the inflamed eye, with burning in the ear, vertigo, and fainting.
10. Ulceration of the conjunctiva, contraction of the pupil, and profuse lachrymation and dimness of the cornea.

Nose.

Burning in the nostrils; inflammation of the nose.

Face and Throat.

Dry, parched lips.
Burning of the lips.
Sensitiveness of the tip of the tongue.
15. White-coated tongue.
Scraping (disagreeable) taste in the fauces.
Burning in the fauces and pharynx.
Constrictive sensation in the throat.

Stomach and Abdomen.

Excessive nausea, with vanishing of sight, sweat on the forehead, distention of the abdomen, excessive gagging, vertigo; worse after drinking.
20. Burning in the stomach.
Sensitiveness of the region of the stomach to the touch.
Abdomen distended; coldness.
Colicky pain in the transverse colon before every stool.
Colic relieved by hot milk.

Stool and Anus.

25. Stools liquid (yellow-colored water), with tenesmus, or with nausea and colic, or coming out like shot.

Stools dark-green or greenish-yellow.
Stools, with burning at the anus.
During stool, perspiration.
Stool as soon as he drinks (the child has a stool and colic as soon as it nurses).
30. At the anus, itching; pulsations; constrictive sensation; stitches; sensation as if a plug lodged in the rectum were pressing out.

Urinary Organs.

Stitches in the region of the kidneys, arresting the breathing.
Increased secretion of (turbid) urine.
Burning in the urethra when urinating.

Sexual Organs.

Men. The left testicle is drawn up; the right testicle is relaxed.
35. *Women.* Catamenia too scanty.
Pain and stitches through the breasts into the chest, and extending to the back, as soon as the child begins to nurse.

Respiratory Organs.

Hoarseness and hollow voice, which obliges him to hawk constantly.
Accumulation of rattling mucus in the larynx.
When coughing, soreness in the abdomen.
40. Cough, morning and evening.
Burning on the chest.
The chest is painful when touched.
Sensation of hollowness in the chest.
Palpitation of the heart, with difficulty of breathing, especially on going up stairs.
45. Stitches in the region of the heart during an expiration.

Extremities.

Upper. Sticking or aching pains in the shoulder-joints.
Lower. Lancinations in the big toes; pricking in the toes.

Sleep.

Drowsiness; the palpitation of the heart prevents him from going to sleep.

Generalities.

Weariness; ill-feeling and irresistible desire to sleep.
50. Fainting spells.
Weakness and bruised feeling through the whole body.

Fever.

Pulse frequent and full.
Chilliness over the back.
Ascension of heat on the body.
55. Heat and fever accompanying the cutaneous eruption.
Perspiration on the forehead.

Skin.

Scarlet redness of the skin (with rash-like vesicles).
Redness, warmth, stinging here and there; pustules running into one, oozing and forming a gray-brown crust, which finally falls off.
Itching, followed by a painful burning.
60. Herpetic eruption on the scrotum.
Painful swelling of the submaxillary glands and tonsils.

Conditions.

Aggravation. Stools, nausea and vomiting, colic, after drinking (and eating).
Amelioration, after sleep (headache, colic, pains).

CUBEBS.

Mind and Disposition.

Exaltation of temper and of the mental faculties.

Stool and Anus.

Diarrhœa, with rumbling and cutting in the abdomen and burning in the rectum.
Suppuration of the rectum.
Burning and itching of the anus.

Urinary Organs.

5. Foaming urine.
Burning and itching in the fossa navicularis.

Sexual Organs.

Discharge from the urethra of a dark-reddish color (gonorrhœa).
Inflammation of the penis.
Sensation of pressure and heaviness in the pelvis.

Extremities.

10. Sensation of heat in the palms of the hands and soles of the feet.

CUPRUM.

Mind and Disposition.

Craziness; attacks with savage malice, with proud bearing, and at times interrupted by clonic spasms.
Great anguish, like fear of death; restlessness, groaning, and desire to escape.
Attacks of rage (wants to bite the bystanders).
Convulsive laughter.
5. Incoherent, delirious talk.

Head.

Vertigo while looking upwards, when reading; the head inclines to bend forward; worse during motion, better when lying down.
Painful hollow sensation in the head.
Tingling in the vertex.
Convulsions of the head; the head is moved from one side to the other; is drawn to one side or falls forward; aggravated or renewed by each contact (hydrocephalus).
10. Headache after an epileptic attack.
The head is twisted to one side; falls forward.
Purplish-red swelling of the head; face purple-red and blue lips; convulsion and twitches in the limbs; worse when touched, which causes the swelling to pain.

Eyes.

Eyes fixed (staring), sunken.
Protruded, glistening eyes.
15. Eyes are turned upward.
Greater immobility of the pupils.
Violent itching in the eyes (evening).
Dim eyes; they feel so weak that they close.

Ears.

Boring pain in and behind the ear.
20. Itching in the ear.

Face.

Distorted muscles of the face; sad, dejected expression.
Paleness of the face; changed features, full of anguish.
Bluish face with bluish lips.

Mouth and Throat.

Spasmodic contraction of the jaws.
25. Difficult dentition in children, with convulsions.
Inability to talk, on account of spasms in the throat.
Foam at the mouth.
Hoarse crying, like a child.
Coldness of the tip of the tongue.
30. Burning in the throat; dryness of the throat, with thirst.
Singultus and spasm of the œsophagus.
When drinking, the beverage descends in the gullet with a gurgling noise.
Excessive thirst, with great dryness of the throat.
Sweet taste in the mouth.
35. Desire for warm food; eats hastily.

Stomach and Abdomen.

Singultus preceding the spasms.
Nausea, ascending from the stomach into the throat.
Vomiting of water containing flakes, offensive smelling; of bile, of blood.
Excessive vomiting accompanied by colic, diarrhœa, spasms.
40. Vomiting is prevented by drinking cold water.
Pressure in the pit of the stomach; worse from pressure.
Gnawing and corroding sensation in the stomach.
Violent colic, with great anxiety.
Pressure in the abdomen, as from a stone; worse from contact.
45. Violent spasms in the abdomen, with convulsions.
Ulcers (corroding, stinging) in the intestines.

Stool and Anus.

Suppressed stool, with general heat.
Violent watery diarrhœa (with flakes; bloody diarrhœa).

Urinary Organs.

Suppressed secretion of urine (and stool).
50. Urine dark-red, turbid, with yellowish sediment; viscous, offensive.
Frequent nocturnal urination.

Respiratory Organs.

Suffocative arrest of breathing.
Asthma increases (at 3 A. M.) when bending the body backwards, when coughing, when laughing.
Painful contraction of the chest, especially after drinking.

55. Hurried breathing, with rattling in the bronchial tubes.
Spasmodic constriction of the chest, obstructing breathing and preventing speech (after fright and anger).
Hooping-cough in long continuing attacks, causing suffocative fits; one swallow of cold water relieves.
Violent palpitation of the heart (before the menses).

Extremities.

Upper. Jerking in the arms and hands.
60. The arms and hands are bluish marbled.
Twitches of the muscles of the forearms and hands (morning).
The fingers twitch.
Herpes in the bends of the elbows, forming yellow scales, itching, especially in the evening.
Inflammation of lymphatic vessels from the hand to the shoulder, with violent swelling of the hand.
65. Coldness of the hands.
Weakness and lameness of the hand.
Lower. In the knee-joint weakness, pain, as if broken.
Twitching of the muscles in the lower extremities.
Painful cramp in the calves.
70. Twitching of the toes.
Burning of the soles of the feet.
Suppressed perspiration of the feet.

Sleep.

Deep sleep, with jerking in the limbs.
Lethargic sleep.
75. During sleep constant grumbling in the abdomen.

Generalities.

Convulsions, with piercing cries.
Clonic spasms.
Epileptic attacks (at night), followed by headache.

Fever.

Pulse small, weak and slow.
80. Chilliness over the whole body, mostly in the extremities.
Chilliness after every attack of indisposition (epileptic attacks).
Debilitating, hectic, internal heat.
Flushes of heat.
Cold perspiration at night.
85. Many attacks (epileptic attacks, attacks of mania) end with (cold) perspiration.

Skin.

Herpes, with yellow scales.
Dry itch.
Old ulcers; caries.

Conditions.

Contact renews and aggravates many complaints.
90. Aggravation from vomiting.
Amelioration after drinking (a swallow of water relieves the cough).

CYCLAMEN.

Mind and Disposition.

Taciturn, depressed, out of humor.
Inclined to internal, undemonstrative grief.
Sudden change of sadness and cheerfulness.
Weakness of the memory.
5. Dulness of the mind and indisposition to perform any sort of labor.

Head.

Vertigo; when leaning against something, he feels as if the brain were in motion.
Vertigo; increasing when exercising in the open air, relieved when sitting in a room.
Stitches in the left temple, the forehead, with dizziness.
Headache in the morning, when rising.
10. Stitches in the head (temples; forehead, when stooping).
Congestion of blood to the head; increased sensation of heat in the head.
The headache is relieved by applications of cold water.
Fine, sharp, itching, stinging in the hairy scalp, which constantly reappears in another place after scratching; worse in the evening and when at rest, better from motion.

Eyes.

Dilatation of the pupils.
15. The eyes lie deep in the orbits, look dim, and are surrounded by blue rings.
Itching of the eyelids.

Swelling of the upper eyelids.
Obscuration of sight.
Double vision; strabismus.
20. Burning in the eyes; worse when reading.

Ears.
Itching in the ears, with increased secretion of wax.
Hearing diminished.

Nose.
Diminished sense of smell.
Fluent coryza (morning).

Face.
25. Pale face.
Small pimples in the face, rapidly filling up and then drying up.

Mouth and Throat.
Dryness of the lips, without thirst.
Increased secretion of tenacious mucus in the mouth.
Mouth and throat redder than usual.
30. Tongue coated white.
Fine stitches in the surface of the tongue.
Redness of the tip of the tongue, with small, burning blister, impeding speech and mastication, with increase of saliva.
The upper lip feels numb, as from an induration.
Burning on the tip of the tongue (evening).
35. Food tastes flat.
Dryness in the throat.
Sensation of painful constriction in the throat.
Burning and scraping in the throat.
The tonsils and palate are shrivelled and white.

Stomach and Abdomen.
40. Aversion to eat bread and butter; less aversion to warm food.
After eating but little, aversion to the rest of the food, with sensation of nausea in the throat.
Thirst during the night.
Thirst and hunger, with dryness in the throat.
Nausea and accumulation of water in the mouth.
45. Nausea and fulness in the chest, with unusual hunger (morning).
Nausea (morning; after eating fat food).
Vomiting of blood.
Nausea caused by eating and drinking; could only drink lemonade without being nauseated.

Vomiting of mucus followed by sleep.
50. Fulness and pressure in the stomach,—pit of the stomach,— as if he had eaten too much.
Stitches in the stomach, region of the liver, navel, abdomen.
Sensitiveness, when moving, of the abdomen to pressure.
Rumbling in the intestines.

Stool and Anus.

Frequent discharge of hard stool (hard lumps).
55. Diarrhœa, watery, papescent, with vomiting at night.
Pressure in the rectum.
Discharge of blood from the rectum.
Drawing, pressing pain in and about the anus and perineum, as from subcutaneous ulceration, when walking or sitting.

Urinary Organs.

Frequent copious emission of whitish urine.
60. Stitches in the urethra, with desire to urinate, followed by a sudden discharge of dark red-yellow urine.
Frequent micturition, with pressure on the bladder and rectum.
Urine dark-colored, with flakes floating in it.

Sexual Organs.

Men. The prepuce and corona glandis feel sore from slight rubbing.
Women. Catamenia too profuse and too frequent.
65. Before menstruation (at night) labor-like pains; the abdomen was bloated and swollen on the previous day; the menstrual blood is black and clotted.
Secretion from the swollen mammæ, like milk.

Respiratory Organs and Chest.

When reading aloud the voice is weak.
Scraping and dryness in the pharynx, causing a suffocative cough.
Oppression of the chest, with impeded breathing.
70. Sensation of great weakness in the chest, as if there was not strength enough to breathe.
Pressure in the sternum.
Palpitation of the heart; stitches in the region of the heart.

Back and Neck.

Dull stitches in the region of the kidney; worse when drawing a long breath.
In the neck stiffness; a paralytic pain.

Extremities.

75. *Upper.* Paralytic hard pressure in the upper and forearm, as if in the periosteum and interiorly in the muscles, extending to the fingers, hindering writing.

Cramp-like, slow contraction of the right thumb and index; they have to be extended by force.

Stinging itching or pricking, as from needles between the fingers, ceasing after scratching.

Sensation of numbness in the right hand.

Lower. Cramp-like pain in the posterior surface of the thigh, above the bend of the right knee.

80. Sensation as if sprained in the left foot.

Soreness in the heels when walking.

Feet (toes) frost-bitten (looking red).

Generalities.

Pressing, drawing pains, generally in the periosteum or where the skin covers the bones.

Weakness, especially in the evening, with ill-humor and sleepiness; better when moving about.

Fever.

85. Pulse double beat.

Attacks of chilliness in the morning or evening.

During the evening chill, great sensitiveness to cold air or to being uncovered.

After the chill heat, especially of the face,—the hands remaining cold for a long time.

Heat after eating.

90. Perspiration at night, during sleep, of offensive smell.

Skin.

Itching; pricking at night, especially at night in bed; disappearing in one place when scratching, but reappearing at once at another place.

Conditions.

Aggravation when at rest and in the evening.

As long as he moves about he feels well, but as soon as he sits down, especially in the evening, he experiences various inconveniences.

Aggravation from eating fat food; while reposing (when sitting, standing).

95. Amelioration from moving (walking).

DAPHNE INDICA.

Mind and Disposition.
Lowness of spirits.

Head.
Feeling of fulness in the head, as if the head would burst.
Heat in the head, especially in the vertex.
Painful pulsation in the temples, with soreness when touched.

Eyes.
5. Contraction of the pupils.
Painful feeling in the eyes, as if pressed into the head.
Eyes inflamed, without lustre; filled with tears.

Ears.
Roaring in the ears.

Face.
Heat and burning of the cheeks.
10. Sensation of swelling; rigidity and tension in the articulation of the jaw.

Mouth.
Ptyalism; saliva hot.

Stomach and Abdomen.
Arthritic pains, which suddenly wander from the extremities to the abdomen.

Urinary Organs.
Frequent and copious micturition.
The urine is turbid, thick, yellowish, like rotten eggs.
15. Fetid smell of the urine.
Red sediment of the urine, which adheres to the sides of the vessel.
After micturition, discharge of prostatic fluid.
Sweating of the scrotum.

Sleep.
Entire sleeplessness.
20. Unrefreshing night-sleep (nightmare).
When falling asleep, starting.

Generalities.
Rheumatic and arthritic pains, especially after suppressed gonorrhœa.

Fever.
Viscid perspiration, having sometimes a putrid smell.

DIADEMA ARANEA.

Head.
Headache, relieved by smoking tobacco and going out in the open air.

Mouth.
Painfulness of all the teeth as soon as he goes to bed in the evening.

Bitter taste, with coated tongue; relieved by smoking.

Abdomen.
Swelling of the spleen (after intermittent fever was suppressed by Quinine).

Respiratory Organs.
5. Hæmoptysis.

Sexual Organs.
Women. Catamenia too early, too profuse, of too long duration.

Metrorrhagia; bright-colored blood.

Extremities.
Upper. Sensation on the ring and little fingers, as if they were asleep.

Lower. Boring and digging in the os calcis, continuing on moving the foot, and disappearing by continuing the motion.

10. Ulcer on the left heel.

Sleep.
As soon as he lies down at night a violent pain in all the teeth.

Generalities.
Hemorrhages from all the organs.

Fever.
Chilliness every day at the same hour (precisely), with sleeplessness, no heat or perspiration following.

Chilliness day and night, even during the summer; worse during rain.

15. Chill and other symptoms are worse every other day, at precisely the same hours.

Conditions.
Aggravation in wet habitations and from being on the water—Daily, at precisely the same hour.

DIGITALIS PURPUREA.

Mind and Disposition.

Great anxiety and inclination to shed tears; apprehension about the future.
Gloomy and peevish.
Indisposed to speak; inclination to lassitude.

Head.

Giddiness, with trembling.
5. Dulness of the head, with limited power of thinking.
Stitches in the temples (evening and night).
Stitches in the forehead, extending into the nose, especially after drinking something cold.
When stooping, sensation as if something fell forward in the head.
Pressure in the forehead, from mental exertion.
10. Sensation of itching in the head (inside, one-sided).
Sudden cracking in the head (during a siesta), with starting, as in a fright.
Hydrocephalus; sensation as if waves or water were beating on the skull; worse while standing, talking, shaking the head and bending the head backward—relieved when lying down or bending the head forward.
The head is inclined to sink backward.

Eyes.

Burning pain in the right eyebrow.
15. Blueness of the eyelids.
Swelling of the lower lid.
Inflammation of the Meibomian glands.
Agglutination of the eyes in the morning.
Lachrymation (tears, acrid); worse in the room than in the open air; worse from bright light and cold air (in the morning).
20. Diminished irritability of the pupil; aversion to light.
Painless obscuration of the lens.
Obscuration of sight.
Dark bodies, like flies, hover before the eyes.
Double vision (diplopia).
25. Things appear green (or yellow).

14

Ears.

Hissing before the ears, like boiling water (with hardness of hearing).
Single stitches behind the ears.
Painful swelling of the parotid gland and behind the ear.

Nose.

Pain above the root of the nose.
30. Coryza, with hoarseness.

Face.

Pale face; bluish hue under the pale skin.
Blue lips (and eyelids).
Lips dry, parched.
Black pores in the skin, which suppurate and become ulcerated
35. Convulsions on the left side of the face.

Mouth and Throat.

Blueness of the tongue.
Swelling of the tongue.
White-coated tongue (morning).
Fetid or sweetish ptyalism (with soreness of mouth, gums and tongue).
40. Ulcer on the tongue.
Mouth and throat rough, sore; scraped feeling of.

Stomach and Abdomen.

Loss of appetite and clean tongue.
Continuous thirst, with dry lips.
Flat, slimy taste; bread tastes bitter.
45. Gulping up of an acrid or tasteless fluid.
Nausea; convulsive efforts to vomit.
Vomiting (morning) of the ingesta, of a green liquid.
Nausea, as if he would die with it; continuous, and not relieved by vomiting.
Nausea and vomiting of food as soon as he eats.
50. If she expectorates she has to vomit at once what she has eaten.
Vomiting of mucus.
Great sensation of weakness in the stomach (sinking), as if he would die, soon after eating.
Burning in the stomach, extending up to the œsophagus.
Colic, with nausea and vomiting.
55. Stitches in the pit of the stomach, extending to the sides and back.

Contractive pain in the abdomen.
Sensitiveness to pressure in the region of the liver.
Distension of the abdomen (ascites).

Stool and Anus.
Stool gray, ash-colored, white as chalk.
60. Watery diarrhœa.
Diarrhœa, consisting of fæces and mucus.
Chilliness previous to stool.

Urinary Organs.
Pressure on the bladder, with the sensation as if it were too full, continuing after micturition.
Continual desire to urinate; each time only a few drops are emitted; the urine is dark-brown, hot, and burning on passing.
65. Frequent emission of small quantities of water-colored urine.
Excessive emission of urine.
While in a recumbent position the urine can be retained for a longer time.
Difficult micturition, as if the urethra were constricted.
Inflammation of the bladder (neck of the bladder).
70. Cutting pain before and after micturition.

Genital Organs.
Men. Hydrocele; the scrotum looks like a bladder filled with water.
Dropsical swelling of the genitals.
Contusive pain in the right testicle.

Respiratory Organs.
Oppressed breathing when walking and in a recumbent position.
75. Hoarseness (in the morning, after a night-sweat).
Tenacious mucus in the throat, detached by coughing.
Hollow, spasmodic cough, from roughness and scraping in the throat; expectoration, only in the evening, of yellow jelly-like mucus, tasting sweet; sometimes small quantities of dark blood are expectorated (expectoration like boiled starch).
Cough worse at midnight and during the morning hours.
The cough is caused by talking, walking, drinking anything cold; when bending the body forward; after eating.
80 Sensation of soreness in the chest.
Increased activity of the heart, with slow pulse.

Violent, audible palpitation of the heart, with sensation of contractive pains on the sternum.
Hydrothorax.

Extremities.

Upper. Heaviness or paralytic weakness of the left arm.
85. The fingers go to sleep frequently and readily.
Lower. Weakness and lassitude of the lower extremities.
Tightness in the bends of the knees; swelling (fatty) of the knee, with stinging pain.
Pain in the hip-joint.
Swelling of the feet during the day (diminished at night).
90. Coldness of the feet (and hands).

Sleep.

Continuous sleepiness during the day (lethargy).
Uneasy, unrefreshing sleep.
Frequent waking at night; starting up from a dream, as with fright, as if one were falling from a height or into water.
Uneasy sleep at night, on account of constant desire to urinate.
95. Feeling of great emptiness of the stomach frequently, previous to falling asleep.

Generalities.

Faintness and debility, with perspiration.
Attacks of great debility, especially after breakfast and dinner.
Great nervous weakness.
Graty nodosities.
100. Prickling pain in the muscles of the upper and lower extremities.
Dropsy of internal and external parts.

Fever.

Pulse very low, especially when at rest (every other beat intermits).
Pulse irregular; intermitting.
While moving about the pulse is accelerated, and soon sinks down again to its accustomed slowness when at rest.
105. Chilliness more internally, with heat of the face; beginning with coldness of the extremities, from them extending over the whole body.
Internal chilliness, with external heat.
Chilliness, with heat and redness of the face.

Coldness of the hands and feet, with cold perspiration.
Sudden flushes of heat, followed by great debility.
110. Increased heat of the body, with cold perspiration on the face.
Heat of one hand and coldness of the other.
Perspiration, generally at night; cold and clammy.
Perspiration after the chill, no heat intervening.

Skin.

Jaundice; cyanosis; dropsy.
115. Elastic white swelling of the whole body.
General paleness of the skin.

DOLICHOS PRURIENS.

Mouth and Throat.

Gums (upper) irritated, tumid, excessively painful; can scarcely take food or drink in the mouth.
Pain in the gums prevents sleep.
Painful sensation of the throat below the angle of the lower jaw on the right side; it was as if a splinter of three-quarters of an inch in length was imbedded vertically in that spot; pain increased by swallowing.

Abdomen.

Bloated, swollen abdomen (with constipation).
5. Worms.
Swelling of the liver.

Respiratory Organs.

Cough most troublesome about bedtime and for a while after going to bed.
Cough, with wheezing and dyspnœa.

Generalities.

Twitching of the muscles.
10. Clonic spasms of the extremities, with loss of consciousness; eyes motionless; eyelids open.

Skin.

Intolerable itching all over the body; worse at night, preventing sleep; scratching increases the itching; there is nothing perceptible on the skin.
Jaundice, with itching of the skin.

DROSERA ROTUNDIFOLIA.

Mind and Disposition.

Anxiety, especially in the evening and when left alone.
Dread of ghosts.
Great mistrust.
Trifles vex him very much.
5. Self-willed; obstinacy; insists upon carrying out his plans.

Head.

Vertigo when walking in the open air.
Pressing headache (temples), with stupefaction and nausea (morning); worse when stooping and from heat; better from motion and in the cold air.

Eyes.

Stitches in the eyes (when stooping).
Presbyopia and weakness of the eyes.
10. Contraction of the pupils.
Gauze before the eyes; when reading, the letters appear blurred and pale.
The eyes are dazzled by day-light and candle-light.

Ears.

Sticking pain and aching, especially when swallowing.
Hardness of hearing, with buzzing in the ears.
15. Roaring, humming, and drumming in the ears.

Face.

Pale face, with sunken eyes.
Small pimples in the face, with fine, sticking, pricking sensations.
Face-ache, aggravated by pressure and contact.
Black pores on the chin.

Mouth and Throat.

20. Sensation of dryness in the throat.
Hemorrhage from the mouth.
Ulceration of the velum.
Stinging in the throat during deglutition.
Sensation in the pharynx as if crumbs of bread had remained behind.

25. Difficulty of swallowing solid food, as if the œsophagus were contracted.
Scraping in the throat from eating salt food.
Hawking up of green or yellow mucus.

Stomach and Abdomen.

Thirst in the morning (during the hot stage of the fever and not during the cold stage).
Aversion to pork.
30. Frequent singultus.
Water-brash.
Vomiting of mucus and food when coughing.
Vomiting of bile (morning); vomiting at night.
Nausea after eating fat food.
35. Vomiting of blood.
Colic after eating sour things.
Sensation of constrictive pain in the hypochondria; he has to press on them with the hand when he coughs.
Clawing sensation in the pit of the stomach.

Stool and Anus.

Diarrhœa, stools consisting of bloody mucus; after the stool, pain in the abdomen and small of the back.

Urinary Organs.

40. Frequent desire to urinate, with scanty urine,—frequently only a few drops.
Frequent urination at night.
Dark urine, of strong smell.
Watery, inodorous urine (with fetid stool of white mucus).

Sexual Organs.

Women. Suppressed menstruation.
45. Menstruation delayed.
Leucorrhœa, with labor-like, spasmodic pains in the abdomen.

Respiratory Organs.

Bad, offensive-smelling breath when coughing.
Oppressed breathing when talking; mostly while sitting.
Sensation of oppression in the chest, as if the voice and breath were retarded when speaking and coughing.
50. Hooping-cough; attacks, every one to three hours, with barking or dull-sounding coughs, choking the breathing, caused by tickling or dryness in the throat, or from a sensation of a soft feather in the larynx; expectoration, only in the morning, yellow and bitter; has to swallow this mucus down.

Aggravation, after lying down, and still more increased after midnight; when at rest; when lying in bed; from heat; from drinking; from singing and laughing; after having had the measles.

Cough, with vomiting first of the food, and later, at the end of the attack, of mucus.

Cough, causing sensation of constriction of the chest; he has to press the hand on it.

Cough, with expectoration of bright red frothy or of black clotted blood.

55. Cough, with the sound of dryness in the pharynx.

Cough when singing, causing smarting in the larynx.

Barking cough.

Dry, spasmodic cough, with gagging.

Hooping cough, with hemorrhage from the mouth and nose, anguish, blue face, wheezing breathing, suffocation.

60. Expectoration green.

Continuous roughness and dryness in the larynx and trachea.

Sensation as if a soft body were lodged in the larynx.

Alternate soft (yellow, green, or gray) or hardened mucus in the trachea.

Inflammation of the larynx and pharynx, causing pain when talking.

65. Deep, cracked voice.

Laryngeal and tracheal phthisis.

Pain (soreness) in the chest, from sneezing and coughing; he has to press his chest with the hand.

The sternum is painful, as from subcutaneous ulceration, when pressing on the part.

Black pores on the chest and shoulder.

Back.

70. The back is painful, as if bruised, particularly early in the morning.

The nape of the neck is stiff and painful to the touch.

Extremities.

Upper. Nightly rheumatic pain in the humeri, going off, during motion, in the day.

Fingers spasmodically contracted; when grasping any thing they are rigid.

Lower. Violent stitch in the os ischium, on rising from a seat.

75. The feet feel constantly chilly; are covered with cold sweat.

Sleep.

Sleepiness at noon and at sunset.
Frequent starting during sleep.
Frequent waking, with perspiration, or as if too wakeful.
On waking great weariness.

Generalities.

80. Rapid emaciation (with acute phthisis laryngealis).
    Epileptic attacks, with twitching of the limbs; after the attack, hæmoptysis and sleep.
    Gnawing, stinging pains in the joints.
    All the limbs feel sore, as from too hard a bed.

Fever.

Chilliness, with coldness and paleness of the face and cold extremities.
85. In the morning hours, coldness of one side (left) of the face, while the other side (right) is hot.
    Chilliness and chill while at rest; finds it everywhere too cold, even in bed.
    Chilliness during the day, heat during the night.
    Heat almost exclusively in the face and on the head.
    Warm perspiration at night, especially after midnight and during the morning hours, mostly in the face.
90. Intermittent fever, with sore throat and nausea.

Skin.

Gnawing-stinging in the long bones; worse during rest.
Violent itching while undressing; when scratching, the skin readily peels off.

Conditions.

Most ailments are worse during the night and towards morning; from heat and during rest (while lying down).
Aggravation from a light (eyes), after undressing (itching); on getting warm in bed (cough; pain in the long bones).

DULCAMARA.

Mind and Disposition.
Great restlessness and impatience.
Inclination to scold. without being angry.

Head.
Painful stupefaction of the head.
Delirium at night with the pain, and during the fever-heat.
5. Vertigo when rising from bed, with darkness before the eyes.
Stupefying headache; heaviness of the head.
Congestion of blood to the head, with humming in the ears and hardness of hearing.
Boring headache, from within to without, in the temples and forehead; worse before midnight and when lying quiet; better when talking.
Sensation of enlargement of the cerebellum.
10. Digging pain in the forehead, with the sensation as if the brain were enlarged; worse in the evening till midnight and when becoming cold; better when lying down.
Unpleasant sensation of chilliness in the cerebellum and over the back, with the sensation as if the hair were standing on end; returning every day in the evening.
Thick crusts on the scalp, causing the hair to fall off.

Eyes.
Twitching of the eyelids in the cold air.
Ophthalmia from catching cold.
15. Dim-sightedness; sees every thing as through gauze (amaurosis).
Sparks before the eyes.
Sensation as if fire were darting out of the eyes, when walking in the sun or in the room.

Nose.
Bleeding of the nose,—the blood is bright-red, very warm,—accompanied with a pressure above the nose.
Dry coryza aggravated in cold air.

Face.
20. Pale face, with circumscribed redness of the cheeks.
Thick herpetic crusts, brown or yellow, on the face, forehead and chin. Crusta lactea.

Humid eruptions on the cheeks.
Warts and eruption in the face.
Twitching movement of the lips when the air is cold.
25. Distortion of the mouth; it is drawn to one side.

Mouth and Throat.

Inflammation of the throat after catching cold.
Dryness (and roughness) of the tongue, with much thirst and increased flow of saliva.
Swelling of the tongue, hindering speech and impeding breathing.
Paralysis of the tongue (in damp and cold weather).
30. Ptyalism; the gums are loose and spongy; saliva tenacious, soap-like.
Continual hawking up of very tough saliva, with much rawness in the fauces.
Itching, crawling on the tip of the tongue.

Stomach and Abdomen.

Strong desire for cold drinks (with dryness of the tongue and increased saliva).
Hunger after the fever-heat.
35. Bitter taste.
Vomiting of (white) tenacious mucus (morning).
Sensation of inflation in the pit of the stomach, with disagreeable sensation of emptiness in the abdomen.
Retraction of the pit of the stomach, with burning pain.
Cutting pain around the umbilicus.
40. Colic from cold, as if diarrhœa would set in.
Dropsy of the abdomen.
Swelling of the inguinal glands.

Stool and Anus.

Diarrhœa, with colic, after a cold.
Diarrhœa, consisting of a green or white mucus.
45. Slimy diarrhœa, with faintness.
Chronic, bloody diarrhœa, with biting at the anus, or with vomiting, eructations and thirst.
Diarrhœa, with colic, particularly in the summer; nocturnal, watery evacuations when the weather suddenly becomes cool,—with prolapsus recti.

Urinary Organs.

Retention of urine; strangury; painful micturition.
Urine turbid and white.
50. Turbid, fetid urine.

Sediment of the urine, mucous.
Involuntary discharge of urine, from paralysis of the bladder.

Sexual Organs.

Men. Tetters on the genitals.
Women. Menstruation too late and of too short duration; blood watery, thin.
55. Suppressed menstruation, from cold.
Rash before menstruation.
Herpes on the mammæ in nursing women.
Suppression of milk from a cold.

Respiratory Organs.

Oppressed breathing, from a cold; from accumulation of mucus.
60. Hooping-cough, with profuse secretion of mucus in the larynx and trachea; during each attack easy expectoration of tasteless mucus, which is often streaked with blood.
Cough, with expectoration of bright blood.
Hoarseness.
Violent palpitation of the heart at night.

Back.

Lameness of the small of the back, from a cold.
65. While at rest, drawing from the small of the back down the thighs; when moving, stitches in it; they are relieved by pressure.
Stiffness of the neck, from a cold.
Swelling of the glands on the neck.

Extremities.

Upper. Paralysis of the arms; they are icy cold, especially during rest.
Herpetic eruptions on the arms and hands.
70. Warts on the hands.
Perspiration in the palms of the hands.
Lower. Herpetic eruption on the knee.
Erysipelas of the feet; they peel off and itch.
Tingling in the feet, as from formication.
75. Burning in the feet.

Sleep.

Restless sleep after midnight.
Wakens early.

Generalities.

One-sided spasms, with speechlessness.
Paralysis of different, single parts.
80. Rheumatic pains and other complaints, from a cold.
Increased secretion of mucus from the mucous membranes and glands, the activity of the skin being suppressed.
Dropsical swelling of the body.

Fever.

Pulse small, hard, tense, especially at night.
Chill extending from the back (towards evening); heat does not relieve it.
85. Chilliness with the pains.
Chill, with violent thirst.
Dry, burning heat over the whole body.
Heat and burning in the back.
Heat, with delirium, without thirst.
90. Fetid perspiration, at night and in the morning, over the whole body; during the day, more on the back, in the armpits and hands.
Perspiration suppressed and entirely wanting.

Skin.

Swelling and induration of the glands.
Redness, dryness, and heat of the skin.
Urticaria (eruption of white blotches, with red areola), stinging, itching and burning when rubbed.
95. Vesicular eruptions.
Herpes, moist, suppurating; pale, oozing water when scratched; red, with a red areola, bleeding when scratched; small, round, yellowish-brown tetters, they bleed when scratched.
Thick crusts all over the body.
Red spots, as if caused by flea-bites.

Conditions.

The conditions are worse in the evening and when at rest.
100. Aggravation in the cold air, in wet weather.
Amelioration from moving about; after rising from a seat; when walking in the warm air.

ELAPS CORALLINUS.

Mind and Disposition.
Absence of mind.
Depression of spirits; desire for solitude.
Fear of being left alone, as if something horrible might happen.
Angry about one's self, and does not wish to be spoken to.

Head.
5. Vertigo; falls forward.
Pain in the cerebellum, right side.
Fulness in the head, as if all the blood were collected in it; fears apoplexy; with cold hands.
Violent pain in the vertex (afternoon), as if the brain were shaking, with nausea, which prevents her from keeping the head quiet.
Congestion of blood to the head on stooping.
10. Stinging headache, with sleeplessness.
Weight in the forehead; pain in the forehead.
Lancinating headache—first in the left side of the head, extending to the right side.

Face.
Dark complexion.
Lancinations from the root of the nose to the ear.
15. Redness and swelling of the right cheek, with chilliness all over the body.
Redness, heat and formication in the right cheek.
Swelling of the face, extending to the right side of the nose.
Red blotches on the bloated face.

Eyes.
Stye at the left eye, with lancination.
20. Tickling and red streaks of the sclerotica.
Large red, fiery spots before the eyes; red bar before the eyes, when opening them.
Dryness and burning in both eyes on waking; bloated around the eyes in the morning.
Eyes red and inflamed; blear-eyed. Glassy look.
When closing the eyes every thing looks red; dotted with black points.
25. Violent itching in the left eye.
Aversion to light. Desire to close the eyes.

Ears.
Buzzing in the right ear.
Crackling in the ears, on swallowing.
Itching in the ear.
30. Cerumen black and hardened.
Illusions of hearing; hears whistling and ringing; imagines he hears some one talk.
Discharge of a serous fluid or greenish-yellow liquid from the (left) ear (in the morning).
Discharge of blood from the ear.

Nose.
Bad smell from the nose.
35. Stoppage of the nostrils; coryza from the least current of air.
White and watery mucus is discharged from the nose.

Mouth and Throat.
Tongue black or dark-red.
Tongue swollen and whitish in the morning.
Pricking at the tip of the tongue.
40. The beverage is arrested in the œsophagus, as from a spasmodic contraction of this organ.
Constriction, with pressure in the throat.

Stomach and Abdomen.
Vomiting of green bile, followed by diarrhœa.
Acidity of the stomach, with nausea and faint feeling; sour eructations.
Violent thirst; cold feeling in the chest after drinking.
45. Hunger, with violent headache if not satisfied at once.
Vomiting of mucus, with fainting.
Fruit and cold drinks feel like ice in the stomach.
Burning in the stomach.
Weight in the stomach, with nausea, after eating.
50. Sudden pains in the stomach, as if she must sink down; worse while sitting, better on walking about.
Lancinations from both groins to the symphysis pubis.
Colic, with urging to stool.
The intestines feel twisted, as if by a cord, and strung together in a knot, with strangulating sensation.
Formication at the anus, as if from worms.
55. Sensation as if the blood in the abdomen were flowing backward.

Stool and Anus.
Diarrhœa, blackish, frothy, yellowish, watery, with mucus and rumbling; bile; bloody mucus.

Discharge of black, liquid blood from the bowels and at stool, with colic and sensation as if the bowels were twisted.
Prolapsus ani.
Constriction of the sphincter, after bloody stool.

Urinary Organs.

60. Red urine, with cloudy sediment.
Thick urine, with red sediment.
Suppression of urine; strangury.
Discharge of mucus from the urethra.

Sexual Organs.

Men. Impotence.
65. Weight and swelling of the testes.
Discharge of prostatic fluid.
The skin of the prepuce is thick and inflamed.
Women. Discharge of black blood between the menses.
Weight at the uterus; at the vagina, after an hysteric attack.
70. Itching in the vagina; formication at the vulva.

Respiratory Organs.

Dry cough, which ends in raising black blood.
Taste of blood in the mouth, before coughing.
Spitting of black blood, with painful tearing, as if proceeding from the heart.
Constriction of the chest.
75. Stitches in the upper part of each lung; better when walking.
Stitches in the left side of the chest; worse when breathing.
Oppressed breathing in the evening.
Palpitation of the heart, with anxiety and trembling of the hands.

Back and Neck.

Lancinations in the whole spinal marrow, from the occiput to the sacrum.
80. Pressure between the shoulders.
Coldness in the back.
Pain in the back, with chilliness, cold feet and strangury.
Stiffness in the right side of the neck.
Lancinations in the left side of the neck.
95. Painful pressure at the nape of the neck.

Extremities.

Upper. Itching under the axilla, with tetter.
The arms and hands are swollen, bluish, covered with red spots; also the right leg and foot.

Crampy constriction at the bend of the elbow, extending to the hand, as if one had carried a heavy weight.
Pricking in the left upper arm.
90. Hot rash on the right wrist.
The right hand feels as if paralyzed.
The tips of the fingers peel off.
Lower. Cramps in the calves.
Icy coldness of the right leg.
95. Rheumatic pains in the left leg.
Sensation of spraining and stiffness in the knee-joint.
The left foot is swollen and blue, with red spots.
Pinking under the toe nails.

Sleep.

Sleeplessness from lancinating headache.
100. Dreams of business, of dead persons.

Fever.

Sensitive to cold.
The arm shudders when dipping the hand into water.
Coldness in the back.
Dry heat, at midnight; cannot endure any cover.
105. With the fever, oppression of breathing.
Flushes of heat in the evening, with redness and heat of the face and ears.
Chill at noon, without thirst, followed by dry heat in the afternoon, without perspiration.
Cold perspiration all over.

Skin.

Red pimples at the tips of the fingers.
110. The tips of the fingers peel off.
Little pimples, followed by desquamation.
Yellow spots on the hands and fingers.
Red tetter from the corner of the right nostril to the cheek.

Conditions.

The rheumatic pains begin on the left side.
115. Fainting, with vomiting of mucus, or on stooping.
A change of position is painful.

ELATERIUM.

Mind and Disposition.
Depression of spirits.
Irresistible propensity to wander from home.

Throat.
A feeling as if the posterior nares and upper part of the œsophagus were enlarged.

Stool and Anus.
Discharges from the bowels of frothy water.
5. Dull olive-green discharges.
Bleeding of hæmorrhoidal tumors.

Sleep.
Incessant gaping.

Fever.
Chilliness, with continued gaping, as if an attack of intermittent fever were approaching.
Before the chill, gaping.
10. During the chill, pain in the head and limbs.
Fever, with violent tearing pains throughout the head; increased pains in the bowels and extremities; pains shooting to the tips of the fingers and toes, and then shooting back into the body.
Perspiration relieves all the symptoms.
If the intermittent fever is suppressed, urticaria break out all over the body.

EUPATORIUM PERFOLIATUM.

Head.
Headache and nausea every other morning, when awaking.
Soreness and pulsation on the back part of the head.
Heat on the top of the head.

Eyes.
Great aversion to light.

Face.
5. Redness of the face, with dry skin.

Mouth and Throat.
Paleness of the mucous membrane of the mouth.
Tongue covered with white fur.
Soreness of the corners of the mouth.

Stomach and Abdomen.
Vomiting immediately after drinking, and preceded by thirst.
10. Vomiting of bile, with trembling and great nausea, causing great prostration.
Tight clothing is oppressive.
Soreness in the region of the liver.

Stool and Anus.
Constipation, with catarrh.
Morning diarrhœa.

Urinary Organs.
15. Dark-brown, scanty urine, depositing a whitish, clay-like sediment.
Itching of the mons veneris.

Respiratory Organs.
Hectic cough, from suppressed intermittent fever.
Cough, with flushed face and tearful eyes.
Difficulty of breathing, attended with perspiration, anxious countenance, sleeplessness.
20. Inability to lie on the left side.

Extremities.
Upper. Heat in the hands, sometimes with perspiration.
Lower. Dropsical swelling of both feet and ankles.
Heat in the soles of the feet, in the morning.

Fever.
The intermittent fever paroxysm generally commences in the morning.
25. Thirst a long time before the chill, which continues during the chill and heat.
At the conclusion of the chill, vomiting of bile, or after every draught.
Pain in the bones (as if broken) all over, before the commencement of the chill.

Headache, backache and thirst during the chill.
Chilliness, with excessive trembling and nausea.
30. Aching pains, with moaning during the cold stage.
During the chill and heat, throbbing headache.
The chill is induced or hastened by taking a drink of cold water.
Great weakness and prostration during the fever.
Headache and trembling during the heat.
35. Vomiting of bile at the close of the hot stage.
The fever goes off by perspiration and sleep.
Coldness during nocturnal perspiration.
Distressing pain in the scrobiculus cordis, throughout the chill and heat.
During the apyrexia, loose cough.

EUPHORBIUM OFFICINARUM.

Mind and Disposition.

Earnest quietness, driving one to occupy himself.
Serious and taciturn.

Head.

Vertigo when standing or walking in the open air.
Sensation of soreness (as if beaten) in the back part of the head; worse in the morning; when lying; from heat; relieved by motion and cooling the head.

Eyes.

5. Smarting of the eyes, with lachrymation.
Pale-red inflammation of the eyelids, with nightly agglutination.
Inflammation of the eyes, with itching of the eyelids and canthi of the eye.
Diplopia; seeing a person walk before him he imagines he sees the same man walking after him.

Nose.

Discharge of a quantity of mucus from the posterior nares.

Face.

10. Red, inflamed, painful swelling of the face, with yellowish blisters secreting a thick yellow fluid.

Erysipelatous, inflammatory swelling of the cheeks, with vesicles full of yellowish humour.
White, œdema-like swelling of the cheeks.

Mouth and Throat.

Toothache increasing when touched or when masticating.
The teeth crumble off.
15. Ptyalism preceded by shivering or with inclination to vomit, shuddering and griping in the stomach, the saliva tastes salt.
Burning in the throat as from hot coal, extending to the stomach with anguish (as if a flame were rushing out).
Dryness of the mouth without thirst.

Stomach and Abdomen.

Great thirst for cool drinks.
Vomiting (with diarrhœa).
20. Nausea with shaking.
Burning (like fire) in the stomach and abdomen.
Spasmodic constriction in the stomach.
Spasmodic flatulent colic (in the morning in bed) with pain as if the abdomen were pressed asunder, relieved by leaning his head upon the elbows and knees.
Sensation of emptiness in the abdomen as after an emetic (morning).

Stool and Anus.

25. Hard stool difficult to pass.
Stool like glue, after previous itching of the rectum.
Violent itching of the rectum during urgent desire for stool, and after the evacuation.
Burning sore pain around the anus.
Diarrhœa, with tenesmus, burning at the anus, and soreness in the abdomen.
30. Stool first thin, then knotty.

Urinary Organs.

Frequent desire to urinate with slight discharge of urine.
White sediment in the urine.
Itching stitch in the external portion of the urethra between the acts of urinating.

Genital Organs.

Men. Erection without sexual desire.
35. Discharge of prostatic fluid from a relaxed penis.
Voluptuous itching of the prepuce.

Respiratory Organs.

Oppression of breathing, as if the chest were not wide enough, with tension in the pectoral muscles, especially when turning the body to the right side.
Stitches in the left side of the chest, during rest; better during motion.
Sensation as if the left lobe of the lung were adhering.
40. Warm feeling in the middle of the chest, as if hot food had been swallowed.
Dry hollow cough from tickling in the chest or throat.
Dry cough day and night, expectoration copious only in the morning.

Extremities.

Upper. Scarlet-red streaks on the (left) forearm, itching when touched.
Paralytic tightness in the shoulder-joint (in the morning) worse on moving the arm.
45. Pain as from a sprain in the (right) upper arm when moving the arm.
Cramp pain in the muscles of the right hand, when writing.
Lower. Pain as if sprained in the hip-joint (on moving).
Burning pain at night in the femur, and hip-joint.
Pain as from a sprain in the left thigh; worse when walking, disappears when standing.
50. Cold perspiration of the legs in the morning.
Great weakness of the legs.
Sore pain in the (right) heel, when walking in the open air.
The feet go to sleep frequently when sitting.

Sleep.

Sleepiness during the day—drowsiness after dinner.
55. Sleeps with his arms extended over his head.

Generalities.

Paralytic weakness in the joints, especially felt when beginning to move.
Burning pain in the internal organs.
Rheumatic pains worse when at rest.

Fever.

Chilliness and coldness predominate.
60. Chilliness when beginning to eat and when walking in the open (not cold) air.
Chilliness with perspiration.
Chill over the upper part of the body with heat of the cheeks.

The body is cold, with internal burning heat.
Heat with aversion to be dressed, the clothing feels too heavy—Heat only on the head.
65. Perspiration in the morning in bed.
Cold perspiration on the legs (in the morning).

Skin.

Burning in the bones.
Caries.
Cold gangrene.
70. Old, torpid ulcers.
Blood-boils.
Warts.
Burning itching which induces scratching.

Conditions.

Aggravation when at rest, while sitting, from contact, or when walking in the open (not cold) air.

EUPHRASIA.

Mind and Disposition.

Inert, hypochondriacal humor, without taking any interest in things around him.
Taciturn, disinclined to talk.

Head.

Headache (in the evening) as if bruised, with coryza.
Pulsating of the head which is felt externally.
5. Headache with dazzling of the eyes from the light of the sun, with sensation as if the head would burst.

Eyes.

Dryness and pressure in the eyes.
Smarting in the eyes, as from sand.
Inflammation and redness of the eye from being wounded.
Stitches in the eyes (ball) from bright light.
10. Inflammation and ulceration of the margins of the eyelids, with headache.
Burning, smarting lachrymation, particularly in the wind.
Swelling of the lower eyelid

Increased secretion of purulent matter and nightly agglutination of the eyes.
Photophobia and pain on looking at the light.
15. Obscuration of and pellicle over the cornea (after mechanical injuries).
Bluish obscurated cornea.
Fine eruption around the eyes.

Nose.

Eruptions on the wings of the nose.
Soreness and painfulness of the inner nose.
20. Bleeding of the nose.
Profuse coryza, with smarting lachrymation and photophobia, or with sneezing and discharge of mucus from the anterior and posterior nares.
Profuse fluent coryza with cough and expectoration in the morning.

Face.

Redness of the face.
Rash on the face, itching in the heat and becoming red and burning when moistened.
25. Stiffness and stitches in the (left) cheeks and lower jaw when talking and chewing.
Stiffness of the upper lip, as if made of wood.

Mouth and Throat.

Stitches in the lower teeth.
Bleeding of the gums.
Lameness and stiffness of the tongue and the cheeks, with impeded speech.
30. Stuttering.
Sensation of gurgling in the throat from below upwards.

Stomach and Abdomen.

Hiccough.
Bitter taste from smoking tobacco in the morning.
Pinching in the abdomen in short paroxysms.
35. The colic alternates with the affection of the eyes.

Urinary Organs.

Frequent emission of clear urine.

Genital Organs.

Men. Spasmodic retraction of the genital organs, with pressure above the ossa pubis (evening).
The testicles are drawn up with tingling in them.

Sycotic excrescence, itching, stinging, with sore and burning pain when touched.
40. *Women.* Menses at the regular period, but they last only one hour.

Respiratory Organs.

Difficulty of breathing, shortness of breath.
The breathing is stopped during a cough (as in hooping-cough).
Stitches under the sternum, especially during an inspiration.
Cough only during the day, with mucus in the chest, which cannot be detached; mucus frequently bloodstreaked, thin; expectoration only in the morning.
45. The cough is worse when at rest or when walking in the wind.

Back.

Attacks of cramp-like pain in the back.

Extremities.

Upper. Painless swelling of the hand and finger-joints on moving.
Cramp pain in the metacarpus.
Numbness of the fingers.
50. *Lower.* Stitches in the hip and knee-joints when walking.
Painful tension in the hamstrings when walking, as if they were too short.
Shocks, like electric shocks, through the thigh upwards, followed by a paralytic numbness.
Cramp in the legs, especially in the calf, particularly when standing.
Cracking in the outer ankle of the left foot, when stepping.

Sleep.

55. Yawning, when walking in the open air.
Frequent waking (as from fright) at and after 3 A. M., lasting till 6 A. M., when he falls in a stupor, from which he wakens with many complaints.

Generalities.

Cramp-like pains in various parts of the body.
Shooting, itching stitches (the whole night).
Crawling as of a fly in one or the other limb, from below upwards in a straight line, with numbness of the part.

Fever.

60. Chill in the forenoon—chilliness predominating.

Attacks of heat during the day, with redness of the face and cold hands.

At night and during sleep, perspiration of strong and offensive smell, principally on the chest.

Skin.

Consequences of blows, bruises and contusions.
Condylomata, itching when walking, burning when touched.

Conditions.

65. Aggravation in the evening.

EVONYMUS EUROPÆUS.

Mind and Disposition.

Vexed, peevish, out of humor, especially when his thoughts vanish while reading.

Head.

Vertigo in the forepart of the head (when sitting) with mistiness of sight.
Stitches in the head (left side).

Eyes.

Obscuration of sight.
5. Dark spots before the eyes.

Face.

Tingling in the left cheek.

Extremities.

Upper. Paralytic pain in the region of the hip, around the pelvis.
Paralytic pains in the knees after sitting.

Conditions.

The pains compel one to lie down; afterwards they are relieved or wander to some other part.

EUPION.

Colliquative perspiration. Perspires from the least exertion; when eating; all night (with tuberculosis.)

FERRUM.

Mind and Disposition.
Anxiety as after committing a crime.
Changeable disposition, one evening low-spirited and melancholy, the next excessively cheerful.
Quarrelsome, disputative.

Head.
Vertigo, particularly when descending and on seeing flowing water; with sickness at the stomach in walking; with the sensation as if the head would constantly incline to the right side.
5. Congestion of blood to the head, with pulsation and hammering in the head, heat and redness of the face, enlarged veins, sensitiveness of the head to the touch; worse after midnight and towards morning; returning periodically.
Pain in the back part of the head when coughing.
Sensitiveness of the head to the touch and falling off of the hair; the hair is also painful to the touch.
Pressure on the top of the head when the cold air touches it.

Eyes.
Dull, lustreless eyes with blue rings around them.
10. Inflammation and redness of the eyes with burning or stinging.
Obscuration of sight in the evening.
Redness and swelling of the upper and lower lids.
Suppurating stye on the upper lid.

Ears.
Stitches in the ear in the morning.
15. Ulcerative pain of the outer ear.

Nose.

Bleeding from the nose (evening).
The nose is continuously filled with clotted blood.

Face.

Earthy, jaundiced color of the face.
Paleness of the face with red spots on the white face.
20. Pale bloated face, especially around the eyes.
Fiery redness of the face; the veins are enlarged.
Pale, dry lips.
Yellow spots in the face.

Mouth and Throat.

Aching, pressing pain in the throat during deglutition, with heat in the fauces.
25. Constrictive sensation in the throat.

Stomach and Abdomen.

Aversion to and bad effects from meat, beer and acids.
Cannot eat or drink any thing hot.
Unquenchable thirst (or thirstlessness). Longing for acids.
Solid food becomes dry and insipid in the mouth during mastication.
30. Every thing he eats tastes bitter.
Sour eructations.
Bitter eructations after fat food.
Vomiting of the ingesta as soon as he eats.
Vomiting of the food tasting sour in the morning or during the night.
35. Every thing vomited tastes sour and is acrid.
Vomiting after eating eggs.
Spasmodic pressure at the stomach after taking the least food or drink, especially after eating meat.
Hardness and distention of the abdomen.
Spasmodic contraction of the abdominal muscles, as if the abdomen were constricted, especially when stooping, so that he can only straighten himself slowly.
40. Painful weight of the abdominal viscera in walking, as if they would fall down.
The bowels feel sore as if bruised, when touching them or when coughing.
Flatulent colic at night (violent rumbling in the abdomen).

Stool and Anus.

Watery diarrhœa with burning at the anus.
Diarrhœa; passes undigested food.

45. Discharge of blood and mucus at every stool.
    With the slimy stool discharge of ascarides.
    Painless diarrhœa (involuntary during a meal).
    Contractive spasm in the rectum.
    Protrusion of large varices at the anus.
50. Itching at the anus from ascarides at night (children).

Urinary Organs.

Involuntary micturition, particularly in the day-time.

Sexual Organs.

Men. Impotence.
Nocturnal emissions.
Discharge of mucus from the urethra.
55. *Women.* Menstruation too early and too profuse.
Suppressed menstruation.
Hemorrhage from the uterus, with labor-like pains in the abdomen and glowing heat in the face; the blood is partly pale, partly clotted.
Miscarriage.
Painfulness of the vagina during an embrace.
60. Swellings and indurations in the vagina.
Prolapsus of the vagina.

Respiratory Organs.

Hot breath.
Oppressed, short breathing.
Fulness and tightness of the chest.
65. Asthma (after midnight), compelling one to sit up.
Asthma most violent when lying, or when sitting still without doing any thing; relieved by walking and talking.
When sitting still loud breathing, as if asleep.
Roughness of the throat, hoarseness.
Stitches and soreness of the chest.
70. Sensation of dryness in the chest.
Spasmodic constriction in the chest.
Spasmodic cough from tickling in the trachea, with expectoration only in the morning of blood-streaked, purulent, albuminous mucus, greenish or frothy, tasting sweetish, putrid or sour.
Cough worse in the evening, till midnight.
Spasmodic cough in the morning relieved by eating.
75. Spasmodic cough after eating and with vomiting of the ingesta.
In the morning, copious expectoration of purulent matter; in the evening, the cough is dry.

Hæmoptysis in the morning and at night.
When coughing, stitches in the chest; sensation of soreness.

Extremities.

Upper. Paralytic tearing pain from the shoulder-joint into the upper arm (left); he cannot raise the arm; slow movement improves it gradually.
80. Cracking in the shoulder-joint.
Nightly tearing and stinging in the arms.
Numbness and contraction of the fingers.
Swelling of the hands (and feet).
Lower. Nightly tearing and stinging from the hip-joint to the thigh, gradually improving from slow motion.
85. Numbness of the thighs.
Painful cramps in the calves, while at rest, especially at night.
Swelling of the feet.
The toes are contracted.

Sleep.

Very sleepy at night, with inability to go to sleep.
90. Can only lie on her back at night.
Anxious tossing about in bed (after midnight).
Vivid dreams.
The child does not sleep, disturbed by the itching caused by the ascarides.

Generalities.

Great emaciation.
95. Weakness of the body almost paralytic; she is so weak that she must lie down.
Restlessness in the limbs.
Contraction of the limbs.
Cramps in the limbs (during the day).
Cracking in the joints.

Fever.

100. Pulse full and hard—Violent ebullitions.
Chilliness in frequent short attacks.
Chill with thirst and red hot face.
Coldness in the evening in bed, frequently continuing all night.
Chilliness and want of animal heat.
105. Dry heat over the whole body, especially in the evening, with very red face and inclination to uncover oneself.
Profuse and long continued perspiration, during the day when moving, and at night, and in the morning hours in bed.

Clammy and debilitating perspiration.
Every other day perspiration from morning till noon.
Cold perspiration (with convulsions).
110. The perspiration is immediately preceded by headache.
Intermittent fevers (consequent upon the abuse of Cinchona) with congestion of blood to the head, distention of the veins, vomiting of the ingesta, swelling of the spleen.

Skin.

Dirty, earth-colored skin.
Dropsy.

Conditions.

Especially suitable after the abuse of Quinine, Tea, and Alcoholic drinks.
115. Aggravation towards and in the morning, and while at rest, especially when sitting still.
Amelioration from slow exercise.

FILIX MAS.

Tænia. Worm fever. Sterility.

FLUORIC ACID.

Mind and Disposition.

Disposition to be exceedingly anxious, causing perspiration.
Sensation as if danger menaced him.
Forgetfulness of dates and of his common employment.

Head.

Vertigo with sickness of the stomach.
5. Congestion of blood to the head—(forehead).
Dulness (towards night) in the occiput.
Sensation of numbness in the forehead.
Heaviness above the eyes, with nausea, worse on motion.
Compressing pain in the temples.
10. Sensation of weakness, like numbness in the head (and hands).
Itching of the head.   Baldness.

Eyes.

Violent itching in the canthi.
Burning in the eyes.
Pressure, as if it were behind the right eyeball.
15. Fistula lachrymalis.
Sensation of sand in the eyes, or as if fresh wind was blowing on them.

Ears.

Itching in the Ears.

Nose.

Red, swollen, inflamed nose.
Obstruction of the nose. Fluent coryza.

Face.

20. Heat in the face; desire to wash it with cold water.
Perspiration particularly in the face.

Mouth and Throat.

The teeth feel warm (left side, upper jaw).
Fistula (dentalis) (near the right eye-tooth) with great sensitiveness of the upper jaw to the touch.
Sensation of roughness (lower incisor teeth).
25. Carious teeth.
Acrid, foul taste from the roots of the teeth.
Increased flow of saliva (with sneezing) (with pricking of the tongue).
In the morning the mouth and teeth are full of mucus.
The posterior nares feel expanded during a walk.
30. Constriction in the throat with difficult deglutition; in the morning hawking up of much phlegm which is mixed with blood.

Stomach and Abdomen.

Aversion to coffee.
Eructation and discharge of flatulency.
Sickness of the stomach, with general heat.
Nausea, eructations and lassitude.
35. Pressure from weight in the stomach, between meals.
Heat in the stomach before the meal.
Pinching in the region of the spleen, (extending to the hips) (11 A. M.)
Pressing pain in the region of the spleen and the left arm.
Sensation of emptiness in the region of the navel, with desire to draw a deep breath; relieved by bandaging and eating.

Stool and Anus.

40. Soft small stools in the morning after drinking Coffee, and again in the evening with protrusion of the hæmorrhoids.

Watery stools in the morning after rising.

Frequent passages of flatus and eructations (with constriction of the anus).

Stool pappy, yellowish-brown, fetid, with tenesmus and prolapsus ani.

Protrusion of the anus during an evacuation.

45. Itching within and around the anus, in the perineum (evening).

Urinary Organs.

Very frequent discharge of light-colored urine (thirst increased).

Whitish purple-colored sediment in the urine.

Genital Organs.

Men. Increased sexual desire (in old men) with violent erections all night.

Sensation of fulness in both spermatic cords.

50. *Women.* Menstruation too early and too copious; the discharge is thick and coagulated.

Chest.

Itching, redness, swelling of (right) nipple.

Itching on the left breast and right side of the nose.

Respiratory Organs.

Itching in the larynx which causes him to hawk and to swallow.

Itches under the ribs (left side).

55. Difficult respiration (afternoon and evening).

During respiration wheezing (Hydrothorax).

In the heart sensation of soreness, jerking.

Back.

Rigidity in the nape of the neck.

Pain (headache) from the nape of the neck extending through the centre of the head to the forehead.

60. Bruised pain in the os sacrum.

Extremities.

Upper. Rheumatic pains in the left arm from the shoulder to the elbow, with lameness.

Trembling in the biceps and triceps of the right arm.

Pain in the right shoulder-joint.
Slight lameness in the right arm (has some difficulty in writing).
65. The left forearm and hand asleep (in the morning).
Numbness and lameness in the left forearm and hand (morning).
Weakness and numbness of the hands and head.
Constant redness of the hands, especially the palms of the hands.
The nails grow more rapidly.
70. Acute prickings, as with needles, in the fingers.
Panaritium.
Lower. Acute stitches in the right hip-bone.
Lameness in the left hip.
Pain in the right knee-joint.
75. The left leg falls easily asleep.
Burning stitches under the soles of the feet (in the morning).
Soreness of all his corns.

Sleep.

Sleeplessness without inclination to sleep; a short sleep suffices and refreshes him.

Fever.

General heat with nausea from the least movement, with inclination to uncover oneself and to wash oneself with cold water.
80. Perspiration, clammy, acid, disagreeably smelling, principally on the upper part of the body, especially on moving in the afternoon and evening, with itching.
The perspiration favors soreness of the skin and decubitus.
Less susceptible to the summer heat.

Generalities.

Limbs go to sleep, although he does not lie on them.
Violent jerking burning pains, confined to a small spot.
85. Increased ability to exercise his muscles without fatigue, regardless of the most excessive heat in summer or cold in winter.

Skin.

Old cicatrices become red around the edges, covered or surrounded by itching vesicles, or they itch violently.
Burning pains on small spots of the skin.
Itching of the skin (in the month of March).
Elevated red blotches.

90. Red, round, elevated blood vesicles, resembling little flesh-warts.
Varicose veins on the (left) leg.
Caries and necrosis.
Ulcerations especially after the abuse of Silicea.

Conditions.
The extreme heat of the summer and the cold of the winter affect him less and he is able to endure more fatigue; tires less easily.
95. Carious ulcers becoming worse from too large or too frequently repeated doses of Silicia are much improved by Fluor. ar.

FRAGARIA VESCA.

Tape-worm.
Pain in the chilblains during the hot season.

GELSEMINUM.

Mind and Disposition.
Great irritability, does not wish to be spoken to.
Vivacity, carelessness, followed by depression of spirits.
Unconnected ideas; cannot follow an idea for any length of time; if he attempts to think consecutively he is attacked by a painful vacant feeling of the mind.
Stupor, cannot open the eyes.
5. Sensation of intoxication with diarrhœa.
Confusion; when attempting to move, the muscles refuse to obey the will; head giddy.
Every exciting news causes diarrhœa; bad effects from fright and fear.

Head.
Staggering as if intoxicated when trying to move.
Giddiness as if intoxicated, as if should fall down.
10. Giddiness with loss of sight, chilliness, accelerated pulse, dulness of vision, double vision.

Fulness in the head with heat in the face and chilliness.
Great heaviness of the head, relieved by profuse micturition.
Pain as from a tape around the head.
Dull pain in the back part of the head after breakfast, worse when moving and stooping.
15. Sensation as if the brain were bruised.
With the headache giddiness, faintiness, pain in the neck, pulsation of the carotid arteries, pain in the limbs, great drowsiness, sneezing, double vision, loss of sight.
Sensation of contraction of the skin in the middle of the forehead.
Itching on the head (face, neck, shoulders), preventing sleep.

Eyes.

Eyes feel bruised.
20. Yellow color of the eyes.
Great heaviness of the eyelids, cannot keep the eyes open.
Fulness and congestion of the eyelids; paralysis of the eyelids.
Double vision controllable by the strength of the will, or when looking sideways, not when looking straight forward. (During pregnancy).
Distant objects look obscure.
25. Appearance like smoke before the eyes.
Dimness of vision (during pregnancy.)
Cannot see any thing (complete blindness.)
Pupils dilated.
Aversion to light,—more to candle-light.

Ears.

30. Sudden loss of hearing (deafness) for a short time.

Nose.

Sneezing followed by tingling and fulness in the nose.
Sneezing with fluent coryza; profuse watery discharge excoriates the nostrils.
Sensation of fulness at the root of the nose extending to the neck and clavicles.

Face.

Heavy, dull expression of the countenance.
35. Yellow color of the face.
Paleness and nausea.
Heat of the face with fulness in the head and cold feet.

Erythema of the face and neck.
The muscles of the face seem to be contracted, especially around the mouth, making it difficult to speak.
40. Stiffness of the jaws, the jaws are locked.
Lips dry, hot and coated.

Mouth and Throat.

Saliva colored yellow as from blood.
Sticky feverish feeling in the mouth.
Putrid taste and fetid breath.
45. The tongue is coated yellowish-white with fetid breath.
Thick coating of the tongue (during the chill).
Tongue red, raw, painful, dry, inflamed in the middle.
Paralysis of the tongue (glottis and eyelids).
Dryness and burning in the throat.
50. Dry roughness in the throat when coughing.
Dryness of the throat with hoarseness.
Sensation of heat and constriction in the throat.
Burning in the mouth extending to the throat and stomach.
Sensation as if a foreign body were lodged in the throat.
55. Difficult deglutition (paralytic dysphagia).

Stomach and Abdomen.

Thirst (during the perspiration).
Increased appetite, or easily satisfied with small quantities of food.
Sour eructations.
Nausea (with giddiness and headache).
60. Sensation of emptiness in the stomach.
Burning in the stomach extending to the mouth.
Gnawing pain in the transverse colon.
Sudden spasmodic pains in the upper part of the abdomen, compelling him to cry, leaving a sensation of contraction.
Sensation of soreness in the abdominal walls.
65. Rumbling in the abdomen with discharge of wind above and below.
Periodical colic with diarrhœa. (Yellow discharges setting in in the evening.)

Stool and Anus.

Frequent discharge of flatulency.
The soft stool is passed with difficulty, as if the sphincter ani resisted the passage by contraction.
Paralysis of the sphincter ani, with disposition to prolapsus ani.

70. Stools loose, color of tea, dark-yellow.
    Diarrhœa with intermittent fever.

Urinary Organs.

Frequent micturition (relieving the headache).

Sexual Organs.

Men. Genitals cold and relaxed.
Involuntary emissions, without erections.
75. Painful redness at the urethra. (Secondary gonorrhœa.)
    Women. Sensation of heaviness in the uterus.
    Suppressed menstruation with convulsions (every evening).
    Rigidity of the neck of the uterus.
    Spasmodic labor-pains.
80. During pregnancy, violent pains in the uterus, headache, drowsiness, double vision, obscuration of sight, giddiness, pulsation of the carotid arteries, small slow pulse.
    Premature labor (abortion) (after fright).

Larynx and Respiratory Organs.

Voice weak.
Paralysis of the glottis with difficult deglutition.
Spasm of the glottis evening, threatening suffocation.
85. Roughness of the throat, raw, as if ulcerated in the larynx —bronchitis.
    Hoarseness with dryness of the throat.
    Burning in the larynx, descending into the trachea.
    Heaviness in the middle of the chest (afternoon).
    Sensation of constriction in the lower thorax.
90. Stitches in the chest (right side), heart.
    Dry cough with soreness of the chest and fluent coryza.
    Pain in the heart when rising from a seat.
    Breathing frequent.

Back and Neck.

Pulsation of the carotid arteries (during pregnancy).
95. The muscles of the neck feel bruised.
    Sensation of constriction in the right side of the neck.
    Pain in the neck, under the left shoulder blade.

Extremities.

Upper. In the shoulders pain during the night.
Sensation as if the right elbow were sprained.
100. Pain in the elbow (left) from draught of air (at night).
    Pain as if sprained in the right wrist.
    Trembling of the hands when lifting them up.
    Coldness of the wrist and hands.

GELSEMINUM.

Hot dry hands, especially the palms of the hands.
105. *Lower.* Unsteady gait.
Loss of the voluntary motion.
Violent lancinating pain in the thigh.
Rheumatic pains during the night in the knees.
Sudden dislocation or slipping of the knee-pan (during breakfast).
110. The calves of the legs feel bruised, pain at night.
Cold feet.
Spasmodic contraction of the toes.

Sleep.

Sleepiness and long continued sleep.
As soon as he goes to sleep he is delirious.
115. Yawning.
Cannot go to sleep on account of violent itching on the head, face, neck and shoulders.
He wakens from headache or colic.

Generalities.

Paralytic affections, muscles weak and will not obey the will.
Rheumatic pains (wandering) in the bones and joint (night).
120. Spasmodic contractive pains.
Sensation as if bruised.

Fever.

Pulse slow, accelerated by motion.
Limbs cold with oppressed breathing. Cold hands and feet.
In the evening, when entering the warm room, thirst, pain in the back and loins and in the lower part of the thigh.
125. Chilliness in the upper part of the body, back.
Chilliness every day at the same hour.
Chilliness especially in the morning.
Nervous chill, the skin is warm; wants to be held that he may not shake so much.
Chill with cold hands, feet and headache.
130. Chill with weak pulse.
Coldness of the feet as if they were in cold water, with heat in the head and face and headache.
Chill followed by heat and later by perspiration.
Heat principally on the head and face.
Profuse perspiration relieving the pains. Perspires freely from slight exertion.

Skin.

135. Papulous eruptions resembling measles especially on the face.

Itching on the head, face, neck and shoulders.
Skin hot and dry.

Conditions.

Smoking tobacco aggravates the headache.
Bad effects from suddenly hearing bad news; from fright; and from thence, diarrhœa, abortion.

GLONOINE.

Mind and Disposition.

Fear, with the sensation of constriction of the chest and as if the neck were swollen, or as if something unpleasant would happen to him.
Unusually bright and loquacious, with great flow of ideas.
Loses his way in the known streets, the walk seems too long; the chin feels too long.

Head.

Unsteady gait.
5. Giddiness when the head is moved.
Heaviness in the head, principally in the forehead.
Dull headache with warm perspiration in the forehead.
Fulness in the head, as if the brain was expanding itself, were moving in waves.
Congestion of blood to the head (apoplexy).
10. Pulsation in the forehead, in the temples, on the vertex; when walking every step is felt in the neck, when moving the head.
Stitches in the temples or the right side of the forehead.
Sore and bruised feeling in the brain, worse when shaking the head.
The pain, heat and fulness in the head ascend from the chest, neck or back part of the head.
Shaking aggravates the headache, as well as stooping motion, ascending steps.
15. External pressure relieves.
Walking in the open air, uncovering the head, relieves.
Headache with accelerated pulse, red face, perspiration on the face; he becomes unconscious.

Eyes.

Eyes dull, staring, sunken.
The whites of the eye is red, the eyes protrude, look wild.
20. Protruding pains.
Heat in the balls of the eyes, lids, around the eyes.
In the eyeballs, stitches, twitchings, soreness, pressure.
Sparks, flashes before the eyes.
The letters appear smaller.
25. Black spots before and obscuration of the eyes, with fainting.

Ears.

Sensation of fulness, in and around the ears.
Stitches in the ears, the ears feel as if closed.
Ringing, singing in the ears.

Nose.

Pain at the root of the nose.
30. The headache extends into the nose.

Face.

Paleness of the face with heat and congestion of blood to the head and chest.
Heat in the face with pulsations in the head and palpitations of the heart.
Redness of the face, especially the upper part of it, with headache.
Itching, especially in the middle of the face.
35. Pain and stiffness of the articulation of the jaw.
Sensation as if the under lip were swollen.

Mouth and Throat.

Pulsating toothache with headache.
Tongue swollen with pricking it, the tongue smarts.
Sensation of soreness and swelling on the roof of the mouth with pulsation.
40. The soft palate feels contracted and dry.
In the throat tickling, heat, soreness.

Stomach and Abdomen.

Nausea causing perspiration.
Nausea with and caused by the headache, with colic; congestion of blood to the head and chest and pale face.
Gnawing in the pit of the stomach.
45. Sensation of emptiness in the pit of the stomach.
Sensitiveness of the pit of the stomach, especially on stooping.

Colic, cutting pain principally below the navel, wakening one in the morning before and after loose stools.

Rumbling in the lower part of the abdomen, principally when lying on the left side.

Stool and Anus.

Diarrhœic stools with rumbling and discharges of flatulency, beginning in the morning and lasting all day.

Urinary Organs.

50. Increased secretion of pale (albuminous) urine; has to rise frequently during the night and must pass large quantities of albuminous urine.

Genital Organs.

Women. Menstruation suppressed by Glonoine. During the menstruation, congestion of blood to the head and chest, headache, fainting.

During pregnancy headache, congestions of blood to the head and chest.

Respiratory Organs.

Constriction of the chest.

Oppression of the chest alternating with headache.

55. Desire to take a long deep inspiration. Sighing.

Congestions to the chest.

Palpitation of the heart with heat in the face, accelerated pulse and pulsation of the carotid arteries.

Severe stitches from the heart, extending into the back.

In the heart sensation of fulness, heaviness and heat, with labored beating of the heart.

Back and Neck.

60. The neck feels weak and tired, cannot support the head.

Stiffness of the neck, clothing seems to be too tight.

On the neck sensation of fulness, tension, pulsation.

Pain in the whole spinal column, or heat and chilliness.

Burning heat between the shoulder-blades.

Extremities.

65. *Upper.* In the arms restlessness, weakness, want of circulation.

Sensation of weakness and numbness in the left arm.

Feels the beating of all the pulses in the tips of the fingers, accompanied by trembling of the fingers.

Lower. Weakness and numbness of the left thigh.

Weakness of the legs, the knees and ankles give way.

70. Restlessness in the limbs causes him to rise.

Sleep.

Yawning with headache, congestion of blood to the head.
Sleepiness early in the evening.
He is difficult to waken.

Generalities.

Weakness as from loss of sleep.
75. Fainting with consciousness.
Unconscious falling down.
Pulsations, tingling, thrills, and a peculiar sensation of warmth through the body, extending from above downward.
Convulsions (from congestions to the head); the fingers are spread apart and stretched out (left side).

Fever.

Pulse accelerated, irregular, intermitting, full and hard, small and rapid.
80. Heat, especially in the face, ascending from the pit of the stomach to the head.
Perspiration principally in the face, after sleeping.
Perspiration relieves the nausea.

Conditions.

Bad effects of mental excitement, fright, fear, mechanical contusions and their later consequences.
Bad effects from having the hair cut.
85. Bad effects from being exposed to the rays of the sun.

GRAPHITES.

Mind and Disposition.

Melancholy with inclination to grief, anxiety about the future, and nightly restlessness driving one out of bed.
Despairing grief with shedding of tears.
Anxious fear of an approaching misfortune.
Irresoluteness and excessive cautiousness.
5. Easily vexed and wrathful.
Want of disposition to work.
Forgetfulness, chooses wrong words in speaking or writing.

Head.

Feeling of intoxication, in the morning on rising, the forehead is contracted, with nausea and vomiting.
Headache every morning on waking, semilateral, with inclination to vomit.
10. Pain in the head as if the head were numb and pithy.
Burning on the top of the head on a small spot.
Fulness in and congestions to the head, the menstruation being suppressed.
Humid, spreading, scurfy eruption on the top of the head, painful to the touch, as if from subcutaneous ulceration, and emitting a disgusting odor; extending down the sides of the head into the whiskers; after scratching, more sore and humid; later drying up to a white scurf.
Smooth large wens on the hairy scalp; the hairy scalp is very hot and itches very much, especially when walking in the open air.
15. The hair becomes gray early and falls out from the top and sides of the head and the whiskers.
Rheumatic pains in the scalp, principally in the sides, extending to the teeth and the cervical glands; worse when walking and becoming cold in the open air, relieved from warmth and while getting warm when walking.
Perspiration smelling acid or very offensive, coloring the linen yellow; on the head (as on the whole body) at night and during the day, from the least exercise; increased even while talking, better when walking in the open air.

Eyes.

Pressure and stinging in the eyes, with lachrymation.
Inflammation of the eyes with photophobia, and red, swollen eyelids.
20. Intolerance to the light (of day).
Short-sightedness.
Sensation of dryness of the eyelids.
Agglutination of the eyes early in the morning.
Dry gum in the eyelashes.

Ears.

25. Dryness of the inner ear.
Sensation as if the (left) ear were filled with water.
Moisture and sore places behind the ears.

Hardness of hearing.
Cracking in the ears when moving the jaw.

Nose.

30. Painful dryness of the nose.   Bleeding at the nose.
Black sweaty pores on the nose.
Dry scurfs in the nose.
Frequent discharge of thick, yellowish, fetid mucus from the nose.
Coryza as soon as he becomes cold.
35. Smell too sensitive (cannot bear the smell of flowers).

Face.

Pale-yellow color of the face.
Flushes of heat in the face.
Swelling and erysipelatous inflammation of the face, burning and stinging; the erysipelas is spreading in rays.
Semilateral (left) distortion and paralysis of the face which impedes the speech.
40. Continued feeling as of cobweb on the face.
Eruption on the face, as if the skin were raw.
Ulcers on the surface of the lips.
Ulcerated corner of the mouth.
Scabby eruptions on the chin and around the mouth.
45. Swelling and induration of the submaxillary glands.

Mouth and Throat.

Lancinating pain in the teeth from cold drinking, and aggravated by warmth.
Swelling of the gums.
The gums bleed readily when rubbing them.
Fetid odor from the gums and mouth.
50. Sensation in the throat (at night) as if a plug had lodged in it.
Constant spasm in the throat, obliging him to swallow as if he were choking.
Swelling of the tonsils, with pain when swallowing.
Accumulation of a great deal of mucus in the throat.
Bitter taste in the mouth, the tongue being much coated.
55. Taste of rotten eggs in the morning, after rising.

Stomach and Abdomen.

Canine hunger (with acidity of the stomach).
Frequent sour eructations, with bitter taste in the mouth.
Morning nausea.
Nausea and vomiting after each meal; sour vomiting.
60. Repugnance to salt food.

Violent thirst, early in the morning.
The abdomen becomes inflated after eating.
Burning in the stomach, causing hunger.
Fulness and heaviness in the abdomen.
65. Distended abdomen with diarrhœa.
Hardness of the abdomen.
Painfulness of the groins, and swelling of the inguinal glands.
Colic and pressure in the stomach with nausea; relieved by heat.
Inflation of the abdomen, owing to an accumulation and incarceration of flatulence.
70. Inflation of the abdomen, with congestion of blood to the head, heaviness in the head and vertigo.
Excessive discharge of fetid flatulence.
Rumbling in the abdomen.
Croaking, as of frogs in the abdomen.
Pinching in the abdomen, previous to every emission of flatulence.

Stool and Anus.

75. Constipation; the stool hard, knotty, the lumps being united by mucous threads; hard, of too large a size.
A quantity of white mucus is expelled with the stool.
Mucous diarrhœa.
Sour-smelling stool with burning at the rectum.
Continuous soft stools of too small a size.
80. With the stool discharge of a little blood; of tape-worm.
Itching and sore feeling of the anus.
Varices of the rectum, and between them burning rhagades at the anus.
Prolapsus recti with the varices, as if the rectum were paralyzed.

Urinary Organs.

Anxious, painful desire to urinate, with discharge of small quantities of brown urine in drops, with a stitch in the
85. urethra, when emitting it.
The urine smells sour.
The urine becomes very turbid, with a reddish sediment.
During micturition pain in the os sacrum.
Wetting the bed at night. Nightly desire to urinate—frequent micturition.

Genital Organs.

Men. Tension and lascivious feeling in the genitals; voluptuous irritation of the genital organs.
90. Immoderate sexual desire; violent erections.

Eruptions on the penis.
Dropsical swelling of the prepuce and the scrotum.
During an embrace painful cramps in the calves; no emission of semen.
After an embrace coldness of the legs, exhaustion, heat of the body and perspiration.
95. *Women.* Soreness of the vagina.
Painful swelling of the (left) ovary.
Menses too late, too scanty and too pale.
The first menses delay.
Suppression of the menses, with heaviness of the limbs and congestions of blood to the head.
100. Before and during the menstruation, fatiguing cough (morning and during the day).
During the menses, colic; violent headache with nausea; morning sickness; soreness between the legs; swelling of the feet; chilliness; pain in the varices.
Profuse white, thin, leucorrhœa, with weakness in the back.

Respiratory Organs and Chest.

Sensitiveness of the larynx; scraping in it and roughness, hoarseness.
Cough, caused by taking a deep inspiration in the evening and at night.
105. Voice (when singing) cracked.
Stitches in the chest and palpitation of the heart from the least exercise.
Oppression of the chest—Asthma in the evening in bed.
Perspiration on the sternum every morning.
Swelling and induration of the mammary glands.
110. Soreness of the nipples with small corrosive blisters.

Back and Neck.

Sensation as if the small of the back were broken or bruised.
Formication in the back.
Contractive pain between the shoulders.
Painful stiffness of the neck, when bending the head and raising the arms.

Extremities.

115. *Upper.* Emaciation of the hands.
Distortion of the fingers.
Gouty nodosities on the finger-joints.
Soreness between the fingers.
The nails are thick and crippled.
120. *Lower.* Soreness between the thighs.

Numbness and stiffness of the thighs (and toes).
Stiffness and contraction of the muscles in the bend of the knee.
Stiffness of the knee.
Stiffness and contraction of the toes.
125. Coldness of the feet (in the evening, in bed).
Stinging pains in the heels.
Between the toes soreness, with violent itching.
On the toes, spreading blisters, ulcers.
Ulceration on the borders of the big toe.
130. Sore pains of the corns.
The nails are thick and crippled.

Sleep.

Unable to fall asleep before midnight on account of a fixed idea.
Perspiration about the head, when falling asleep.
Bleeding from the nose at night.
135. Wakens at night with a suffocative attack.
During sleep frightful, vexatious dreams.
Constant talking during sleep.
Bleeding from the nose at night.
Wetting the bed at night while asleep.

Generalities.

140. Great emaciation.
The limbs go to sleep.
Drawing through the whole body, with inclination to stretch.
Contractions of the muscles.
Pulsation through the whole body whenever he moves.
145. Sensation of debility, without pain, compelling one to groan.

Fever.

Pulse full and hard, but not accelerated.
Chill and chilliness, principally in the evening, after 4 P. M.
General dry heat, evening and night, preceded by a chill.
Heat when riding in a carriage.
150. Perspiration from the least exercise.
Perspiration sour, coloring the linen yellow, of offensive smell.
Night-sweat, offensive smelling.
Inability to perspire.
Quotidian fever; shaking chill in the evening; an hour afterwards heat in the face and cold feet, without any subsequent perspiration.

Skin.

155. Swelling and induration of the glands.
Dryness of the skin and want of perspiration.
Erysipelatous inflammation.
Humid tetters and eruptions.
Soreness and rawness of the skin (in the bends of the limbs, groins, neck, behind the ears), especially in children.
160. Unhealthy skin; every little injury causes suppuration.
Ulcers, with fetid pus; proud flesh; itching, stinging.
Burning pain in an old cicatrix.
Itching of the varices on the lower limbs.
Itching-stinging on the surface of a mole.

Conditions.

165. Liability to take cold; has to avoid a draught of air.
Dread of the open air (in the morning), sensitiveness to a draught of air.
Aggravation, at night; from becoming cold; during and after menstruation; from suppressed menstruation.
Amelioration from eructations.

GRATIOLA OFFICINALIS.

Mind and Disposition.

Serious, taciturn, absorbed in reverie.
Irresolute, want of perseverance.
Ill-humor, tired of life, apprehensive of the future.

Head.

Vertigo, while reading; on rising from a seat.
5. Intoxicated feeling during and after a meal.
Pressure in the forehead, with vertigo.
Sensation of heaviness in the forehead, as if the brain would fall forward, with stoppage of the nose.
Heat in the head, on raising the head.
Tightness in the forehead with wrinkles in the skin.
10. The headache is aggravated by rising from the seat and by walking in the open air.
The head is very sensitive to cold.
Itching of the scalp.

17

Eyes.

Itching of the eyelashes.
The eyes feel dry and as if sand were in them.
15. Mist before the eyes, when reading or writing.
Short-sightedness, with burning heat in the face.

Ears.

Itching of the ears.

Nose.

Smarting-itching in the left nostril.
Pressure at the upper part of the nose.

Face.

20. Burning heat in the face.
Tingling-burning in the malar bones.
Sensation of tension in the face; it feels swollen.
Swelling of the upper lip (every morning) (with stinging).

Mouth and Throat.

Accumulation of clear water in the mouth.
25. Tongue rough, coated with mucus.
Fetid breath on waking
Pain in the throat obliging one to swallow constantly; the swallowing is difficult, as if the throat were contracted; worse during empty deglutition.
Stinging in the throat (left side).
Phlegm in the throat, with inability to throw it off.

Stomach and Abdomen.

30. Hunger without appetite.
Violent thirst.
Hiccough.
Gulping up of bitter substances.
Paroxysms of inclination to vomit, relieved by eructations.
35. Empty retching.
Pressure in the stomach after every meal.
Empty or cold feeling in the stomach.
Gnawing, as from hunger after eating.
In the left hypochondrium heating pain, burning.
40. Pinching in the umbilical region, relieved by emission of flatulence.
Cold feeling in the abdomen.
Rumbling, with nausea, eructations, and vertigo.

Stool and Anus.

Diarrhœa; stools, watery yellow-green, succeeded by burning at the anus; green frothy, coming out with great force.
Stools with burning and protrusion of large, stinging-burning tumors.
45. Passage of feces without being conscious of it.
Discharge of ascarides.
In the rectum soreness; burning during and after stool.
In the anus stinging, itching.

Urinary Organs.

Scanty, reddish urine, becoming turbid while standing.
50. Floculent sediment in the urine.
Burning in the urethra during and after micturition.

Genital Organs.

Man. Stitches in the left spermatic cord, ascending through the abdomen up to the chest.
Involuntary emission succeeded by a painful erection.
Women. Menses too early and too profuse.
5. Nymphomania.
Dartings in the right mamma.

Respiratory Organs.

Heat in the chest, then in the head and hands, with redness of the face.
Violent palpitation of the heart, particularly immediately after stool, and with oppression of the chest.

Back and Neck.

Sensation as if the neck were seized with the hand.
60. Darting from the left scapula to the shoulder and mamma.

Extremities.

Upper. Rheumatic pains in the shoulders, arms, fingers, particularly in the elbow and wrist joint.
Itching in the palms of the (right) hand.
Lower. Bruised pain in the thigh, after a short walk.
Lancinating tearing in the tibia when sitting, disappearing when walking.
65. Smarting-itching on the tibia.

Sleep.

Irresistible drowsiness with yawning.
Deep sleep, like stupor.

Fever.

Pulse small, intermittent.
Chilliness in a warm room, during sleep, after an evacuation; with the hair standing on end.
70. Heat, ascending to the face, with redness and increased external warmth.
Constant vaporous exhalation from the body.

Generalities.

Physical and mental depression.
Great languor and prostration.
Tetanic condition, without loss of consciousness, while lying down after a meal, followed by a deep sleep with emission of semen; bruised feeling of the body, back and left arm on waking.

Skin.

75. Itching, with burning after scratching.

Conditions.

Aggravation on sitting, or on rising from a seat; in the afternoon; after a meal.
Amelioration by contact.

GUAJACUM OFFICINALE.

Mind and Disposition.

Forgetfulness, especially of names.
Thoughtless staring during the morning.

Head.

Violent sharp stitches in the brain.
Rheumatic pains in one side of the head, extending to the face.
5. External headache, with the sensation as if the blood-vessels were overfilled.
Pulsative throbbing in the outer parts of the head, with stitches in the temples; removed for a short time by external pressure and by walking, increased by sitting and standing.

Eyes.

Swelling of the eyes.
Sensation of swelling and protrusion of the eyes; the eyelids appeared too short to cover the eyes.

Ears.

Violent otalgia, with tearing (left ear).

Face.

10. Redness and painful swelling of the face.
Lancinations and painful stitches in the right malar bone and cheek, as if knives were plunged in.

Mouth and Throat.

Tearing pain in the teeth, ending with a stitch.
Violent burning in the throat.

Stomach and Abdomen.

Aversion to milk.
15. Violent hunger (afternoon and evening).
Much thirst.
Frequent empty eructations.
In the morning violent vomiting of watery mucus.
Nausea occasioned by the sensation of accumulated mucus in the throat.
20. Pinching in the abdomen (as from incarcerated flatulence), receding towards the rectum until flatulence was emitted.
Sensation of constriction in the stomach, with oppression of breathing and anguish.
Twitches in the abdominal muscles (right side).
Inguinal hernia.

Stool and Anus.

Constipation; stools hard and crumbling, very offensive.

Urinary Organs.

25. Continuous desire to urinate (even after urinating), with profuse emission of very fetid urine.
Cutting pain in the urethra when urinating.
Stitches in the neck of the bladder after ineffectual pressure to urinate.

Sexual Organs.

Men. Nocturnal emissions without lascivious dreams.

Respiratory Organs.

Stitches in the left side of the chest, worse from breathing deep.

30. Dry cough with shortness of breathing till expectoration sets in.
Cough with copious expectoration of fetid pus.

Back and Neck.

Contractive pain between the scapula.
Corrosive itching in the back (by day).
When moving, excessive stiffness of one side of the back, from the neck extending to the small of the back.
35. Chilliness in the back, in the afternoon.

Extremities.

Upper. Sharp stitches in the top of the right shoulder.
Rheumatic pains in the left arm, from the shoulder to the wrist.
Lancinating rheumatic pains from the elbow to the wrist (left arm).
Rheumatic pains in the left wrist-joint.
40. Stitches in the right thumb.
Lower. Exhaustion in the lower limbs.
Pricking in the nates, as if sitting on needles.
Tearing, drawing lancinations in the leg, from the right tarsus to the knee.
Tension in the thighs, especially the right, as if the muscles were too short, with languor when walking; worse by contact, better when sitting.

Sleep.

45. Nightly restlessness and sleeplessness.
Feels unrefreshed in the morning when waking.
Nightmare when lying on the back, waking with screams.

Generalities.

Tearing-pricking pains in the muscles of the extremities, with heat of the parts.
Immovable stiffness of the contracted limbs.
50. The limbs go to sleep.
Great emaciation.

Fever.

Pulse small, weak, soft, accelerated.
Chilliness internally, even near the warm stove, principally in the afternoon and evening.
Heat in the face, especially in the evening.
55. Perspiration, principally on the head and on the forehead (when walking in the open air).
Night-sweats, smelling very offensively.

Skin.
Swelling and softening of the bones. Caries.

Conditions.
Yawning and stretching relieves the general ill-feeling.
Most ailments begin in the morning and forenoon, and while sitting.
60. The affected parts are very sensitive to contact.
Aggravation in the open air.

GUMMI GUTTI.

Mind and Disposition.
Cheerful, talkative, feeling of ease, great lightness of all his motions.

Head.
Heaviness in the head with drowsiness and pain in the back.
Heat rises to the head, with perspiration.
Pain in the vertex, as if bruised, in the forenoon; relieved in the open air.

Eyes.
5. Itching of the inner canthi, with discharge of acrid, corrosive tears after rubbing; relieved in the open air.
Nightly agglutination.
Itching of the eyes in the evening.
Burning of the eyes, relieved by walking in the open air.

Ears.
Lancination in the ears.

Nose.
10. Ulceration of the right nostril, with burning pain.
Dryness of the right nostril.
Sneezing (in day-time).
Much mucus in the nose, smelling like pus.

Mouth and Throat.
Feeling of coldness in the points of the incisors.
15. Dry mouth.
Burning of the anterior half or only of the tip of the tongue, which feels hard.

Sore pain in the throat, which is felt when even touching the outer side of the neck.
Stinging in the right side of the throat during and between the acts of deglutition.
The throat feels swollen.

Stomach and Abdomen.

20. Bitter taste in the mouth.
Nausea, with accumulation of water in the mouth and gulping up of sour water.
Violent empty eructations.
Horrid vomiting and purging, with fainting.
Empty feeling in the stomach and abdomen.
25. Ulcerated pain in the stomach, relieved by eating.
Dartings in the stomach, causing one to start.
Inflation and tension in the abdomen.
Burning in the region of the liver.
Gnawing, in a small spot below the umbilicus.
30. In the groins sticking, tension.
Rumbling in the bowels.

Stool and Anus.

Frequent emission of flatulence.
Hard, insufficient stool, with violent urging, pressing, and protrusion of the rectum.
Hard stool, succeeded by burning at the anus.
35. Diarrhœa, with burning pain and tenesmus, protrusion of the anus, pinching around the umbilicus.
Watery diarrhœa, with colic and tenesmus.
Stools yellow or green, mixed with mucus.

Urinary Organs.

Emission of a few drops at a time, then intermitting, and finally returning, with burning at the orifice.

Sexual Organs.

Women. Menses too early and too profuse.

Respiratory Organs.

40. Sensation of soreness in every part of the chest.
Pressure in the middle of the chest.
Stitches going from both sides of the chest towards each other.

Back.

Pain in the small of the back, as if bruised or as if sprained.
Gnawing in the os coccygis.

Extremities.

45. *Upper.* Stitch on the top of the right shoulder.
Stinging and numb feeling in the ball of the right thumb.
Lower. Cramp in the calf, with contraction of the toes.
Heaviness and languor of the feet.

Sleep.

Drowsiness the whole day.

Generalities.

50. Itching and formication in various parts.
Pains, as if bruised.
Burning-stinging pain.
Gnawing.

Fever.

Chill, proceeding from the back, with coldness of the whole body from evening till morning.
55. Chilliness is accompanied by empty eructations, yawning, thirst, pain in the small of the back, biting as of ants over the whole body (by night), excessive stitches in the ears.
Increased warmth, with anxiety and perspiration.
Night-sweat all over.
Violent thirst in the evening.

Skin.

Intolerable itching and formication in various parts.
60. After scratching, burning and ulcerative pain.
Itching blisters on both hands, first pale, then red.

Conditions.

The majority of ailments come on while sitting, and go off during motion in the open air.
Aggravation in the evening and at night.

GYMNOCLADUS CANADENSIS.

Mind and Disposition.

Indifference to what happens around him.
Cannot think, comprehend or study; forgets every thing.

Head.

Dizziness with dimness of sight; nausea, belching.
Head feels full, tight, as if bound up.

5. Fulness and pressure in and over the eyes, extending to the top of the head.
Throbbing headache over the left eye.
Pain in the head and back.
Pain in the left temple to the ear and top of the head.
Bruised feeling of the head (left side).
10. Desire to lean the head on something.

Eyes.

Pain in the left eyeball and temple.
Eyes feel as if pushed forward.
Eyes feel sore in the morning.

Face.

Sensation as if flies were crawling over the right side of the face.
15. Erysipelatous swelling of the face and head; hot face; it feels swollen; is compelled to rub the eyes.

Nose.

Frequent violent sneezing, originating very high up in the nose.

Mouth and Throat.

Great sensibility of the teeth; more on the left side and in the upper teeth; the slightest draught of cold air causes toothache; cold drink is very painful.
Tongue coated bluish-white.
Burning, drawing and scraping; burning in the roof of the mouth, extending to the uvula and tonsils.
20. Inflammation and purple color of the right tonsil.
Sticking and shooting in the throat.
Burning in the œsophagus and stomach.
Mucus in the throat and frequent hawking.

Stomach and Abdomen.

Nausea after eating, with pain and fulness in stomach and belching.
25. Belching of sour water.
Burning in the stomach (circumscribed, the size of a dollar).
Heat in the stomach and sour watery eructations.
Pain in the left side, as if the spleen were swollen.
Stitches in the bowels and umbilical region.
30. Soreness and tenderness of the abdomen.

Stool and Anus.

Constipation, with ineffectual disposition to go to stool.
After stool, aching fulness in the rectum.

Urinary Organs.

Pressure on the bladder and frequent desire to urinate; the urine is passed in a small stream.

Sexual Organs.

Man. Itching of the glans penis and prepuce.

Respiratory Organs.

35. Smarting in the larynx.
In the morning, tickling in the throat, causing a cough, increasing through the day; cough hard, dry and racking.
Pressure on the chest and sternum.
Stitches in the right breast and intercostal muscles.

Extremities.

Upper. Perspiration of the axillary region and palms of the hands.
40. Violent pain in the left forearm, in the radius, as if the bones were crushed and broken.
Pulsation in the left index, as if a panaritium were forming.
Lower. Stinging pain in the left knee-joint.

Fever.

Pulse small and quick.
Cold chills and pains in the bowels (in the descending colon).
45. Desire for increased heat; wants to be near the fire.

Conditions.

Aggravation in the evening.
Repugnance to motion; a short walk fatigues him much (afternoon).
The whole body feels numb.

HÆMATOXYLUM CAMPECHIANUM.

Head.

Pain in the forehead, and disposition to vomit on stooping.

Eyes.

Redness of the eyes, with blue margins.
Contraction of the pupils and dimness of sight.

Ears.

Violent pain in the right ear, extending to the throat; throat feels contracted, with burning pain during deglutition.

Face.

5. Pale face, with desponding expression.

Pain in the lower jaw, with stinging in the teeth and cheek.

Throat.

Contraction of the throat, with desire to swallow.

Stomach and Abdomen.

Tympanitic distention of the abdomen and rising of air.

Cutting colic, with distention; relieved by a soft stool.

10. After the colic ceases, chilliness, with burning in the palms of the hands.

Urinary Organs.

Small quantity of red, burning urine.

Chest.

Constriction of the chest down to the pit of the stomach.

Pain in the region of the heart, as if a bar were extending from the heart to the right side, with oppressive anxiety, palpitation of the heart, small pulse, hot hands and general chilliness.

Extremities.

The limbs are painful and languid.

15. Pain and chilliness between the shoulders.

Pain in the shoulder, as if inflamed.

Suppression of the habitual sweat of the feet.

Sleep.

Irresistible drowsiness.

Fever.

Chilliness, with goose-flesh.
20. Dry skin.

HELLEBORUS NIGER.

Mind and Disposition.

Silent melancholy, with great anguish, much moaning, thoughtless staring and inability to think.
Home-sickness.
Sadness, despair of his life.
Dulness of the internal senses.
5. Diminished power of the mind over the body; the muscles do not act properly, if the will is not strongly fixed upon their action; if he talks he lets fall what he holds in the hand.
Weakness of memory.

Head.

Giddiness on stooping.
Stupefying headache, with coryza (4 to 8 P. M.); worse from stooping, relieved at rest and in the open air.
Pressing headache from outward to inward, with stupefaction and heaviness of the head; worse on moving the head, from exertion; better in the open air and from distraction of the mind.
10. Inflammation of the brain, with stupefaction; heat and heaviness of the head; boring with the head in the pillows, with chilliness of the whole body; coldness of the fingers; worse from thinking of the pain.
Hydrocephalus with stupefaction; stupor; boring with the head in the pillows; coldness of the body; aggravated from stooping.
Sensation of soreness of the head, as if bruised, especially in the back part of the head, with stupefaction worse on stooping.
Burning heat in the head, with paleness of the face.
Boring with the head in the pillows, with the sensation as if the scalp on the occiput were pulled down tight.
15. Falling off of the hair (on the head and on the whole body), with pricking pain on the scalp, especially on the occiput, with pale, dropsical swelling of the face and body.
Humid scurf on the scalp.

Eyes.

Inclination to stare.
Photophobia without inflammation.

Sensation as if the eyelids were pressed down.
20. Pupils dilated.
Twitching in the levatores palpebrarum and the cheeks, with heat in the face.

Face.

Pale-yellowish color of the face.
Œdematous pale swelling of the face.
The forehead is full of wrinkles.
25. Soreness of the corners of the mouth, with continuous flow of saliva.
White blisters (vesicles) on the swollen lips.
The upper lip is cracked.
Dull pain in the right malar bone.

Mouth and Throat.

In the evening and at night pricking toothache in the molars; can bear neither cold nor heat.
30. Vesicles in the mouth and on the tongue.
Ptyalism, with soreness of the corners of the mouth.
Aphthæ in the mouth.
Swelling of the tongue.
Pimple on the tip of the tongue, painfully stinging when touched.
35. Insensibility and numbness of the tongue.
Dry, white tongue (in the morning).

Stomach and Abdomen.

Nausea, sensation of hunger with repugnance to food.
Vomiting of green-blackish substances, with colic.
Fulness and distention of the pit of the stomach.
40. Burning and scraping in the stomach.
Painfulness of the stomach when coughing and walking.
Gurgling in the bowels, as if full of water.
Distention of the abdomen (Ascites).
Sensation of coldness in the abdomen.

Stool and Anus.

45. White, jelly-like stools, with tenesmus.
Frequent watery stools.
Stools consisting of pure, tenacious, white mucus.
After an evacuation, burning hot smarting at the anus.

Urinary Organs.

Frequent desire to urinate, emitting but a small quantity.
50. Dark urine, feeble stream.
A large quantity of pale, watery urine is emitted.

Sexual Organs.
Suppressed sexual desire.

Respiratory Organs.
Suffocative attacks, as from constriction of the lungs.
Constriction of the throat, nose, chest.
55. Hydrothorax.
Dry cough while smoking tobacco.

Back.
Stiffness of the cervical muscles as far as the occiput.
Swelling of the cervical glands.

Extremities.
Upper. Boring-sticking pain in the wrist and finger-joints.
60. Humid, painless vesicles between the fingers.
Ulceration around the nails.
Lower. Stiffness of the hip and knee-joints.
Pricking pain in the left hip.
Boring-stinging in the knee and foot-joints.
65. Humid, painless vesicles between the toes.

Sleep.
Stupor, sopor.
Lies in a stupor, with the eyes half open and with the pupils turned upward.
Confused, anxious dreams, which cannot be recollected.

Generalities.
Sudden relaxation of all the muscles.
70. The muscles refuse their services, if not governed by strong attention and will.
Convulsive twitching of the muscles (during sleep).
Stinging-boring pains in the coverings of the bones; worse in the cool air.

Fever.
Pulse, small, slow, almost imperceptible.
Chilliness predominates during the day, as long as he remains out of bed, with heat of the face and drowsiness.
75. Chill with goose-flesh and pain in the joints.
The chill begins and spreads from the arms.
After lying down in bed, the heat comes on immediately, generally accompanied by perspiration.
In the evening, in bed, burning heat over the whole body, with internal chilliness and aversion to drink; when attempting to drink, very little can be taken at a time.

Heat followed by chill, with colic.
80. Perspiration while in bed with the heat; worse towards morning.
Cold, at times clammy perspiration.

Skin.
Pale color of the skin.
Sudden dropsical swelling of the skin; Anasarca.
The hair and nails fall off.
85. Desquamation all over the body.

Conditions.
The pains (pricking, tearing, pressing) run across the parts.
Aggravation, in the evening (4 P. M.), in the cold air, and from bodily exertion.
Amelioration in the warm air.
In the open air he feels better, with the sensation as if he had been sick for a long time.

HEPAR SULPHURIS CALCAREA.

Mind and Disposition.
Great anguish in the evening, almost driving one to commit suicide.
Over-sensitiveness and irritability, with quick, hasty speech.
The slightest cause irritates him and makes him extremely vehement.
Dejected, sad, with inclination to shed tears.

Head.
5. Fainty giddiness when riding in a carriage or when shaking the head, with headache and obscuration of sight.
Boring headache from without to within, in the right temple; on one side of the head; the root of the nose, when waking from sleep; aggravated by motion and stooping.
Pressure in the head, semi-lateral, as from a plug or dull nail, at night and when waking in the morning; aggravated when moving the eyes and on stooping; relieved when rising and from binding the head up tight.
Aching in the forehead, like a boil, from midnight till morning.
Lancinating headache; better when walking in the open air.

10. Sense of swashing in the head.
 Boring headache in the root of the nose, every forenoon.
 Morning headache, aggravated from every contusion.
 Humid eruption over the whole head, feeling sore, of fetid smell; itching violently on rising in the morning; burning and feeling sore on scratching.
 Boils on the head and neck, very sore on contact and when lying on them.
15. The head is bent backwards, with swelling below the larynx, with violent pulsation of the carotid arteries and rattling breathing (in croup).
 Falling off of the hair, with very sore, painful pimples and large bald spots on the scalp; sensitiveness of the scalp to contact, with burning and itching in the morning after rising (after abuse of mercury).
 Burning-itching on the scalp, from the forehead to the back part of the head.
 Cold, clammy perspiration, smelling sour, principally on the head and face, with aversion to be uncovered; worse from the least exercise and during the night; better from warmth and when at rest.
 Nodosities on the head, sore to contact; better from covering the head warm and from perspiration.
20. Disposition to catch cold when uncovering the head.

Eyes.

Inflammation of the eyes and eyelids; they are sore to the touch, with lachrymation.
Pressure in the eyes, as from a foreign body (sand).
The eyes are protruded.
Spasmodically closed eyelids (at night).
25. Photophobia.
 Ulcers and spots on the cornea.
 Obscuration of sight when reading.
 The eyes ache from the bright light of day, when moving them.
 The objects appear to be red.

Ears.

30. Darting pain in the ears.
 Itching of the external ear.
 Discharge of fetid pus from the ear.
 Scurfy eruption on and behind the ear.
 Whizzing and throbbing in the ears, with hardness of hearing.

18

35. Detonation in the ear when blowing the nose.
Increase of cerumen.

Nose.

Inflammation (redness and heat) of the nose.
The nose feels sore, as if bruised.
Sore pain on the dorsum of the nose when touching it.
40. Very sensitive smell.
Coryza, with inflammatory swelling of the nose, which feels as sore as a boil.

Face.

Heat and fiery redness of the face.
Erysipelatous swelling of the face.
Yellow color of the face, with blue border around the eyes.
45. Pain in the bones of the face on touching them.
Boils on the lips, chin and neck, very painful to the touch.
Eruption in the corners of the mouth.
Itching around the mouth.
Ulcer in the corner of the mouth.
50. Eruption in the face, scurfy, very painful to the touch.
Itching pimples on the chin.
The middle of the lower lip becomes chapped.
Sore and smarting pimple in the vermilion border of the upper lip.

Mouth and Throat.

The gums and mouth are very painful to the touch and bleed readily.
55. Toothache worse in the warm room; increased when pressing the teeth against one another.
Looseness of the teeth.
The hollow teeth feel too long and painful.
Ulcer on the gums and in the mouth, with a base resembling lard.
The tip of the tongue is very painful and feels sore.
60. When swallowing, sensation as if a plug were in the throat, or as if splinters were sticking in it.
Scraping in the throat when swallowing saliva.
Hawking up of mucus.
Swelling of the tonsils and glands of the neck.
Dry throat.
65. Stitches in the throat, extending to the ear.

Stomach and Abdomen.

Longing for acids, wine, sour and strong-tasting substances.
Unusual hunger (in the forenoon).
More thirst than hunger; much thirst.

HEPAR SULPHURIS CALCAREA.

Aversion to fat.
70. Distention of the pit of the stomach, compelling one to loosen the clothing.
Burning in the stomach.
Heaviness and pressure in the stomach after moderate eating.
Pressure in the stomach, as if lead were in it.
Spasmodic contraction in the abdomen.
75. Sensation of soreness (as if bruised) in the abdomen (in the morning).
Cutting pain in the abdomen.
Vomiting (every morning).
Stitches in the region of the liver, when walking.
Splenetic stitches when walking.
80. Rumbling in the abdomen (incarceration of flatulence).
Swelling and suppuration of the inguinal glands (buboes).

Stool and Anus.

Constipation; hard, dry stool.
The feces are not hard, but are expelled with great difficulty.
Sour-smelling, whitish diarrhœa, in children.
85. Clay-colored stool.
Dysenteric stools; difficult evacuation of soft stool, or of bloody mucus, with tenesmus.
Hemorrhage from the rectum, with soft stool.
Soreness of the rectum after stool, with ichor.
Burning at the rectum.
90. Protrusion of the varices.
Perspiration on the perineum.

Urinary Organs.

The urine is passed slowly, with difficulty; drops out perpendicularly.
Sharp, burning urine, corroding the prepuce.
Burning in the urethra during micturition.
95. Urine dark-red, hot.
Bloody urine.
Stitches in the urethra.
Inflammation and redness of the orifice of the urethra.
Discharge of mucus from the urethra.
100. Wetting the bed at night.

Sexual Organs.

Men. Itching of the penis (glans, frænulum).
Ulcers like chancres on the prepuce.
Humid soreness on the genitals, scrotum, and the folds between the thigh and the scrotum.
Diminished sexual instinct. (Feeble erections).

105. Discharge of the prostatic juice during the hard stool and after urinating.
Women. Congestion of blood to the uterus.
Menstrual discharge delayed and diminished.
Discharge of blood between the times of menstruation.
Itching nipples.
110. Scirrhous ulcer on the mamma, with stinging-burning of the edges, smelling like old cheese.

Respiratory Organs.

Rattling breathing (during sleep).
Dry, hoarse cough.
Titillation, as from dust in the throat, inducing cough, which is deep, wheezing, with expectoration only in the morning of mucus, bloody or like pus, generally tasting sour or sweet.
Cough worse from evening till midnight.
115. Cough caused by a limb becoming cold; from eating or drinking any thing cold; from cold air; when lying in bed; from talking, crying.
Sneezing or crying, after the attacks of cough.
Anxious wheezing breathing.
Suffocative attacks, compelling him to raise himself up and to bend the head backwards.
Wheezing in the larynx and painfulness of a small spot in the larynx.
120. Swelling below the larynx.
Roughness in the throat.
Hoarseness.
Sensitiveness of the larynx to cold air.
Croup, with swelling under the larynx.
125. Cough, with expectoration of blood.
Bronchitis.
Soreness in the chest.
Weakness of the chest; cannot talk from weakness.
Tenacious mucus in the chest.
130. Spasmodic constriction of the chest.
Violent palpitation of the heart, with fine stitches in the heart and the left half of the chest.

Back and Neck.

Violent pulsation of the carotid arteries.
Sensation as if bruised in the small of the back and thighs.
Stitches and rheumatic pains in the back.

HEPAR SULPHURIS CALCAREA.

Extremities.

135. *Upper.* Suppuration of the axillary glands.
Fetid sweat in the axilla.
Pain, as from bruises in the humeri.
Red, hot swelling of the joints of the hands and fingers.
Cold perspiration of the hands.
140. Deadness of the fingers.
Tingling in the tips of the fingers.
Itching in the palms of the hands.
Steatoma at the point of the elbow.
Rough, dry, grating, cracked skin of the hands.
145. Panaritium.
Lower. The hip-joint feels sore, as if sprained when walking.
Sensation of soreness in the thighs.
Swelling of the knee.
Pain, as from bruises in the knee.
150. Cramp in the soles and toes.
Tickling in the soles of the feet.
Prickings in both heels.
Swelling of the feet around the ankles (with difficult breathing).
Tingling in the toes.
155. Burning, stinging pain in the toes.
Cracked skin of the feet.

Sleep.

Sleepiness during the day (morning and evening) with spasmodic yawning.
Restless, soporous slumber, with the head bent backwards.
Starts up from sleep with the feeling as though he would suffocate.
160. Wakes at night with an erection and an urgent desire to urinate.
The side on which he lays at night becomes painfully sore; he must change his position.

Generalities.

Fainting (evening) from slight pains.
Rheumatic pains in the limbs and stitches in the joints.
Weakness in all the limbs; they feel bruised.

Fever.

165. Pulse hard, full, accelerated; at times intermitting.
Chill in the evening, 6 or 7 P. M.

Chilliness and heat alternating during the day, with photophobia.
Chilliness at night; in bed aggravating all the symptoms.
Great chilliness in the open air.
170. Dry, burning heat, with redness of the face and violent thirst all night.
Flushes of heat with perspiration.
Profuse perspiration day and night.
Perspiration easily excited through the day, especially from exertions of the mind.
Night and morning sweat, with thirst.
175. Cold, clammy or sour or offensively smelling perspiration.
Intermittent fever; first chills, then thirst and, an hour later, much heat, with interrupted sleep.
Violent chill, 8 P. M., with chattering of teeth; hands and feet are cold; followed by heat with perspiration, especially on the chest and forehead, with slight thirst.

Skin.

Inflammation, swelling and suppuration of the glands.
Caries.
180. Erysipelatous inflammation on external parts.
Suppurations, especially after previous inflammation.
Ulcers very sensitive to contact, easily bleeding, burning or stinging, with corrosive pains.
Eruptions very sensitive and feeling sore when touched.
Burning-itching in the skin after scratching; white vesicles.
185. Nettle-rash.
Unhealthy skin; the slightest injuries produce suppuration and ulceration.
Promotes suppuration.
Yellow skin and complexion.

Conditions.

Great sensitiveness of the affected parts to contact.
190. *Aggravation*, at night; from cold air; from lying on the painful side; from external pressure; from touching the parts; during sleep; when swallowing food.
Amelioration from warmth; from wrapping oneself up warmly.

HIPPOMANE MANCINELLA.

Mind and Disposition.

Sudden vanishing of thought. Thoughtlessness.
Vivacity, looks on the bright side of everything; is inclined to sing.
Bashful and taciturn.

Head.

Pulsating pains in the head and neck preventing one from writing.
5. The whole head feels sore as if bruised, or as if it had been exposed to the sun.
Stitches in the head with nightly sleeplessness.
Heaviness in the head.
Vertigo with loss of consciousness.
Vertigo in the morning, on rising from the bed.
10. Stitches over the left eye.

Eyes.

Blue circle around the eyes.
Burning in the eyes, compelling one to close them.
Sensation of heaviness of the eyes.
Sensation of dryness of the eyelids.

Ears.

15. Redness and heat in the ears.
The ears feel as if closed.

Nose.

Pressure at the root of the nose.
Dryness of the nose.

Face.

Bloated, yellowish face.
20. Heat rises to the face followed by violent itching, stinging, and burning, the face swells up and on it are formed small vesicles filled with yellow fluid, they finally disappear with peeling off of the skin.
A large number of small vesicles on the skin, they peel off.
Pricking pains in the lips.
The lips are pale.
The lower lip hangs down.

Mouth and Throat.

25. Dryness of the mouth.
Burning in the mouth not relieved by cold water.
The whole mouth and tongue are full of small vesicles, he can only take fluid nourishment.
The mouth bleeds.
Burning on the tongue.
30. Dry tongue.
Tongue coated white as in aphthæ.
On the white-coated tongue numerous small circumscribed red, not coated spots.
Bloody taste.
Bitter taste, worse after sleeping.
35. Increased saliva, fetid, yellowish, burning.
Burning at the soft palate and the roof of the mouth.
Burning in the throat.
Aversion to meat and bread.
Longing for water and aversion to wine and alcoholic drinks.
40. Great thirst for water, but a constrictive sensation ascending from the stomach prevents her swallowing it.
Inflammation and suppuration of the tonsils with wheezing breathing and suffocative attacks.
Sore throat during scarlet fever.
White yellowish burning ulcers on the tonsils and in the throat.
Palate much elongated.
45. Great dryness of the throat on waking.
Stitches in the throat.
Sensation of constriction in the throat ascending from the stomach, caused by accumulation of air, with palpitation of the heart and great sensation of weakness, impeding speech.

Stomach and Abdomen.

Violent vomiting, bitter, watery, green, of the ingesta.
Vomiting at night of a greasy watery substance, a white substance like hardened fat swims on the top of it.
50. The vomiting relieves the headache.
Burning in the stomach and throat with nausea.
Burning in the pit of the stomach.
Swelling of the pit of the stomach with tenderness to the touch.
Distended abdomen.
55. Sensation of soreness, as if bruised, of the abdominal walls.
Eruptions of rash on the abdomen.

Rumbling in the abdomen renewed by every motion and when taking a deep inspiration, with headache which is much increased near the warm stove.
Colic after drinking water.
Colic and diarrhœa (at midnight).

Stool and Anus.

60. Sudden desire to go to stool (in the morning) and after stool tenesmus.
Diarrhœa with much discharge of flatulence.
Diarrhœa with burning in the stomach and anus.
Bloody evacuations with colic, sleepiness and giddiness.
Stools, painful, black, fetid, bloody, with tenesmus.
65. Sensation of fulness in the rectum.
After stool pulsation in the anus; discharge of fetid blood from the hæmorrhoidal tumors.

Urinary Organs.

Stitches in the bladder before and at the beginning of micturition.
Burning in the urethra.

Genitals.

Men. Itching in the scrotum.
70. *Women.* Before menstruation congestions of the head.
Pale menstrual blood.
Colic during menstruation.

Respiratory Organs.

In the larynx scraping; cutting as with a knife; tension.
Cough, after drinking, at night (midnight).
75. Suffocative attacks with pulsation in the chest, while coughing or as soon as he begins to talk.
Oppression of the chest relieved by expectorating.
Rattling of mucus on the chest when breathing.
The breath is very offensive, perceptible to oneself.
Pulsations in the chest.
80. Constriction in the chest.
Stitches in the middle of the sternum.
Frequent hawking with nausea.
Stitches in the heart as from needles.
Palpitation of the heart in the evening, as from eating.

Back and Neck.

85. Stiffness of the neck in the morning.
Backache with nausea and tenesmus.

Stiffness in the small of the back (and the fingers).
Soreness in the region of the kidneys.
Stitches in the left shoulder-blade and the left breast at intervals.

Extremities.

90. *Upper.* Trembling and heaviness of the arms.
When waking the hands feel as if asleep and numb.
Trembling of the hands.
Blue finger nails.
Lower. Trembling of the legs.
95. Cramps in the legs and feet.
Tingling in the feet when sitting.
Stitches in the heels.

Generalities.

Convulsions.
Stitches here and there.

Fever.

100. Pulse feeble, accelerated.
Coldness of the hands and feet.
Flashes of heat, as if flames were spreading from the pit of the stomach, uncovers himself to become cooler.
Fever heat with tingling in the skin and desire to cover oneself with loss of consciousness, painful deglutition, reslessness, profuse micturition.
Typhus fever with tympanitis and sensitiveness of the abdomen aggravated by drinking water.

Sleep.

105. Great sleepiness.
Wakens as from electric shocks on the neck (above the larynx).

Skin.

Redness of the skin (hands).

Conditions.

Most symptoms are aggravated from anger and after eating.
Aggravation at night.
110. Amelioration from heat and when lying down.

HIPPOMANES.

Head.

Headache, with giddiness, heat in the head, sleepiness, yawning, thirst.
Violent headache; heaviness on the vertex; when walking, it feels as if the head would fall forward.
The head feels so heavy that it falls forward if he raises himself.
Pressing pain in the temples.
5. The headache is worse when walking in the sun.
The headache is lighter, when lying on the painful side.
Sensation of lightness in the head.
The hair becomes nearly dry; falling off of the hair.

Eyes.

Painfulness of the eyes when moving them, with headache.
10. Stitches in the eyes (with headache).
The light of the candle looks blue.

Nose.

Sensation of coldness, when drawing the air in.
Bleeding of the nose in the morning.

Face.

Involuntary twitching of the under lip.

Mouth and Throat.

15. Increased secretion of saliva, with headache or sore throat.
Tongue coated white, with redness of the tip of the tongue.
Bitter taste in the mouth.
Painfulness of the left tonsil.
Sensation of plug in the throat (left side).

Stomach and Abdomen.

20. Desire for acids, and aversion to sweet things; the tongue being coated white with redness on the tip of it.
Nausea, especially in a draft of air, with headache.
Icy coldness in the stomach.
Sensation of emptiness in the stomach (and head).

Stool and Anus.

Soft stool, with vomiting and discharge of prostatic fluid after micturition.
25. Hard stool, in balls.
Spasmodic contraction of the sphincter ani.

Urinary Organs.

Frequent discharge of watery urine.
Drawing pain from the anus through the urethra.
The urine is discharged in a small stream, and with straining,—it feels as if a swelling retarded it (prostatitis).

Sexual Organs.

30. *Men.* Sexual desire increased.
Drawing pain in the testicles.
Women. Menstruation too early.

Respiratory Organs.

Larynx feels raw, as if the air were too cold.
Tickling in the throat when breathing.
35. Cough, barking, during sleep.
Stitches in the left side of the chest.

Extremities.

Upper. The left arm feels as if paralyzed.
Formication on the right hand.
Paralysis of the right wrist (in the morning).
40. Great weakness of the hands and fingers, so that he cannot hold any thing.
In the wrist (especially the left) sensation as if sprained.
Lower. Weakness and sensation of dryness in the foot-joints and soles of the feet.
Sensation of weakness, and as if sprained, in the knees.
Cramps in the soles of the feet (in the evening).
45. Cold feet.

Generalities.

Heaviness in the limbs.
Desire to lie down, which does give no relief.
Great weakness and debility, with pale face.

Fever.

Chill relieved by being warmly covered in bed.
50. Chill, beginning in the back.
Heat in the evening, with dull headache.

Skin.

Itching on the chest, between the shoulders.

Conditions.

More symptoms appear while sitting.
Aggravation in the sun (headache).
55. Amelioration when covering up warm in bed (chill).

HYDROPHOBIN.

Mind and Disposition.

Ill-humor; irritable; inclined to use offensive language, to scold his friends, to beat those near him, and to abuse them.

Face.

Heat and redness of the face.
The articulation of the jaw feels stiff; imagines he cannot open the mouth.

Mouth and Throat.

Large quantities of tough saliva in the mouth and throat.
5. Continued spitting.
Sensation of constriction of the throat.
Sensation of elongation of the palate.
Imagines that he cannot swallow any thing.
Sensation of a lump in the throat, and desire to swallow.

Appetite and Taste.

10. Aversion to water; says he is thirsty, but cannot look at the water nor hear it poured out.
Swallows very small quantities of warm chocolate.

Stool and Anus.

Discharge of bright red blood from the rectum with burning and stinging, as from thorns in the anus.
Dysenteric stools with tenesmus; renewed as soon as he hears or sees the water run.
Discharge of blood from the rectum during the menses.

Sexual Organs.

15. *Men.* The testicles shrink and become softer.
Hydrocele.
Women. Pressing downwards in the region of the uterus (prolapsus uteri).

Chest.

Stitches in the heart.

Generalities.

Aversion to water; cannot drink water; imagines he cannot swallow it.
20. When he hears the water poured out, or if he hears it run or if he sees it, he becomes very irritable, nervous it causes desire for stool, and other ailments.

Conditions.

Natrum muriaticum follows well after Hydrophobin.

HYDROCYANIC ACID.

Mind and Disposition.

Despondency; oppression.
Anguish in the pit of the stomach.
Inability to think.

Head.

Dizziness with feeling of intoxication.
5. Vertigo with reeling.
Headache with giddiness.
Stupefying headache.
Pricking in various parts of the head.

Eyes.

Protruded eyes.
10. Distorted, half open eyes.
Pupils dilated, immovable, insensible to the light.
The lids immovable, they seem paralyzed.
Dimness of sight; gauze before the eyes.

Ears.

Roaring and buzzing in the ears.
15. Hardness of hearing.

Nose.

Enlarged, bluish wings of the nose.
Dryness of the nose.

Face.

Face bloated.
Pale-bluish face, looks old.

20. Sallow and gray complexion.
    Distortion of the corners of the mouth.
    Distortion of the facial muscles.
    Lock-jaw.
Mouth and Throat.
Increased secretion of saliva.
25. Tongue coated white.
    Cold feeling of the tongue.
    Burning on the tip of the tongue.
    Lameness and stiffness of the tongue; tongue protruded.
    Loss of speech.
30. Spasm in the pharynx and œsophagus.
    Heat and inflammation of the throat.
Stomach and Abdomen.
Taste acrid, sweet or fetid.
Absence of thirst, with heat of the whole body, or violent thirst.
Vomiting of a black fluid.
35. Cold feeling in the abdomen with stitches.
    Spasmodic contraction of the stomach.
    Inflammation of the stomach and bowels.
    Coldness in the abdomen alternating with burning.
Urinary Organs.
Retention of urine.
40. Copious emission of watery urine.
Stool and Anus.
Involuntary stools.
Respiratory Organs.
Sensation as if the larynx were swollen.
Scraping and burning in the larynx.
Short, hacking cough, caused by a pricking in the larynx and trachea.
45. Rattling, moaning, slow breathing.
    Arrest of breathing caused by stitches in the larynx.
    Tightness in the chest, sensation of suffocation.
    The heart beats irregular, feeble.
Sleep.
Irresistible, constant drowsiness.
50. Sleeplessness.
Generalities.
Languor and weakness of the limbs.
Paralysis first of the lower then of the upper limbs.

Nervous weakness.
Irregular pulsation of the heart.

Fever.

55. Coldness within and without.
Heat in the head with coldness of the extremities.
Heat and perspiration over the whole body.

Skin.

Dryness of the skin.
Paleness with a blue tinge.

HYOSCYAMUS NIGER.

Mind and Disposition.

Jealousy, with rage and delirium.
Fright, followed by convulsions and starts from sleep.
Unfortunate love with jealousy, with rage and incoherent speech.
Delirium without consciousness; does not know any body and has no wants (except thirst).
5. Unconscious delirium, with closed eyes; talks of business; fears to be poisoned or to be sold; scolds, raves.
Melancholy from unfortunate love, with rage or inclination to laugh at every thing.
Delirium tremens, with clonic spasms; unconsciousness and aversion to light and company.
When spoken to, the answer is properly given, but immediately unconsciousness and delirium return.
Indomitable rage.
10. Mania with lasciviousness and occasional muttering; sings amorous and obscene songs; uncovers his whole body.

Head.

Loss of memory.
Vertigo, with obscuration of sight, as from intoxication.
Unconsciousness, from congestion of blood to the head, with delirium; answering all questions properly; pupils dilated.

Congestion of blood to the head; red, sparkling eyes; face purple-red; worse in the evening.
15. Inflammation of the brain, with unconsciousness; heat and tingling in the head; violent pulsations in the head, like waves; the head shakes; worse from becoming cold and after eating; relieved by bending the head forward (stooping) and from heat.

The brain feels as if it were loose.

Hydrocephalus, with stupor; the head is shaken to and fro; sensation of swashing in the head.

Pressing, stupefying pain in the forehead.

The head is shaken or is drawn to one side, with loss of consciousness and red, sparkling eyes.
20. Heat of the head and face, with general coldness of the body, without thirst.

Liability to catch cold in the head, principally from dry, cold air.

Eyes.

Red, sparkling eyes.

Spasmodic closing of the lids; inability to open the eyelids.

Staring, distorted eyes.
25. Squinting.

Contortion of the eyes.

Pupils dilated.

Quivering in the eye.

Optical illusions; every thing looks red as fire; things look too large; dim-sightedness; double vision.
30. Night-blindness.

Face.

Heat and redness of the face.

Swollen, brown-red face.

Distorted, bluish face, with the mouth wide open.

Lock-jaw.

Mouth and Throat.

35. Soreness; sensation as if bruised in the soft parts between the gums and the cheeks.

Toothache, with congestion to the head.

Pulsating toothache, as from inflammation of the periosteum.

He closes the teeth tight.

Foam at the mouth.
40. Constriction of the throat, with inability to swallow, especially fluids.

Saliva tasting salt; bloody saliva.

Tongue red.

Loss of speech; utters inarticulated sounds. Paralysis of the tongue.
Parching dryness of the fauces. Elongation of the palate.

Stomach and Abdomen.

45. Voracious appetite and thirst, with inability to swallow.
Thirst, with drinking but little at a time.
After drinking, convulsions; dread of drink.
Hiccough (with spasms and rumbling in the abdomen).
Bitter eructations.
50. Vomiting of blood and bloody mucus.
Vomiting and retching after coughing.
Sensitiveness and tenderness of the pit of the stomach to the touch.
Burning in and inflammation of the stomach.
Colic relieved by vomiting.
55. Distention of the abdomen, with pain when touched.
Pain, as from soreness in the abdominal walls, when coughing.

Stool and Anus.

Frequent urgent desire for stool, with but small discharge.
Involuntary stools, from paralysis of the sphincter ani.
Watery, painless diarrhœa.
60. Diarrhœa of lying-in women.
The stool is small-shaped.
Hæmorrhoids profusely bleeding.

Urinary Organs.

Frequent desire to urinate, with scanty discharges.
Involuntary micturition, as from paralysis of the bladder.
65. Retention of urine, with pressure in the bladder.
Frequent emission of urine (as clear as water).

Sexual Organs.

Menstruation too profuse (with delirium).
Before menstruation, hysterical spasms; uninterrupted loud laughing.
During the menses, convulsive tremblings of the hands and feet; severe headache; profuse perspiration.
70. Metrorrhagia, the blood pale, with convulsions.
Suppressed menstruation; suppressed lochia.
Spasms of pregnant women, especially during parturition.
Puerperal fever.

Respiratory Organs.

Slow, rattling breathing.
75. Spasms of the chest, with arrest of breathing, compelling one to lean forward.

Stitches in the sides of the chest. (Inflammation of the lungs.)
Violent, spasmodic cough; short consecutive coughs, caused by a tickling sensation in the throat, as if some mucus were lodged in it; during the day, expectoration of saltish tasting mucus, or of bright-red blood, mixed with clots.
Dry, spasmodic cough at night (in old persons), from continuous tickling in the throat (as if the palate were too long).
Hæmoptysis, blood bright-red, with spasms.
80. The cough is worse, at night (after midnight), when at rest, during sleep, in the cold air, from eating and drinking.
The cough is relieved by sitting up.
Rough voice, from mucus in the trachea and larynx.

Extremities.

Upper. Painful numbness of the hands.
Trembling of the arms.
85. Rigor of the hands.
Swelling of the hands.
Hands closed, with clenched thumb.
Floccillation—picking of the bed-cover or of the face.
Lower. Cramps in the anterior part of the thigh.

Sleep.

90. Coma vigil.
Deep, heavy sleep, with convulsions.
Nightly sleeplessness, with convulsions and concussions, as if by fright; starting from sleep.
Sleeplessness from nervous irritation.

Generalities.

Spasms and convulsions (with watery diarrhœa).
95. Epileptic attacks, ending with deep, heavy sleep.
Apoplexy with snoring.
Uncommon sinking of strength.
Fainting, repeated attacks of.
Subsultus tendinum.

Fever.

100. Pulse full, hard, accelerated; distended arteries.
Chilliness over the whole body, with heat in the face, ascending from the feet.
Nightly coldness, extending over the back from the small of the back.
Burning heat of the body every evening.

292   HYPERICUM PERFOLIATUM.

Heat (in the evening) with congestion of blood to the head and putrid taste.
105. Debilitating perspiration during sleep.
Cold, sour-smelling perspirations.
Perspiration, principally on the legs.
Intermittent fever, quartan, with short, dry, hacking cough at night.
Afternoon fever; coldness predominates, with pain in the back.

Skin.

110. Hot, dry, brittle skin.
Brown or gangrenous spots on the body (as in typhus).
Frequent large blood-boils.
Rash, from the abuse of Belladonna.
The ulcer is very painful and bleeds.

Conditions.

115. Bad effects from getting cold and cold air; from the abuse of Belladonna; from jealousy, unhappy love.
Aggravation in the evening; after eating and drinking; during menstruation.
Amelioration by stooping (head, breathing).

HYPERICUM PERFOLIATUM.

Head.

Great heaviness in the head.
Pulsation, heat and burning in the vertex (afternoon).
Sensation in the forehead as if touched by an icy cold hand.
Sensation as if the head became elongated.

Eyes.

5. Stitches in the right eye.

Ears.

Shooting through the ear.

Face.

The face feels hot, bloated.
Tension in the cheek.

HYPERICUM PERFOLIATUM.

Mouth and Throat.
Dryness of the lips and mouth.
10. Dry, burning heat in the mouth.
Tongue, white or coated foul; yellow.
Thirst, with feeling of heat in the mouth; violent thirst.

Stomach and Abdomen.
Eructation on drinking water.
Pressure at the stomach on eating but little.
15. Sticking in the stomach; right hypochondrium.
Tympanitic distention of the abdomen; relieved by a stool.

Stool and Anus.
Constipation; violent tenesmus, with discharge of a hard little ball; with nausea.

Urinary Organs.
Nightly urging to urinate, with vertigo.
Desire to urinate, with violent tearing in the genital organs.

Sexual Organs.
20. *Women.* Menses too late.
Tension in the region of the uterus, as from a tight bandage.
Leucorrhœa.

Respiratory Organs.
Hoarseness.
Stitches in the chest, below the breasts.
25. Pressure and burning in the chest.

Back.
Aching pain and sensation of lameness in the small of the back.
Stitches in the small of the back.

Extremities.
Upper. Stitches on the top of the shoulder at every inspiration.
Tension in both arms and in the hands.
30. *Lower.* Sensation as if the left foot was strained or dislocated.
The feet feel pithy, as if pricked with needles.

Sleep.
Constant drowsiness.

Generalities.
Sensation of lameness of the left arm and right foot.
Feeling of weakness and trembling of all the limbs.

Fever.

35. Pulse hard, accelerated.
Shuddering over the whole body, with desire to urinate.
Heat, with delirium; wild, staring look; hot head; throbbing of the carotids; bright-red, bloated face; moist hair on the head; burning heat of the skin; great oppression and anguish.

Skin.

Smarting eruption, like nettle-rash, on the hands.
Mechanical injuries, wounds by nails or splinters in the feet, needles under the nails, squeezing, hammering; of the toes and fingers, especially the tips of the fingers; when the nerves have been lacerated, wounded, torn, with excruciating pains; it prevents lock-jaw from wounds in the soles of the feet, or of the fingers and palms of the hands.

Conditions.

40. Sensitiveness to cold.
Violent, excruciating pains from laceration of the nerves are readily subdued by the internal administration alone.

IGNATIA AMARA.

Mind and Disposition.

Sensitiveness of feeling; delicate conscientiousness.
Fearfulness, timidity.
Irresoluteness; anxious to do now this, now that.
The slightest contradiction irritates.
5. Intolerance of noise.
Taciturn, with continuous sad thoughts; still, serious melancholy, with moaning.
Anger, followed by quiet grief and sorrow.
Inclination to grief, without saying any thing about it; keeping it to himself.
Great tenderness.
10. Changeable disposition; jesting and laughing, changing to sadness, with shedding of tears. (Hysteria.)
Inclination to start.

Head.

Heaviness in the head.
Pressing, stinging pain, from within to without, in the forehead and root of the nose.
Headache, as if a nail were pressing from within to without, in the temples and sides of the head; relieved when lying on the painful side.
15. Pressing headache in the forehead and vertex.
Sensation as if sore; bruised in the head (morning).
The headache is aggravated in the morning, from coffee, tobacco, alcohol, noise; from reading and writing; from the sunlight; from moving the eyes; and is relieved when changing the position and when lying on the painful side.
Trembling and shaking of the head; the head is bent backward (during spasms); relieved by heat.

Eyes.

Acrid tears in the eyes during the day; agglutination during the night.
20. Pressing in the eyes, as if grains of sand were lodged under the upper lids.
Swelling of the upper eyelid, with bluish veins; the eyelid is turned upwards.
Inflammation of the upper part of the eyeball as far as it is covered by the upper lid.
Convulsions of the eyes.
Cannot bear the glare of light.
25. Flickering zigzags before the eyes.

Ears.

Itching in the ears.
Hard hearing, except for speech.
Noise before the ear, as from strong wind.

Nose.

Soreness and sensitiveness of the inner nose, with swelling of it.
30. Ulcerated nostrils.
Stoppage of one nostril. Dry coryza.

Face.

Alternate redness and paleness of the face.
Redness and heat of one cheek (and ear).
Clay-colored, sunken face, with blue margins around the eyes.
35. Perspiration only in the face.

Convulsive twitchings in the muscles of the face.
Twitching of the corners of the mouth.
Spasmodic closing of the jaws (lock-jaw).
Lips dry, cracked, bleeding.
40. Ulceration of one of the corners of the mouth.

Mouth and Throat.

Toothache from cold in the molars, as if they were crushed.
Difficult dentition, with convulsions.
Redness, inflammation and soreness of the inner mouth.
Stitches in the soft palate, extending to the ear.
45. Stitches in the throat, when not swallowing (only between the acts of deglutition).
Sensation as from a plug (lump) in the throat, when not swallowing.
When swallowing, sensation as if one swallowed over a lump, causing soreness and a cracking noise.
Inflamed, hard, swollen tonsils, with small ulcers.
Accumulation of much acid saliva in the mouth.
50. When talking and masticating, he bites his tongue easily.
Pain in the submaxillary glands, when moving the neck.
Trembling, low voice.

Stomach and Abdomen.

Sour taste in the mouth.
Food has no taste.
55. Feeling of hunger in the evening, which prevents one going to sleep.
Desire for a variety of things, but when they are offered the appetite fails.
Aversion to tobacco, warm food, meat and brandy.
Hiccough from smoking.
Taste flat, like chalk.
60. Gulping up of a bitter fluid.
Regurgitation of the ingesta.
Hiccough after eating and drinking (evening).
Nausea without vomiting.
Vomiting of food at night.
65. Sensation of emptiness in the stomach.
Sensation of weakness (sinking) in the pit of the stomach.
Spasmodic pains in the stomach.
Stitches in the region of the stomach.
Burning in the stomach, especially after brandy.
70. Heaviness and pressure in the pit of the stomach.
Fulness and swelling in the epigastrium.
Swelling and induration of the spleen.

IGNATIA AMARA.

Periodical abdominal spasms.
Drawing and pinching in the region of the navel.
75. Spasmodic pains, cutting-stinging, like labor pains.
Pulsation (throbbing) in the abdomen.
The colic pains are aggravated by brandy, coffee and sweet things.
Sensation of protrusion in the umbilical region.
Protrusions on various parts of the abdomen.
80. Rumbling in the bowels, as from hunger.
Flatulent colic (at night).
Increased accumulation of flatulence and an increased discharge of it.
The flatulence presses on the bladder.

Stool and Anus.

The stool is of too large a size, soft, but difficult to discharge.
85. Diarrhœa, with smarting in the rectum.
Unsuccessful urging to stool, felt mostly in the upper intestines.
Constipation from taking cold and riding in a carriage.
Stitches from the anus up the rectum.
Itching and creeping (as from ascarides) in the rectum.
90. Prolapsus ani, with smarting pain, from slight pressure to stool.
Constriction of the anus after stool.

Urinary Organs.

Sudden irresistible desire to urinate.
Frequent discharge of watery urine.
Pressure to urinate, from drinking coffee.
95. Burning and smarting in the urethra during micturition.
Itching in the forepart of the urethra.

Genital Organs.

Men. Violent itching of the genitals in the evening; relieved by scratching.
Lasciviousness without erections.
Contraction of the penis; it becomes quite small.
100. Erections during stool.
Perspiration on the scrotum.
Women. Menstruation too early (and too profuse).
Menstrual blood, black, of putrid odor, in clots.
Metrorrhagia.
105. During menstruation uterine spasms, with crampy pressing (relieved by pressure and in a recumbent posture).
Uterine spasms with lancinations or like labor pains.

Respiratory Organs.

Impeded breathing and suffocative attacks.
Desire to draw a long breath.
Slow breathing.
110. Oppression of the chest at night (after midnight).
Oppressed breathing, alternating with convulsions.
Arrest of breathing when running.
Spasmodic constriction of the chest.
Sensation of soreness in the larynx.
115. Constrictive sensation in the trachea and larynx.
Low voice.
Hollow spasmodic cough, caused in the evening from a sensation of vapor of sulphur or dust in the pit of the throat; in the morning, from a tickling above the pit of the stomach, with expectoration in the evening difficult, tasting and smelling like old catarrh. (Hooping-cough.)
Dry spasmodic cough.
The longer he coughs the more the irritation to cough increases.
120. Stitches in the chest, from flatulent colic.
Palpitation of the heart at night, with stitches in the heart.

Back and Neck.

Painless glandular swellings on the neck.
The back is bent forward.
Lancinating stitches in the back through the loins, extending to the legs, as from a sharp-cutting knife.
125. Pain in the os sacrum in the morning, when lying on the back.
Stitches in the small of the back, in the nape of the neck.

Extremities.

Upper. Lancinating, cutting pain in the shoulder-joint, when bending the arm forward.
Pain in the shoulder-joint, as if dislocated, on moving the arm.
Twitching, jerking in the deltoid muscle; arms; fingers.
130. Sensation of numbness of the arms, at night in bed, with the sensation as if something living were running in the arm
Warm perspiration in the palm of the hand and fingers.
Lower. Lancinating, cutting pain in the hip-joints.
When walking the knees are involuntarily drawn up.
Convulsive jerking of the lower limbs.
135. Cracking in the knee.
Heaviness of the feet.

Sensation as if bruised or stinging in the soles of the feet.
Burning in the heels at night; when they come in contact they are cold to the touch.
Coldness of the feet and legs, extending above the knee.

Sleep.

140. Spasmodic yawning, with pain in the lower jaw, as if dislocated, with running of the eyes.
Light sleep; hears every thing that happens around him.
Restless sleep, and great restlessness at night.
Dreams with fixed ideas, continuing after waking.

Generalities.

Convulsive twitchings, especially after fright or grief.
145. Convulsions alternating with oppressed breathing.
Hysterical spasms.
Trembling of the limbs.
Pressing pains, as from a hard-pointed body pressing from within to without.
Sensation as of dislocation in the joints.
150. Lancinating stitches, as from a sharp knife.

Fever.

Pulse hard, full and frequent, or very variable.
Chill and coldness, causing the pains to increase.
Chill with thirst, and relieved by external heat.
Chill, frequently only of the back part of the body.
155. External coldness with internal heat.
External heat with internal coldness.
Only external heat without thirst, with aversion to external heat.
Flushes of heat externally.
Burning heat of the face, only on one side.
160. Very little perspiration or only in the face.
Perspiration while eating.
Intermittent fever; chill with thirst, followed by heat without thirst; redness of the cheeks, or first heat (without thirst), followed by chill with thirst, or afternoon fever; shiverings with colic (and thirst), afterwards weakness and sleep, with burning heat of the body.
During the fever violent itching; nettle-rash over the whole body.

Skin.

Itching over the whole body, which disappears on scratching.
165. Itching when becoming heated in the open air.
Great sensitiveness of the skin to a draught of air.

Conditions.

The symptoms are renewed after dinner, in the evening after lying down, and in the morning as soon as awaking; they are relieved when lying on the back or on the painful side, or from a change of position.

Aggravation from tobacco, coffee and brandy.

INDIGO.

Mind and Disposition.

Melancholy, sadness.

Head.

Flushes of heat from the abdomen to the head.
Sensation as if the head were tightly bandaged around the forehead.
Tearing in the vertex.
5. Sensation as if a cluster of hair were pulled out from the vertex.

Eyes.

Violent jerking and twitching in the lids.
Pressure in the ball of the eye.
Inflammation of the Meibomian glands on the lower lids.

Nose.

Excessive continued sneezing, succeeded by violent bleeding of the nose.

Face.

10. Pricking in the right malar bone.
Pain in the submaxillary glands, extending to the teeth.

Mouth and Throat.

Vesicles on the tip of the tongue.
Numbness of the inner mouth.

Stomach and Abdomen.

Retching and vomiting of watery fluid.
15. Vomiting of glue-like mucus.
Tingling pain in the pit of the stomach.

Stool and Anus.

Emission of an excessive quantity of flatulence.
Diarrhœa; stool liquid, with flatulence; creeping over the skin and cold hands and colic.

Urinary Organs.

Renal colic.
20. Frequent desire to urinate, with burning in the fundus of the bladder; painful emissions of small quantities of turbid urine.
Increased emission of turbid urine, containing much mucus, without thirst, with violent contraction of the urethra and pain in the bladder.

Sexual Organs.

Men. Depressed sexual desire.
Itching of the urethra, glans and scrotum.
Women. Menstruation too early.
25. Stinging in the mamma, going off momentarily by rubbing.

Respiratory Organs.

Violent cough, inducing vomiting; bleeding of the nose.
Suffocative cough in the evening and after going to bed.

Back.

Stitch between the scapula.
Stitch in the small of the back, going off after an evacuation.

Generalities.

30. Excessive nervous irritation.
Subsultus tendinum.
Illusory sensations.

Fever.

Chilliness, with cold hands and violent headache, with constant desire to urinate; urine turbid.
Great heat, particularly in the face, with increased secretion of urine.

Conditions.

35. Aggravation, in the afternoon and evening, during rest and when sitting.
Amelioration of pain by rubbing, pressure, motion.

IPECACUANHA.

Mind and Disposition.

Irritability; restlessness, impatience.
Ill-humor and despising every thing.
Cannot endure the least noise.

Head.

Vertigo, when walking and when turning round.
5. Stitches, in the vertex (or forehead).
Headache, as if the skull and brain were bruised, with nausea and vomiting.
Pain in the occiput and nape of the neck.

Eyes.

Twitching of the eyelids.
Pupils dilated.
10. Obscuration of sight; red, inflamed eyes.

Ears.

Coldness and chilliness of the ears (during the febrile heat).

Nose.

Bleeding of the nose.
Loss of smell.
Coryza, with stoppage of the nose.

Face.

15. Pale face with blue margins around the eyes.
Convulsive twitches in the muscles of the face and lips.
Red skin around the mouth.
Smarting eruption and aphthæ on the margin of the lips.
Rash in the face.

Mouth and Throat.

20. Pain in a hollow tooth, when biting on it, as if it were extracted.
Smarting in the mouth and on the tongue.
The tongue is coated yellowish or white.
Spasmodic contractive sensation in the throat.
Fauces, stinging, rough, sore and dry.
25. Copious secretion of saliva.

Stomach and Abdomen.

Want of appetite; the stomach feels relaxed.
Aversion to all food.
Desire for dainties and sweet things.
Thirstlessness.
30. Bad effects from eating pork.
Sweetish, bloody taste in the mouth.
Nausea, as if proceeding from the stomach, with empty eructations and accumulation of much saliva.
Nausea and retching from drinking any thing cold and from smoking tobacco.
Vomiting of all the ingesta.
35. Vomiting of bile; green, jelly-like mucus.
Vomiting of blood; black, pitch-like substances.
Sensation of emptiness and relaxation of the stomach.
Horrid, indescribable pain and sick feeling in the stomach.
Cutting and pinching (as if grasping with the hands) around the umbilicus; aggravated by motion, ameliorated by rest.
40. Flatulent colic, with frequent diarrhœic stools.

Stool and Anus.

Diarrhœa; stools as if fermented with nausea and colic; stools green as grass.
Dysenteric stools, with tenesmus.
Feces covered with bloody mucus.
Bloody stools.
45. Stools smelling putrid.

Urinary Organs.

Scanty urine, dark-red.
Unsuccessful urging to urinate.
Hæmaturia, with cutting in the abdomen and in the urethra.
Turbid urine, with brick-dust sediment.

Sexual Organs.

50. *Women.* Menstruation too early and too profuse.
Metrorrhagia; blood bright-red, clotted, with oppressed breathing.

Respiratory Organs.

Quick, anxious breathing.
Sighing breathing.
The breath smells fetid.
55. Suffocative attacks in the room; better in the open air.
Suffocative feeling from the least motion.

Spasmodic asthma, as from constriction in the chest and throat.
Contraction of the chest, with short and panting breathing.
Dry cough, caused by a tickling, especially in the upper part of the larynx.
60. Frequent attacks of spasmodic cough, shaking, racking, hollow, quickly following coughs from tickling in the upper part of the larynx, as from vapor of sulphur; with expectoration of blood with mucus in the morning.
Suffocative cough; the child becomes quite stiff, and blue in the face.
Suffocative cough in the evening; continuous cough, with perspiration on the forehead, shocks in the head, retching and vomiting.
Hæmoptysis from the slightest exertion.
Rattling noise in the bronchial tubes when drawing breath.

Back and Neck.

65. Swelling and suppuration in the throat-pit.
Opisthotonos and emprosthotonos.
Cramp pain between the scapula during motion.

Extremities.

Upper. Coldness of one hand while the other is hot.
Lower. Convulsive twitching in the lower limbs and feet (not in the upper).
70. Cramps in the thighs, at night, with lump in the thighs.
Itching of the calves.
Ulcers on the foot with a black base.
Sensation in the femur, as if dislocated on sitting down.

Sleep.

Sleeplessness.
75. Sleeps with the eyes half open; moans and groans.
Starts frequently in his sleep.

Generalities.

Great weakness and aversion to all food; nausea, with almost all ailments.
Hemorrhages from all the orifices of the body.
Sensation as if the joints had gone to sleep.
80. Over-sensitiveness to heat and cold.
Twitching in the limbs.
Spasm, bending the body forward or backward.
The body is stretched out stiff.

Skin.

Rash (in lying-in women); suppressed rash.
85. Itching of the skin, with nausea; has to scratch till he vomits.

Fever.

Pulse very frequent, but at times scarcely perceptible.
Chill of short duration and soon changing to heat.
Internal chilliness, as if under the skin, aggravated from heat.
Chill with thirst.
90. Damp coldness of the hands and feet.
After a short chill dry heat, with parchment-like skin.
Sudden attacks of general heat, with cold hands and feet.
During the heat no thirst.
Violent perspiration, principally during the night.
95. Perspiration smelling sour (with turbid urine).
Sudden attacks of hot perspiration (in the room).
Intermittent fever; nausea and vomiting predominate: slight chills are followed by much heat, with thirst and no subsequent perspiration,—consequent upon the abuse of Quinine; slight chilliness without thirst; afterwards violent heat, with thirst, nausea and vomiting, dyspnœa, stitches in the chest, finally copious perspiration.

IRIS VERSICOLOR.

Mind and Disposition.

Low-spirited; discouraged.
Fear of an approaching illness.

Head.

Fulness in and heaviness of the head.
Head and face are cold.
5. Headache (temples and eyes), with distressing vomiting (of a sweetish mucus, occasionally with a trace of bile).
Sensation of constriction around the forehead (when trying to cough).
Stitches in the lower part (right side) of the cerebellum.

Eyes.

Redness of the conjunctiva.
Inflammation of the eyelids.

20

Mouth and Throat.

10. Toothache in the warm room.
    The tongue and gums feel as if covered by a greasy substance (in the morning on rising).
    Dry, cracked lips.
    Roughness in the throat.
    Burning in the mouth and fauces.
15. Increased flow of saliva.

Stomach and Abdomen.

Bitter, putrid taste.
Nausea and empty eructations.
Nausea and vomiting of a watery and very acid substance.
Vomiting of food, sour; bilious.
20. Pain in the stomach before breakfast and from drinking water.
    Pain in the region of the liver; worse from motion.
    Colic relieved by bending forward; relieved by discharge of flatulence.
    Cutting pain in the lower part of the abdomen.
    Fetid flatulence.

Stool and Anus.

25. Diarrhœa, with colic and rumbling in the bowels.

Urinary Organs.

Cutting and pricking in the urethra while urinating.

Genital Organs.

Coldness and itching of the genitals.

Extremities.

Acute rheumatic pain in the right shoulder; worse from motion, especially on raising the arm.
Pain in the fingers on writing.

Sleep.

30. Great sleeplessness.
    Starts up in his sleep.

Generalities.

Great debility.
Gastric symptoms predominate (with headache).

Fever.

Pulse accelerated,
35. Chilliness during the whole night.

Heat over the whole body, followed by chilliness, with cold hands and feet.
Perspiration over the whole body, but principally in the hypochondria.

Skin.

Small blood-boils, face, hands and back.

Conditions.

Most symptoms appear in the evening and at night.
40. The right side is principally affected.
Aggravation of the pains by motion.

JACARANDA CAROBA.

Head.

Dull pain between the forehead and right temple, shifting to the other side and then disappearing.
Fulness in the head.
Fulness first in the right, later in the left temple, going to the nape of the neck, where it disappears.
Pain, as if a plug were pressing on the right side of the forehead.

Ears.

5. Flapping in the ears, as of wings.
Stoppage and heat in the left ear, with burning, digging pain extending to the left nostril.

Nose.

Sneezing and fluent coryza.
Coryza, with heaviness and weariness at the vertex, forehead and eyes.

Mouth and Throat.

Food tastes flat or acid.
10. Dry mouth in the morning, in bed.
Raw pain at the left side of the tongue.
Mouth dry and clammy.
Sore throat, with constriction of the pharynx and difficult deglutition.
Constrictive sensation at the throat.

Stomach and Abdomen.

15. Nausea when eating.
Fulness at the pit of the stomach, with hurried breathing.
Pressure at the pit of the stomach.
Painful stitch between the pit of the stomach and the umbilicus.
Painful stitch in the left side of the navel.
20. Swelling of the right groin painful to the touch.
Acute pain at the hypogastrium when pressing upon it.

Stool and Anus.

Constipation.
Itching at the anus while sitting.
Acute pain, with lancination in the anus.
25. Prickings around the anus.
Excrescence at the anus.

Sexual Organs.

Men. Heat and pain of the penis.
The orifice of the urethra looks like two inflamed lips, itching on being touched.
Discharge of yellowish-white liquid from the prepuce.
30. Prickling in the prepuce.
Pain in the prepuce, as if a small bundle of fibres were seized.
Phymosis—The prepuce cannot be drawn back.
Suppuration between the glans and prepuce.
Itching and pricking at the margin of the prepuce.
35. Itching pimple at the glans, suppurating like a chancre, and leaving a red point when dry.
Acute pain in the left testicle when walking.
Heat and swelling of the scrotum.
Painful erections caused by the swelling of the prepuce.
The contact of the urine causes tearing pains, which affect the whole organism. Syphilis.

Respiratory Organs.

40. Dull pain under the sternum on raising the head and drawing breath.
Prickings under the sternum.
Sensation as if the heart beat in the pit of the stomach.
Lancing pain in the region of the heart.
Painful stitch at the heart, extending to the right side.
45. Stitch at the heart, which seems to beat slowly.

Extremities.

Upper. Rheumatic pains in the left arm in the morning.
Pain from the left elbow through the forearm.
Red spot with a yellowish pellicle on the wrist.
Lower. Ulcers on the legs.
50. Rheumatic pain in the right knee, disappearing on motion.

Sleep.
Restless sleep with frightful dreams.

Fever.
Internal chill.
Dry, pricking heat all over.

JATROPHA CURCAS.

Mind and Disposition.
Anxiety, with burning in the stomach and coldness of the body.
Quietude of mind; indifference to pain.

Head.
Giddiness, followed by unconsciousness and delirium.
Heat and heaviness of the head.
5. Head hot; stupefaction, with yawning and nausea.
Heat in the head, face and ears.
Headache, with nausea and vomiturition, beginning in the morning.
Violent pressing pain in the temples, ceasing in the open air and reappearing when entering the room.
Stiffness of the muscles on the forehead and neck.

Eyes.
10. Itching and smarting of the edges of the eyelids.
Twitching of the left upper eyelid.

Ears.
Burning in the ears, with heat in the head.
Burning hot ears, with heat in the back part of the head.

Nose.
Itching of the nose while eating.
15. Ulcers in the nose (and mouth).

Face.

Hot face and head; chilliness in the back.
Pale face with blue margin around the eyes.
Painful cracked lips.

Mouth and Throat.

Metallic-bloody taste, with much spitting of saliva (in the morning).
20. Long-continued pain and burning of the tongue.
Numbness of the tongue, with heat and dryness of the mouth.
Dryness of the mouth and tongue, without thirst (at night); the mouth feels as if scalded.
Dryness of the throat.
Burning in the mouth and throat, followed by dryness.
25. Spasmodic constriction in the throat, ascending from the stomach.
Increased accumulation of thin saliva.

Stomach and Abdomen.

Violent, irresistible thirst, when drinking cold water.
Eructations of air.
Vomiting of a large mass of dark-green bile.
30. Vomiting of large quantities of watery, albuminous substances; at the same time watery diarrhœa, with spasmodically contracting pains in the stomach, burning in the stomach, cramps in the calves and coldness of the body. (Cholera.)
Vomiting of pregnant women.
Heat and burning in the stomach.
Sensation of sinking, with nausea in the pit of the stomach.
Pain deep in the abdomen, behind the navel.
35. The abdomen is swollen and is sore to the touch.
Lancinating, stinging pain with the colic.
Tympanitis.
Rumbling in the abdomen, with colic; better when walking in the open air.
Noise in the intestines, as if a bottle were emptied, or as if a fluid were running in the intestines; not relieved by a loose stool.

Stool and Anus.

40. Watery diarrhœa; it gushes from him like a torrent.
Cholera—Stool watery and in gushes.
Stitches at the anus and in the rectum.

Urinary Organs.

Frequent desire to urinate; urine, pale-yellow, frothy.

Extremities.

Cramps in the muscles of the (upper) arms.
45. Cramps in the calves of the legs. (Cholera.)
Tingling in the toes.
Itching between the toes at night.
The heels are very sensitive when walking on them.

Fever.

Chilliness in the back, with heat in the face and head.
50. Chilliness with cold hands and blue nails.
Coldness of the whole body; chilliness and clammy perspiration.
Cold hands, with heat in the mouth and throat.
Cold, clammy perspiration.

JODIUM.

Mind and Disposition.

Excessive excitability; irritability and sensitiveness.
Restlessness, with inclination to move about, not permitting one to sit or to sleep.
Despondency, with disposition to weep.
Fixed, immovable thoughts.

Head.

5. Congestions to and pulsations in the head.
Headache, as if tape or a band were tightly drawn around the head.
Pressure on a small spot, above the root of the nose.
Throbbing in the head at every motion.
The headache is aggravated in the warm air, or when riding a long time in a carriage or walking fast.

Eyes.

10. Smarting in the eyes.
The white of the eye is of a dirty-yellow color.
Watery white-swelling of the eyelids.
Obscuration of sight.
Twitching of the eyes; the lower eyelids.
15. Double vision.

Ears.
Sensitiveness to noise.
Hardness of hearing; buzzing in the ears.

Nose.
Small scab in the right nostril.
Dry coryza, becoming fluent in the open air.

Face.
20. Complexion pale, yellow, or soon changing to brown.
Convulsive twitching of the facial muscles.
Suppurating ulcer on the (left) cheek, with swelling of the submaxillary glands.

Mouth and Throat.
The teeth are colored yellow and are covered with mucus in the morning.
Gums puffed up, red, inflamed, painful to the touch and bleed easy.
25. Ulcers in the mouth, with putrid smell from the mouth.
Aphthæ in the mouth, with ptyalism.
Thickly-coated tongue.
Dryness of the tongue.
Swelling and elongation of the uvula.
30. Inflammation of the throat, with burning pain; burning in the fauces.
Constriction of the throat, with impeded deglutition.
Increased secretion of watery saliva.

Stomach and Abdomen.
Taste salt, sourish or sweet on the tip of the tongue.
Unusual appetite; feels much better after having eaten a good deal.
35. Eats too often and too much; rapid digestion, but losing flesh all the time.
Alternate canine hunger and want of appetite.
Thirst increased, day and night.
Heartburn, after heavy food.
Sourish eructations, with burning.
40. Hiccough.
Qualmishness, nausea (with spasmodic pain in the stomach).
Violent vomiting; renewed by eating.
Vomiting of bile, with violent colic.
Gastric derangement, with constipation.
45. Spasmodic pains in the stomach renewed by eating.

Swelling and distention of the abdomen; when assuming a wrong position he is threatened with suffocation (has to lie on the back).
Pulsations in the pit of the stomach.
Swelling of the mesenteric glands.
Labor-like spasms in the abdomen.
50. Pulsations in the abdomen.
Incarceration of flatulence (left side of the abdomen).
Scirrhous swelling of the inguinal glands.

Stool and Anus.

Stools hard, knotty, dark-colored.
Constipation alternating with diarrhœa (whitish).
55. Dysenteric mucous stools without feces.
Copious papescent stools.
Itching and burning of the anus (in the evening).

Urinary Organs.

Retention of urine.
Urine yellowish-green, or acrid; dark; turbid; milky; with a variegated cuticle on its surface.

Sexual Organs.

60. *Men.* Increased sexual desire.
Swelling and induration of the testicles and of the prostate gland.
Women. Menstruation irregular, sometimes too early, at other times too late.
Menses premature, violent and copious (Metrorrhagia).
Leucorrhœa, corroding the linen; acrid; profuse.
65. Induration and swelling of the uterus and ovaries.
The mammæ dwindle away, become flabby.

Respiratory Organs.

Inflammation of the larynx and trachea.
Pain in the larynx, with discharge of hardened mucus.
Contraction and heat in the larynx.
70. Increased secretion of mucus in the trachea.
Hoarseness in the morning and insupportable tickling and tingling in the larynx.
The voice becomes deeper.
Dry morning cough, from tickling in the larynx.
Dry cough, with stitches and burning in the chest.
75. Cough with expectoration of large quantities of mucus, which is frequently bloody.
Rattling of mucus in the chest, with roughness under the sternum and oppression of the chest.

Burning-stinging tension in the integuments of the chest.
Difficulty of expanding the chest on taking an inspiration.
Sensation of weakness in the chest (and heart).
80. Violent palpitation of the heart; increased from the least exertion (from walking or going down stairs).
Sensation as if the heart were squeezed together.

Back and Neck.

Swelling of the neck.
The neck swells up when talking.
Struma; enlargement and painful induration of the goitre.
85. Sensation of constriction in the goitre.
Swelling of the glands of the neck.
Swelling of the thyroid gland.

Extremities.

Upper. Pain in the bones of the arm on which he lies at night.
Trembling of the arms and hands.
90. Subsultus tendinum in the hands.
Coldness of the hands.
The fingers go to sleep.
Lower. White swelling of the knee.
Hot, bright-red swelling of the knee, with inflammation, pricking and burning; aggravated by touch and pressure.
95. Subsultus tendinum in the feet.
Œdematous swelling of the feet.
Acrid sweat of the feet, corroding the skin.
Pain in the corns.

Sleep.

Restless sleep with vivid or anxious dreams.

Generalities.

100. Great irritability of the whole nervous system.
Great emaciation (with good appetite).
Great debility, even talking causes perspiration.
Twitching of the muscles; subsultus tendinum.
Trembling of the limbs.
105. Chronic rheumatism in the joints, with violent pains at night, without swelling.

Fever.

Pulse large, hard, quick, or accelerated, weak, thread-like
The pulse becomes much quicker as soon as one moves about

KALI BICHROMICUM.

Chill alternating with heat.
Cold feet all night.
110. Chill, with shaking even in the warm room.
Flushes of heat over the whole body; ebullitions and pulsations over the whole body.
Internal dry heat, with external coldness.
Profuse night-sweat.
Very debilitating perspiration in the morning hours, smelling sour, with much thirst.

Skin.

115. Swelling and induration of the glands (after bruises).
Pain in the bones at night.
Dirty, yellow, clammy, moist skin.
Rough, dry skin.
Itching and itching pimples on an old cicatrix.

Conditions.

120. *Aggravation* at night, in the evening; before eating; from fasting; when lying on the painful side; from pressure; from warmth; in a warm room; from wrapping the head up warm; on walking quickly.
Amelioration from cold; in a cold room; on getting cold; from uncovering the head; after eating; after rising from bed.

KALI BICHROMICUM.

Mind and Disposition.

Ill-humor; low-spirited; indifferent.
Aversion to mental (and bodily) exertion.

Head.

Sudden attacks of giddiness, when rising from a seat.
Vertigo, with nausea, inclination to vomit; retching up of sour watery fluid.
5. Headache in the forehead, often only over one eye.
In the morning, when waking, pain in the forehead and vertex; later, extending to the back part of the head.
Violent pricking, stinging pain, from the root of the nose, extending over the (left) orbital arch to external angle of the eyes, with obscuration of sight, as if scales were

before the eyes; beginning in the morning, increases at noon and disappears towards the evening.

Complete obscuration of sight (blindness) is followed by violent headache, compelling one to lie down; with great aversion to light and noise; the sight returns with the increasing headache.

Stinging headache (in one temple).

10. Periodical attacks of semi-lateral headache, on small spots that could be covered with the point of the finger.

Morning headache.

Headache from suppression of the discharge from the nose (Ozœna).

The bones of the head feel sore.

Stitches in the bones of the head, as from a sharp needle.

15. Lancinating stitches in the right side of the head, lasting but a short time.

Pressure on the vertex, as from a weight.

Eyes.

Heaviness of the upper eyelid on waking; it requires an effort to open it.

Eyelids burning, inflamed, much swollen.

Watering, itching and burning in the eyes; heat in the eyes and desire to rub them, with redness of the conjunctiva.

20. The eyes are glued in the morning; accumulation of yellow matter in the angles.

Œdematous swelling of the eyelids.

Itching and redness of the eyelids; tender to the touch; the tarsi seem rough, causing the sensation of friction, as from sand on the eyeballs when moving them; feeling of sharp sand in the eyes.

The conjunctiva is reddened and traversed by large red vessels.

The albuginea is dirty-yellow and appears puffy, with yellowish-brown points, like pin-heads.

25. Soreness in the right caruncula.

Photophobia; when opening the eyes twitching of the eyelids; lachrymation and burning of the eyes.

Small white, granular pustules on the (left) cornea, with pricking pain.

Brown spots on the conjunctiva.

Obscuration of sight; objects appear yellow.

Ears.

30. Stinging in the ears; from the external meatus into the internal ear.

Violent stitches in the (left) ear, extending into the roof of the mouth, into the corresponding side of the head and the same side of the neck, which was painful to the touch and the glands swollen.
The external meatus of the (left) ear swelled and inflamed.
Stitches in the left ear and left parotid gland, with headache.
Discharge of fetid, thick, yellow pus from both ears (after scarlet fever).
35. Itching of the lobe of the (right) ear (waking him at night).

Nose.

Nose painfully dry; the air passes with great ease through it.
Tickling, like a hair moving or curling itself in the top of the left nostril.
Sneezing (in the morning).
Coryza, fluent; worse in the evening, in the open air; obstruction in the morning and bleeding of the nose (right nostril).
40. Profuse secretion from the right nostril; a spot in the right lachrymal bone is swollen and throbbing.
Flow of acrid water from the nostril, excoriating the nostrils and burning the upper lip (right).
Pressure at the root of the nose.
The nose is stuffed up.
The sensation of a hard substance compels one to blow the nose, but there is no discharge from the dry nose.
45. When blowing the nose violent stitches in the right side of the nose, and the sensation as if two loose bones rubbed one against the other.
The exposed air feels hot in the nose.
Scab on the septum.
The septum ulcerates—Round ulcer in the septum.
Small ulcers on the edge of the (right) nostril, violent, burning when touched.
50. Discharge of large masses of thick, clean mucus from the nose; if that ceases he has violent headache; pain from the occiput to the forehead.
Watery secretion with great soreness and tenderness of the nose.
Discharge of tough green masses from the nose.
Discharge of hard, elastic plugs (clinkers) from the nose.
Sensation of fetid smell before the nose—Loss of smell.
55. Fetid smell from the nose.

Face.

Pale, yellowish complexion.

Pain in one side of the face, especially in the malar bone.
Sensitive painfulness, as if bruised, of the bones of the face.
Perspiration on the upper lip.
60. Digging pain in the rami of the lower jaw.

Mouth and Throat.

Dryness of the mouth and lips only for a short time relieved by drinking cold water.
Accumulation of saliva in the mouth; saliva bitter, viscid, frothy, tasting salt.
Tongue coated, thick brown, as with thick yellow felt, at the root; papillæ elevated.
Tongue dry, smooth, red, cracked (in dysentery).
65. Ulcers with hard edges, smarting, at the mucous surface of the lips.
Painful ulcer on the tongue.
Stinging pains in the tongue.
Sensation of a hair on the back part of the tongue and velum; not relieved by eating or drinking.
Erythema of the fauces and soft palate, bright or dark-red or of a coppery color.
70. The soft palate slightly reddened; uvula relaxed, with the sensation of a plug in the throat, which is not relieved by swallowing.
Deep-excavated sore, with a reddish areola, containing a yellow, tenacious matter at the root of the uvula; the fauces and palate presenting an erythematous blush.
The posterior wall of the pharynx dark-red, glossy, puffed, showing ramifications of pale-red vessels; on the middle, towards the left side, a small crack, from which blood exudes.
Sharp, shooting pain in the left tonsil, towards the ear; relieved by swallowing.
Burning in the pharynx, extending to the stomach.
75. In the forepart of the palate are single circumscribed spots, of the size of a barley-corn, colored red, as if little ulcers were about to form.
Ulcer on the roof of the mouth, with sloughing (Syphilis).
Ulceration of the uvula and tonsils.
The throat pains more when the tongue is put out.
Sensation as if an acid, acrid fluid were running through the posterior nares over the palate, causing cough.
80. Discharge of thick yellow matter through the posterior nares.
Taste coppery; sweetish; sour.

Stomach and Abdomen.

Loss of appetite; increased thirst.
Longing for beer or acidulated drinks.
Eructations of air.

85. Nausea, with feeling of heat over the body, with giddiness, rush of blood to the head; aggravated by moving about; in the morning at sight of food; after meals; after stool; excited by drinking and smoking; relieved by eating; better in the open air.

Nausea and vomiting of mucus.

Vomiting of undigested food, sour; of bile, bitter; of pinkish, glairy fluid; of blood; with cold perspiration on the hands; burning in the stomach; heat of the face.

After eating a full meal, which was relished. a sensation as if digestion were suspended; the food lies in the stomach like a heavy load.

Pressure and heaviness in the stomach after eating.

90. Giddiness, followed by violent vomiting of a white, mucous, acid fluid, with pressure and burning in the stomach.

Colic alternating with cutting pain at the umbilicus, during the night.

Swelling of the stomach (in the evening), with fulness and pressure; cannot bear tight clothes.

Sensitiveness of the abdomen to the least pressure.

Dull, heavy pressure or stitches in the region of the liver.

95. Stitches in the region of the spleen, aggravated by motion and pressure.

Tympanitis; the whole abdomen feels bloated; followed by eructations.

Cutting in the abdomen, as from knives, soon after eating.

Attacks of periodical spasmodic constriction of the intestines, with nausea, followed by a papescent stool and burning in the anus, with tenesmus.

Stitches through the abdomen, extending to the spinal column.

Stool and Anus.

100. Constipation, with debility, coated tongue, headache and coldness of the extremities.

Scanty, knotty evacuations, followed by burning in the anus.
Stools dry, with burning at the anus.
Constipation, with painful retraction of the anus.
Very painful evacuation of extremely hard feces.

105. Periodical constipation (every three months).
Stools slate-colored, bloody.

Papescent evacuations, with much rumbling in the intestines.
Morning diarrhœa; wakes from urgent pressure to stool; the watery contents gush out, followed by violent tenesmus; she cannot rise on that account; later, burning in the abdomen, nausea and violent straining to vomit.
Frequent bloody evacuations, with gnawing pain about the umbilicus with tenesmus; tongue smooth, red, cracked.
110. Dysenteric evacuations of brownish, frothy water, with violent painful pressing, straining and tenesmus.
Pressing and straining in the anus, with tenesmus.
Periodical dysentery every year in the early part of the summer.
Sensation of a plug in the anus (can scarcely sit down).
Soreness at the anus, making it very painful to walk.
115. Fulness in the hæmorrhoidal vessels.

Urinary Organs.

During micturition heat in the urethra.
During and long after micturition burning in the glandular portion of the urethra.
After micturition burning in the back part of the urethra, with the sensation as if one drop of urine had remained behind with unsuccessful effort to void it.
Stitches in the urethra, especially after micturition.
120. Frequent discharge of watery urine of strong smell (wakens him at night).
Continuous desire to urinate during the day.
Painful drawing from the perineum into the urethra.
Urine with white film and deposit, with mucous sediment.
Violent pain in the os coccygis; worse when rising, after he sat long, to urinate.

Sexual Organs.

125. *Men.* Stitches in the prostate gland (when walking; must stand still).
Itching in the hairy parts of the genitals; the skin becomes inflamed and small pustules of the size of a pin's head are formed.
Constrictive pains at the root of the penis (in the morning on waking).
Pricking and itching at the glans penis.
Women. Menstruation too early, with giddiness, nausea and headache.
130. Swelling of the genitals.
Soreness and rawness in the vagina.

Fluor albus, yellow, ropy; pain and weakness in the small of the back and dull pain in the upper part of the abdomen.

Respiratory Organs.

Sensation as from ulceration in the larynx.
Accumulation of mucus in the larynx, causing hawking.
135. Hoarse, rough voice.
Hoarseness (in the evening).
Tickling in larynx; every inhalation causes cough (with hoarseness).
Cough in the morning, with viscid expectoration.
Dry cough, with stitches in the chest.
140. Violent, rattling cough, lasting some minutes, with an effort to vomit and expectoration of viscid mucus, which can be drawn in strings to the feet.
Cough, with thick, heavy expectoration; bluish lumps of mucus.
Hawking up of copious, thick, bluish mucus.
Expectoration with traces of blood.
Cough, with pain in the sternum, darting to between the shoulders.
145. Sensation of dryness in the bronchi (in the morning).
Dry cough after dinner.
Cough, with pain in the loins, vertigo, dyspnœa, shootings in the chest.
Stitches below the sternum, extending to the back.
Pressure and heaviness on the chest, as from a weight; wakens with this sensation at night and is relieved after rising.
150. Sensation of pressure on the heart (after eating).
Pricking pain in the region of the heart.

Back and Neck.

Stiffness of the neck when bending the head forward.
Sharp, stinging pain in the region of the kidneys.
Pain, as from a knife, through the loins; cannot walk.
155. Pain in the sacrum; cannot straighten himself.
Pain in the os coccygis (in the morning); worse from walking and touching it.

Extremities.

Upper. Rheumatic pain in both shoulders (worse at night).
Stitches at the lower angle of the left shoulder-blade.
Stiffness of the shoulder-joint.

160. Sensation of lameness of the right arm (as if it had gone to sleep).
Burning pain in the middle of the forearm, extending to the wrist.
Painful stiffness of the right arm.
Stinging pain in the left elbow.
Rheumatic pains in the joints, especially the wrists.
165. Great weakness in the hands.
Spasmodic contraction of the hands.
Rheumatic pains in the fingers.
Cracking of all the joints from the least motion.
Lower. Rheumatic pains in the hip-joints and knees on moving, and more especially during the day.
170. Pain in the course of the left sciatic nerve, extending from behind the great trochanter to the calf of the leg.
Pain in the tendons of the muscles of the calf, as if stretched, causing lameness.
Soreness in the heels when walking.
Heaviness of the legs.
Pain in the right hip, extending to the knee.
175. Pain in the middle of the tibia.
Sensation of dislocation in the left ankle.

Generalities.

Pains which wander quickly from one part of the body to another.
Periodical wandering pains in all the limbs.
Sensitive painfulness of the whole body in the morning on rising.
180. The gastric symptoms supersede the rheumatic symptoms.
Great debility, with desire to lie down.

Sleep.

Unrefreshing sleep; feels very debilitated, especially in the extremities.
Wakens in a start, with nausea or headache (2 A. M.), with heat and perspiration, accelerated pulse, palpitation of the heart and dyspnœa; with anxiety, heat in the pit of the stomach and spitting of blood; from frequent desire to urinate.

Fever.

Pulse accelerated; irregular, small, contracted.
185. Great inclination to yawn and stretch.
Chilliness in the back and sleepiness; seeks a warm place.
Chilliness alternating with flushes of heat.

Chilliness, with giddiness and nausea, followed by heat with the sensation of coldness and trembling, and periodical stinging pain in the temples; without thirst.

Attacks of chilliness, extending from the feet upwards, and sensation as if the skull on the vertex became contracted, in frequently returning paroxysms.

190. Chill, followed in an hour by heat, with dryness of the mouth and lips, which have to be moistened all the time; followed in the morning with great thirst but no perspiration.

Chilliness, especially on the extremities, and flushes of heat alternating with general perspiration.

Heat of the hands and feet; nausea; pain in the upper part of the abdomen; dryness of the mouth; sleeplessness, followed by perspiration of the hands, feet and thighs; ceasing for two hours, when they reappear.

Giddiness; violent, painful vomiting is followed by pain in the forehead, burning of the eyes, great burning heat of the upper part of the body and face, with internal chilliness and violent thirst.

Perspiration on the back during effort to stool.

Skin.

195. Hot, dry and red skin all over the body.

Dry eruption, like measles, over the whole body.

Small pustules over the whole body, similar to small-pox; they disappear without bursting open.

Pustules over the whole body, appearing on inflamed parts of the skin, as large as a pea, with a small black scab in the middle.

Blood-boil on the right thigh; on the right side of the spine, near the last rib; painful on the least motion.

200. Small pustules on the roots of the nails, spreading over the hands to the wrist; the arm became red and the axillary glands suppurated; the small pustules on the hands secreted a watery fluid when they were broken; if they were not touched the fluid became thickened to a yellow, tough mass.

The eruption begins in hot weather.

Suppurating tetter (Ecthyma).

The pustulous eruption resembling small-pox, with a hair in the middle, is more prominent on the face and on the arms.

Brown spots (on the throat) like freckles.

205. Blister, full of serum, in the sole of the (right) foot.

Scabs (fingers and corona glandis).
Ulcers, dry, form oval; have overhanging edges, a bright-red, inflamed areola, hard base; movable on the subjacent tissues; dark spot in the centre; after healing the cicatrix remains depressed.
After an abrasion, a swelling like a knot, forming an irregular ulcer, covered with a dry scab and painful to the touch; under the skin is felt a hard, movable knot, like a corn, with a small ulcerated spot in the middle, where it touches the cuticle; the hard, knotty feel remains after the healed ulcer is covered with white skin.
The ulcers corrode and become deeper, without spreading in the circumference.

210. Ulcers on the previously inflamed feet.
Ulcers on the fingers, with carious affection of the bones.
The hands become covered with deep-stinging cicatrices.

Conditions.

Periodically appearing complaints (dysentery every year in the beginning of the summer; headache in the morning); at the same hour daily.
The symptoms alternate (Rheumatism and gastric affections).

215. The pains will fly rapidly from one place to another, not continuing long at any place, and intermit.
Aggravation in the morning (headache; nausea); from cold (the open, moderately cold air affects him painfully); after eating; during the summer.
Amelioration from heat.
Fat and light-haired persons are more affected by it.
The best antidote for too large doses or too intense symptoms is its relative Pulsatilla, which can also be given before or after it to advantage. An interesting group for study are Kali bichr., Pulsat. and Thuya.

KALI CARBONICUM.

Mind and Disposition.

Angry and irritable.
Anxiety with fear.
Becomes easily startled; great tendency to start when touched.

KALI CARBONICUM.

Vexed and irritated mood; trifles vex one; noise is disagreeable.
5. Dread of labor.

Head.

Sudden attack of unconsciousness.
Giddiness, as if proceeding from the stomach.
Dulness of the head; confused, stupid feeling, as after intoxication.
Vertigo when rapidly turning the head or body.
10. Vertigo, mostly in the evening and morning.
Congestions of blood to the head, with throbbing and humming in it.
One-sided headache, with nausea.
Stitches in the temples and forehead; worse from stooping and moving the head, eyes and the lower jaw; ameliorated when raising the head and from heat.
Pressing pain in the back part of the head.
15. Headache from riding in a carriage; from coughing and sneezing.
Pressure over the eyes, with violent pain in the whole forehead.
Liability of the head to take cold, especially when exposed to a draught after being heated (from it headache or toothache).
Painful tumors on the scalp, like beginning blood-boils; more painful from pressure and motion, and less so from external heat; accompanied by itching, as if in the bones of the head, with great dryness of the hair.
Falling off of the hair, especially on the temples, of the eyebrows and the beard, with great dryness of the hair, with violent burning-itching of the scalp in the morning and evening; the scalp oozes if scratched.

Eyes.

20. Stitches in the eyes.
Pimples in the eyebrows.
The white of the eye is red; the capillaries are injected.
Swelling of the eyelids and agglutination of the eyes early in the morning.
The corners of the eyes ulcerate.
25. Sensation of coldness of the eyelids.
Swelling (like a bag) between the upper eyelids and eyebrows.
Inclination to stare.

While reading or looking in the bright light moving spots, gauze and points before the eyes.
Bright sparks, blue or green spots before the eyes.
30. Painful sensitiveness of the eyes to the light of day.

Ears.

Stitches out of the ears (from within to without).
Inflammation and suppuration of the ear.
Itching and tickling in the ears.
Redness, heat and violent itching of the external ear.
35. Cracking in the ears.
Discharge of a yellow, liquid cerumen or pus from the ear.
Inflammation and hard swelling of the parotid gland.
Dulness of hearing.
Singing, whizzing and roaring in the ears.

Nose.

40. Redness and swelling of the nose, with internal soreness.
Burning in the nose.
Sore, scurfy nostrils.
Ulcerated nostrils.
Bloody, red nostrils (every morning).
45. Dull smell.
Obstruction of the nose.
Fluent coryza, with excessive sneezing; pain in the back and headache.

Face.

Face bloated.
Yellow color of the face.
50. Swelling and redness of the cheeks.
Swelled, ulcerated lips.
Swelling and rhagades of the upper lip; it bleeds readily.
Chapped lips, peeling off.
Freckles.

Mouth and Throat.

55. Toothache, only when eating (throbbing in all the teeth); the teeth are painful when touched by either cold or warm substances.
Stitches in the teeth, with swelling of the cheeks (with stinging pain).
Looseness of all the teeth.
Bad smell from the teeth.
Tearing, lancinating toothache, with pain in the facial bones.
60. Sensation of dryness in the mouth, with increased secretion of saliva.

Painful vesicles all over the inner mouth, with burning pain.
Burning of the tip of the tongue, as if raw or full of vesicles.
Swelling of the tongue, covered with small painful vesicles.
Painful pimple on the tip of the tongue.
65. Bitter taste in the mouth.
Soreness of the frænum linguæ.
Stinging pain in the throat when swallowing.
Difficult deglutition; the food descends very slowly in the œsophagus, and small particles of food easily get into the windpipe.
Tenacious mucus in the posterior part of the pharynx (early in the morning); difficult to hawk up or to swallow, with the sensation as if a lump of mucus were in the throat.—Hawking of mucus.
70. Dryness in the posterior part of the throat.

Stomach and Abdomen.

Great desire for acids or sugar.
Aversion to rye bread.
Milk and warm food disagree.
Sleepiness during a meal.
75. Distention of the abdomen after a meal.
Sour eructations (after a meal).
Nausea from mental emotions.
Nausea, as if he would faint; also with anxiety.
Retching for several evenings.
80. Sour vomiting, or of food.
Tension across the abdomen.
Colic renewed after each meal.
Stitches in the pit of the stomach and hypochondria, preventing breathing.
Hard, distended abdomen, with painfulness of the umbilical region to the touch.
85. Cutting and drawing in the abdomen, resembling false labor-pains.
Inactivity and coldness in the abdomen.
Stitches in the right side of the abdomen (liver).
Heaviness in the abdomen.
Labor-like colic, with pain in the back.
90. Ascites.
Stitches and painful bloatedness in the groins.
Excessive emission of flatulence.
Incarceration of flatulence, with colic.

Stool and Anus.

Constipation, with difficulty of emission of too large-sized feces.
95. Retarded stool from inactivity of the rectum.
Stool resembling sheep's dung.
White mucus before and during stool.
Painless diarrhœa, with rumbling in the abdomen.
Diarrhœa, with smarting pain at the anus.
100. Discharge of blood with the stool.
Continual burning at the anus after stool.
Itching and tingling of the anus
Ulcerated pimples at the anus.
Protrusion and distention of the varices during stool, with pricking and burning.
105. Protrusion of the varices during micturition, emitting first blood, afterwards white mucus.
Inflammation, soreness, stitches, and tingling, as from ascarides in the varices.

Urinary Organs.

Frequent micturition, with discharge of small quantities of fiery urine.
Burning in the urethra during and after micturition.
The urine is discharged slowly.
110. After micturition discharge of prostatic fluid.

Sexual Organs.

Men. Sexual desire excessive or deficient.
Swelling of the testes and the spermatic cord.
Copious painful pollutions, with subsequent painful erections.
Pollutions with voluptuous dreams.
115. *Women.* Difficult first menstruation.
Menstruation suppressed; too early or too scanty
Suppression of menses, with anasarca and ascites.
The menstrual blood is acrid; makes the thighs sore and covers them with an eruption.
During the menses (morning) headache; cutting pain in the abdomen; pain in the small of the back, like a weight; stitches in the ears; coryza; itching of the whole body.
120. During pregnancy discharge of blood (clots of coagulated blood).
Labor-pains (false); violent pains in the small of the back, extending to the uterus.

KALI CARBONICUM.

Yellowish leucorrhœa (burning), with pain in the small of the back; labor-like pain; and itching and burning in the pudendum.
Tearing stitches in the milk-breasts.

Respiratory Organs.

Difficult wheezing breathing.
125. Spasmodic asthma (in the morning); relieved by sitting up and bending forward, resting the head on the knees.
Roughness of the throat.
Complete hoarseness (aphonia), with violent sneezing.
Spasmodic cough, in short but frequently returning attacks, caused by a tickling in the throat and larynx; during the morning and day the cough is loose, but the yellow pus and tough mucus has to be swallowed again.
Night cough; worse from 3 to 4 A. M.
130. Cough with sourish expectoration, or of blood-streaked mucus, or of pus.
Spasmodic cough, with retching and vomiting.
During cough, rough pain in the larynx; stinging in the throat; stitches in the right side of the chest (lower part); sparks dart from the eyes; wheezing in the chest; asthma.
The cough is worst after midnight (3 to 4 A. M.); from motion; when sitting erect; from cold; after eating (warm food, milk, bread); fasting (better after breakfast); while lying on the side.
Hooping-cough (with inflammation of the lungs; with swelling between the upper eyelid and the eyebrows), and worse from 3 to 4 A. M.
135. Arrest of breathing awakes him at night.
Pain in the chest, especially when talking.
Stitches in the sternum and right side of the chest through to the back, when taking an inspiration.
Tearing in the sides of the chest.
Inflammation of the lungs (and liver), with stitches in the chest (right side).
140. Suppuration of the lungs; abscesses of the lungs.
Weakness and faintness in the chest from walking fast.
Palpitation of the heart in the morning (when hungry).
Frequent intermissions of the beats of the heart.
Burning in the region of the heart.
145. Crampy pain in the region of the heart.
Hydrothorax.

Back.

Stiffness between the shoulder-blades.
Pain in the small of the back, with labor-like pains in the abdomen.
Pain in the small of the back after a fall.
150. Stiffness of the back; unable to stoop.
Stitches in the region of both kidneys.
Gnawing pain in the os coccygis.
Pain in the small of the back; worse after standing or walking.
Pain (during pregnancy) in the small of the back, drawing up to the middle of the back.
155. Stiffness of the nape of the neck, with elongation of the uvula (in the morning when in bed).
Congestion of blood to the neck; the neck appears larger and the neck-cloth too tight.
Hard swelling of the submaxillary gland.
Swelling of the cervical glands.
Tickling in the glandular swelling of the neck; relieved by pressing on the part with the cold hand.

Extremities.

160. *Upper.* The arms feel numb in the cold and after violent exercise.
Swelling and sore pain of the axillary glands.
Perspiration in the axilla.
Cracking in the shoulder-joint, when moving or raising the arm.
Pain, as from blows and bruises, under the right shoulder-joint, especially when moving and touching it.
165. Weakness and want of strength in the arms (in the morning).
Cold hands.
The hands tremble (in the morning) when writing.
Itching of the palms of the hands; itching vesicles in the palms of the hands.
The tips of the fingers go to sleep (early in the morning).
170. *Lower.* Nightly rheumatic pains in the legs.
Burning and stinging in the legs.
Restlessness of the legs in the evening.
The lower limbs frequently go to sleep; the feet go to sleep after a meal.
Itching of the tibia.
175. Heaviness and stiffness of the feet.
Profuse fetid sweat of the feet.

Cold feet in bed.
Swelling of the feet up to the ankles.
Swelling and redness of the soles of the feet.
180. Inflamed, red chilblains on the toes (ball of the big toe).
Stitches in the painful and sensitive corns.
Sensation as if the nail of the big toe would grow into the flesh.

Generalities.

Stinging pains, in the muscles, joints and inner parts.
Rheumatic pains with swelling; more when at rest.
185. Twitching of the muscles.
A short walk fatigues much.
Dropsical affections and paralysis of old persons.

Sleep.

Great drowsiness in the day-time and early in the evening.
Starting when asleep.
190. Gnashing of the teeth at night while asleep.
Arrest of breath rouses him from sleep at night.
At night the left leg and the right arm go to sleep.
Sleep disturbed by horrid dreams.

Fever.

Pulse very variable; frequently more rapid in the morning than in the evening; strong pulsations in the arteries.
195. Chilliness generally in the morning.
Frequent shudderings during the day.
The chilliness in the evening is relieved near the warm stove and after lying down.
Chill very frequently after the pains.
Heat in the morning hours in bed.
200. Internal heat with external chilliness.
Perspiration every night.
Morning perspiration.
Perspiration easily excited during the day by exercise and exertion.
Perspiration more on the upper part of the body and increased by warm drinks.
205. Perspiration is fetid or smells sour.
Entire want of perspiration and inability to perspire.
Intermittent fever; constant chilliness, with violent thirst from internal heat; hot hands; loathing of food.
Long yawning, with heat; pain in the chest and head; pulsations in the abdomen, 9 A. M. and 5 P. M.

Chills and heat alternate in the evening, followed by perspiration during the night.
210. Evening fever; first, chilliness with thirst (for one hour), then heat without thirst, accompanied by violent, fluent coryza; afterwards slight perspiration with sound sleep.
Chill and fever, with oppression of breathing, constriction of the chest, pain in the region of the liver; most of the thirst during the chill.
Intermittent fevers, with hooping-cough.

Skin.

Burning and stinging-itching on the skin.
Dryness of the skin; deficient perspiration.
215. Painful skin, as from subcutaneous ulceration, when pressing on it.
Yellow, scaly, violent itching spots over the abdomen and around the nipples.
Burning-itching herpes,—when scratching them they become moist.
Ulcers bleeding (at night).
Fissure in the cicatrix of an old issue.
220. Warts itching.
Ascites and anasarca.
Chilblains purple-red.
Swelling and indurations of the glands, after contusions.

Conditions.

The ailments are worse in the morning (2 and 3 A. M.) and when at rest, than during the day and while exercising.
225. He feels better in the open air than in the room, but the fever is worse in the open air.
After taking a walk, faint-like weakness and trembling.
Great liability to catch cold after being heated and aversion to the open and cold air and draughts.
Aggravation from cold air; from becoming cold; when lying on the side.
Amelioration from eructations, on getting warm; in the warm air.

KALI CHLORICUM.

Head.

Vertigo, with congestion of blood to the head, after violent exercise.
Easily intoxicated from small quantities of beer or wine.
Vertigo, with headache.
Tightness in the sinciput, with sneezing and coryza.
5. Headache extending into both jaws.

Eyes.

Luminous appearance before the eyes when coughing or sneezing.
Redness in the eyes (in the evening).

Nose.

Bleeding of the nose (at night) (only from the right nostril).
Violent coryza, with much sneezing and profuse secretion of mucus.
10. Tension and tensive drawing in the cheeks, inducing a desire to sneeze, with cramp in the malar muscles.
Cramp-like drawing in the cheeks, extending to the articulation of the jaw, with stinging in the jaw and teeth.
Twitching of the muscles of the lower jaw.
Swelling of the lips.
Pimples on the lips.

Mouth and Throat.

15. Dulness of the teeth.
The gums bleed readily when cleaning them.
Coldness on the tongue and in the pharynx.
Stinging-burning on the tongue.
Tongue coated white or white only in the middle.
20. Dryness of the fauces. Cynanche tonsillaris.
Stinging-burning; sour taste in the mouth.
Violent hunger between the regular meals.

Stomach and Abdomen.

Empty or sourish eructations.
Pressure in the pit of the stomach, with chilliness and listlessness.
25. Colic, with diarrhœa and shifting of flatulence.

Congestions (and obstructions) to the portal system and liver, with hæmorrhoidal complaints.

Stool and Anus.

Hard, dry stool,—the latter part is mixed with mucus.
Painful diarrhœa, passing at last nothing but mucus.
Continuous pain in the rectum.

Urinary Organs.

30. Turbid urine.
Itching in the urethra.

Respiratory Organs.

Dryness of the throat and chest, with violent cough, as from the vapor of sulphur.
Violent cough, with coryza.
Oppression of the chest, with violent palpitation of the heart.
35. Constriction in the chest, as from the vapor of sulphur.
Palpitation of the heart, with sensation of coldness in the region of the heart.

Extremities.

Upper. Coldness of the arms.
Lower. Cold feet, with palpitation of the heart.

Generalities.

Convulsions followed by delirium.
40. Rheumatic pains.
Twitchings, especially about the head.
Pulse accelerated, or soft and sluggish, not synchronous with the beats of the heart.

Fever.

Chilliness in the open air.
Chilliness over the back and neck, with warm feet.
50. Chill in the afternoon.
Intolerable heat in the head.

Skin.

Violent itching of the whole body.
Numerous small red papulæ.

KALI HYDRIODICUM

Mind and Disposition.
Great talkativeness and inclination to jest.
Every little noise makes one start.

Head
Heat in the head, with redness and burning of the face.
Headache and heaviness in the head (5 A. M.); better after rising.
5. Feeling of heaviness in the forehead (in the afternoon).
Lancinations and dartings over the left eye and in the left temple.
The scalp feels as if ulcerated when scratching it.

Eyes.
Burning in the eyes; they secrete a purulent mucus; the eyes and lids are red with lachrymation.
Painful twitching of the lower eyelids.
10. Œdematous swelling of the eyelids, with lachrymation.
Dimness of the eyes.

Ears.
Boring pain in the ears.
Darting in the ears (right).

Nose.
Violent bleeding of the nose.
15. Redness and swelling of the nose, with constant discharge of watery, acrid, colorless liquid.
Inflammation of the mucous membrane of the nose and the eyelids.
From the least cold repeated attacks of violent, acrid coryza, with bloated eyelids, stinging pain in the ears, redness of the face, white-coated tongue, nasal voice, violent thirst, alternate heat and chilliness, dark, hot urine, headache, and great soreness and tenderness of the nose (in persons who have previously taken much mercury).

Face.
Swelling of the face and tongue.
Painful stinging and darting in the left cheek.

Mouth and Throat.

20. Ulcerative pain and swelling of the gums.
    Swelling of the gums around a decayed tooth.
    Gum-boils.
    Sensation as if the teeth were elongated.
    Dry, chapped lips.
25. The lips are covered with viscid mucus in the morning.
    Burning of the tip of the tongue.
    Burning vesicles on the tip of the tongue.
    Ulceration of the tongue and mouth, without ptyalism.
    Ulceration of the mucous membrane of the mouth.
30. Ptyalism; the saliva is viscid and saltish (during pregnancy).
    Bloody saliva, with sweetish taste in the mouth.
    Dryness and bitterness in the pharynx and mouth.
    Increased secretion of mucus in the throat.
    Goitre (sensitive to contact).
35. Swelling and suppuration of the submaxillary glands.

Stomach and Abdomen.

The food has no taste; tastes like straw.
Continual excessive thirst, day and night.
Great bitterness in the mouth and throat, going off after breakfast.
Rancid taste in the mouth after eating or drinking.
40. Hiccough.
    Gulping up of large quantities of air.
    Rumbling and shrill noises in the stomach.
    Inflammation of the stomach.
    Phlegmasia of the stomach (and intestinal canal).
45. Sudden painful bloating up of the whole abdomen, or only the umbilical region, followed by diarrhœa.
    Burning in the pit of the stomach.
    Cutting and burning round the umbilicus.

Stool and Anus.

Hard, very scanty stool is passed with great difficulty.
Discharges of serous mucus from the rectum.
50. Diarrhœa, with pain in the small of the back.

Urinary Organs.

Painful urging to urinate.
Increased secretion of urine, with unquenchable thirst.
Frequent and copious emission of pale and watery urine.
Urine red as blood.
55. Discharge of mucus from the urethra.

Genital Organs.

Men. Atrophy of the testicles.
Sexual desire diminished.
Women. Suppressed menstruation.
Frequent urging to urinate when the menses appear.
60. During the menses, chilliness with goose-flesh and heat in the head.
Thin, watery, acrid, corrosive leucorrhœa.
Discharge of mucus from the vagina.
Atrophy of the mammæ.

Respiratory Organs.

Nasal, catarrhal voice.
65. Hoarseness, with pain in the chest, cough, oppression of breathing, and pain in both eyes.
Short, dry cough, occasioned by roughness in the throat.
Dry, hacking cough; afterwards copious, greenish expectoration.
Stitches deep in the chest while walking.
Stitches in the left side of the (upper) chest when sitting bent.
70. Stitches in the middle of the sternum, extending to the back.
Darts in the region of the heart.

Back.

Pain in the os coccygis, as from a fall.
Stitches in the small of the back when sitting.
Pain in the small of the back, as if bruised (when sitting bent).

Extremities.

75. *Upper.* Bruised pain in the left shoulder.
Tearing in the shoulder, followed by tearing in the ear.
Lower. Gnawing in the hip-bones.
Dart in the left hip, at every step, obliging one to limp.
Tearing and pain in the left femur.
80. Tearing in the right thigh, extending below the knee, waking one at night and becoming insufferable when lying on that side, or on the back.
Tearing in the left knee, as if in the periosteum; the knee feels swollen (during the night).
Pain as if bruised in the left instep.
Ulcerative pain in the heels and toes.

Generalities.

Spasmodic contraction of the muscles.
85. Subsultus tendinum.

Irresistible desire to go into the open air.
Hemorrhage from the nose, lungs, rectum.
Paralysis.

Sleep.

Restless confused sleep.   Sleeplessness.
90. Weeping during sleep.

Fever.

Pulse accelerated—frequent.
Chilliness with drowsiness, proceeding from the lower part of the back extending upwards and through the whole body (6 to 8 P. M.)
Chilliness not easily removed by external warmth.
Chilliness with thirst (4 to 7 P. M.)
95. Chilliness all night with shaking and frequent waking.
Flushes of heat, with dulness of the head.
At times chilly with dry skin, at other times profuse perspiration.

Skin.

Profuse papulous eruption in the face, on the shoulders, and over the whole body.
Itching herpes in the face.
100. Pustulous eruption.
Small boils (like furuncles) on the neck, face, head, back, and chest.
Purpurea hemorrhagica.

Conditions.

Most symptoms appear during rest and are relieved during motion, especially when walking in the open air.
Constant irresistible desire to walk in the open air, it does not fatigue him.
105. After abuse of Mercury—pain in the bones—catarrh:—against the abuse of Kali hydriodicum in massive doses. Hepar s. c. is the best antidote.

KALMIA LATIFOLIA.

Head.

Giddiness, with headache and nausea.
Giddiness when stooping and looking downwards.
Sensation of heat in the head in the morning.
Pain in the forehead in the morning when waking, after rising and then increasing.
5. Pulsating headache as if a pulse were beating in the forehead.
Pressing pain on a small spot on the right side of the head.
The headache is worse in the evening and in the open air.

Eyes.

Everything is black before the eye when he looks downward; with nausea and eructations of wind (in the morning).
Dull weak eyes.
10. Pressure in the right eye (evening).
Pressure above the right eye.
Sensation of stiffness around the eyes and in the eyelids.
Stitches in the eyes (ears, fingers, feet).
Itching in the eyes, and when rubbing them they sting.
15. The eye symptoms are worse in the evening and in the open air.

Ears.

Stitches in the right ear (ears), behind the right ear, neck and thighs (at night).

Nose.

Coryza, with increased sense of smell.

Face.

Stitches and tearing in the lower jaw.
Fothergill's faceache.
20. Paleness of the face.
Itching in the face at night.
Roughness of the cheeks (during every summer).

Mouth and Throat.

Lips swollen, dry and stiff (morning).
Cracked lips with dry skin.
25. Tongue white, dry.
Stitches in the tongue.
Increased secretion of saliva.

The throat feels swollen.
Sensation as if a ball were rising in the throat.
30. Sensation of dryness in the throat, with difficult deglutition and thirst.
Pressure in the throat, stitches in the eyes, and nausea.

Stomach and Abdomen.

Nausea, everything becomes black before the eyes, with pressure in the throat, incarcerated flatulence, oppression of breathing, and rheumatic pains in the limbs.
Pressure in the pit of the stomach, worse when sitting in a stooping position, better when sitting erect, with the sensation as if something should be pressed off below the pit of the stomach.
Pains in the region of the liver.
35. Incarcerated flatulence, with nausea.
Sensation of weakness in the abdomen extending to the throat, relieved by eructation.

Stool and Anus.

Stool like mush, easily discharged, as if glazed, followed by pressure on the rectum.

Urinary Organs.

Frequent micturition of large quantities of yellow urine.

Sexual Organs.

Women. Menstruation insufficient and too late.

Respiratory Organs.

40. When breathing, a noise as from spasm in the glottis.
Pain in the chest as from a sprain.
Difficult and oppressed breathing; the throat feels swollen, nausea; with rheumatism.
Cough caused by scraping in the throat.
Hypertrophy of the heart; palpitation of the heart.

Neck and Back.

45. Violent pain in the upper three vertebræ, extending through the shoulders.
Pain in the back during menstruation.
Sensation of lameness in the back.
Sensation as if the spinal column would break from within.

Limbs.

Upper. Pain in the right shoulder.
50. Stitches in the lower part of the left shoulder-blade.
Rheumatic pains in the arms (right).

Cracking in the elbow-joint.
Stitches in the hands; stitches in the fingers.
The hands feel as they had been sprained.
55. Pain in the left wrist, causing the hand to feel paralyzed.
Erysipelatous eruption on the hands and extending further.
Weakness in the arms; the pulse being slow.
Lower. Tearing pain from the hip down the leg, extending to the feet.
Stitches externally on the knee: in the feet, soles of the feet, toes, left big toe.
60. Pain in knee (the left).
Sensation of weakness in the calves.
The feet feel sprained.
Rheumatic pains in the extremities.

Sleep.

Restless sleep, turns often.
65. While sleeping he stands up and walks about.
Talking during sleep.

Fever.

Pulse slow, weak.
Chilliness.
Cold limbs, the pulse is scarcely perceptible.
70. Heat with burning and pain in the back and loins.
Cold perspiration.

Skin.

Pricking sensation in the skin and moderate perspiration.
Dry skin.
Erysipelatous, inflamed eruption on the hand, similar to the eruption caused by Rhus tox., with oppressed breathing.
75. Eruption like itch.

Conditions.

Motion increases especially the great weakness and tired feeling in all the muscles.
The head and eye symptoms are worse in the evening and in the open air.
Bending forward increases the sensations in the pit of the stomach.
Stooping and looking downwards increases the giddiness.
80. The rheumatic pains are mostly in the upper arms and lower parts of the legs; and are worse when going to sleep.
Amelioration when lying down.
The rheumatism often attacks the heart, and generally goes from the upper to the lower parts.
Wine relieves the vomiting.

KINO.

Stitches in the ear (right).
Suppuration after inflammation of the ear.

KOBALTUM.

Mind and Disposition.
Great exhilaration of spirits.
Great vivacity and rapid flow of thoughts (evening).
More disposed to study.
Feeling of great uneasiness, had to move about and could not keep still (with pain in the stomach and abdomen).

Head.
5. Dizziness during stool.
Dulness in the head, with hard stools.
Fulness in the head; feels too large, worse from stooping and bending forward.
Pain in the forehead soon after rising.
Bruised pain in the head.
10. Headache as if it would burst, had to lie down, with sour stomach after supper.
As if the top of the head would come off.
When stepping, sensation as if the brain went up and down.
Headache worse in the room, going off in the open air.
Headache, with severe pain in the small of the back.
15. Great itching in the hairy scalp, in the beard and under the chin.

Eyes.
Loss of vision on writing, dimness of sight; while reading the letters look blurred.
The eyes smart in the light.
On writing, dartings in the eye.
Pain in the back part of the eyes, with headache.
20. Darting pains in the eyes on coming to the bright sunshine.
The eyes ache at night.

Profuse lachrymation in the open air with water from the nose, with pain in the eyes in the cold air.
Sensation as if something (sand) were under the upper lid, obliging him to rub it.

Ears.

Stinging through the left ear from the roof of the mouth.

Nose.

25. Putrid, sickish smell before the nose.
Thin discharge from the nose, water from the nose.
The nose feels obstructed.

Face.

A large, very painful boil on the right side of the chin.
Peeling of the lips with soreness, they bleed easily.
30. Disposition to keep the jaws tightly closed.

Mouth and Throat.

Flat mucous taste in the mouth.
Tongue coated white with cracks across the middle (morning).
Stinging pain in the roof of the mouth.
Constant secretion of water in the mouth with swallowing.
35. Throat feels dry and raw.
The throat is filled with white mucus.
Soreness of the throat when hawking.
Sensation of fulness in the throat from the stomach.

Stomach and Abdomen.

Hiccough, after eating, with soreness in the pit of the stomach.
40. Belching of wind (in the morning), (during stool).
Rising of bitter water, with pain in the stomach, afterwards dryness in the throat.
Feeling in the stomach as if it contained undigested food.
Fulness of the stomach as if it were filled with air.
Soreness in the pit of the stomach caused by hiccough.
45. Shooting pain in the region of the liver.
Sharp pain in the region of the spleen, worse on taking a deep inspiration.
Feeling of emptiness in the abdomen and umbilicus.
Colic (5 A. M.) followed by watery stool and tenesmus.
Rumbling in the bowels (before stool).
50. Fulness in the abdomen after a slight meal.

Stool and Anus.

Constant desire for stool while walking, worse when standing still, followed by diarrhœa.
Soft, thin stool with severe colic in the lower bowels, followed by tenesmus, pain in the sphincter ani and headache.
Small, hard, dry stool.
Feces like hazel-nuts, with dulness in the head.
55. Pressure in the rectum.
Constant dropping of blood from the anus (no blood with the stool).

Urinary Organs.

Increased secretion of pale urine, frequent micturition, after drinking coffee early in the morning.
Frequent discharge of small quantities of urine.
Scanty urine with a greasy pellicle and yellow, flocculent sediment and strong pungent smell.
60. Smarting in the end of the urethra during micturition.
Burning in the urethra.
(Secondary) gonorrhœa, with a greenish discharge.

Sexual Organs.

Men. Frequent nocturnal seminal emissions with lewd dreams, waking him up from sleep; with headache.
Impotence and nocturnal emissions without erections.
65. Severe pain in the right testicle; better after passing urine.
Yellow brown spots on the genitals (and.abdomen).

Respiratory Organs.

Frequent sighing.
On taking a deep inspiration, stitches in the chest, soreness in the stomach and pain in the spleen.
Cough with soreness in the throat and rawness when hawking.
70. Stitches in the anterior part of the larynx.
Short hacking cough, with frequent eructation of a quantity of bright red blood, it feels as if it came from the larynx.
Raising of much thick, tough mucus mixed with a considerable quantity of bright red blood; with the sensation of fulness and pressive pain in the larynx, accompanied by a sensation of scratching and rawness, with occasional burning pains, and a disposition to keep the jaws closed tightly: these sensations are increased by pressure, empty deglutition and cold water.
Copious expectoration of frothy white mucus.

Back.

Pain between the shoulders, in the lumbar region and small of the back.
75. Aching pain in the small of the back, worse when sitting, going off when rising, walking or lying down.
Pain in the back (spine), increasing while sitting, better on walking or lying down.
Backache with seminal emissions.

Extremities.

Upper. Stitches in the arms (wrist joints).
Aching pain in the wrist joints.
80. *Lower.* Shooting in the thighs from the liver.
Excessive weakness of the knees.
Foot-sweat, mostly between the toes, smelling sour or like sole-leather.
Flushes of heat along the legs.
Stitches in the legs.
85. Bruised pain in all the limbs.
Jerks in the limbs when falling asleep.
Trembling of the limbs, especially the legs, aching when sitting.

Sleep.

Difficulty of falling asleep.
When falling asleep jerks in the limbs.
90. Wakens from lewd dreams and pollutions.
Can do with less sleep than usual, wakefulness.
Unrefreshing sleep.

Fever.

Chilly from 11 to 12 A. M.; headache with nausea and languor from noon to 2 P. M.; followed by fever and perspiration.
Chilliness with yawning from 4 to 5 P. M.; feels dull and weak with aversion to mental exertion.
95. Flushes of heat with perspiration.
Flushes of heat along the legs.

Skin.

Itching all over when getting warm in bed.
Itching of the shoulders; outside of the knee.

Conditions.

Bending forward increases the headache.
100. Sitting increases and causes pain in the spine.
Cold water increases the pain in the larynx.

LACHESIS TRIGONOCEPHALUS.

Mind and Disposition.

Loquaciousness, with mocking jealousy, with frightful images, great tendency to mock, satire and ridiculous ideas.

Perfect happiness and cheerfulness followed by gradual fading of spirituality, want of self-control, and lasciviousness; felt as if she was somebody else and in the hands of a stronger power.

Nervous irritability.

Discouragement; distrust; easily affected to tears.

Head.

5. Giddiness (after resting.)

Pulsating, beating headache with heat in the head, especially on the vertex or on the right side or over the eyes, preceding a cold in the head with stiffness of the neck.

Pressing headache in the temples as if the brain were pressing out, in the morning after rising, from motion, from stooping; aggravated from pressure and while ascending; relieved from lying down after eating.

Cutting headache as if a part of the right side of the head were cut off, worse after rising or ascending; relieved from heat and after belching up wind.

Headache preceding coryza.

10. Headache in the sun.

Falling off of the hair, especially during pregnancy, with great aversion to the rays of the sun.

Eyes.

The eyes water with headache from a cold.

Itching and burning of the eyes.

Yellow color of the white of the eyes.

Ears.

15. Dryness with want of wax and hardness of hearing.

Nose.

Redness of the point of the nose.

Bleeding of the nose (blood dark) and blowing of blood from the nose, especially in the morning.

Discharge of blood and matter from the nose.

Coryza with discharge of thin water and red nostrils.

20. Scabs in the nose.

Face.
Paleness, yellowness or lead-like color of the face.
Heat and redness of the otherwise pale face.
Erysipelatous inflammations of the cheeks.

Mouth and Throat.
Crumbling off of the decayed teeth.
25. Difficulty of moving the tongue, with impossibility of opening the mouth wide.
Tongue dry, red, black, cracked, especially on the tip.
Swelling of the tongue.
Much slimy saliva, especially in the back part of the mouth.
Sensation of a plug in the throat, or as if a lump of mucus had collected in the throat, with continued painful desire to swallow.
30. The fluid which is swallowed escapes through the nose.
Ulcers in the throat and on the inflamed tonsils.
Empty swallowing aggravates the pain in the throat more than the swallowing of food, or fluids are swallowed with less pain then solids.
Cannot swallow the food after masticating it, because it rests on the back part of the tongue, and produces a thrilling pain there.
Tonsils swollen, mostly the left one.
35. When swallowing the pain extends to the (left) ear.
The inflammation and ulceration of the throat begin on the left side and extend later to the right side: (vide Lycopodium.)
Much hawking up of mucus, which is excessively painful.
The external throat is very sensitive to the touch.

Stomach and Abdomen.
Desire for wine; desire for oysters.
40. Great thirst.
Nausea and vomiting of food.
Vomiting of bile or mucus.
The pit of the stomach is very painful to the touch.
Heat in the abdomen.
45. Inflammation and abscess of the liver.
Great discomfort from having the clothes tight around the waist.

Stool and Anus.
Constipation, with ineffectual effort to evacuate.
Stools excessively offensive.
Diarrhœa and constipation in alternation.
50. Constriction in the rectum, or sensation of a plug in the anus.

The desire to evacuate continues after a pappy, offensive stool.
Stitch in the rectum when laughing or sneezing.
Hæmorrhoidal tumors protrude after the stool, with constriction of the sphincter.
Large hæmorrhoidal tumors (in persons addicted to spirituous drinks).

Urinary Organs.
55. Urine foaming.
Sensation as if a ball were rolling in the bladder.

Sexual Organs.
Men. Great excitement of the sexual desire.
Induration of the prepuce.
Mercurio-syphilitic ulcers.
60. *Women.* Menstruation suppressed.
Menstruation too scanty (blood black).
Menstrual colic, beginning in the left ovary.
During menstruation labor-like pain, as if everything were pressed downward, followed by a slight flow.
The uterus feels as if the os were open.
65. Redness and swelling of the external parts (with discharge of mucus).
Swelling, induration, pain and other anomalies of the left ovary.
Mammæ swollen.
Nipples swollen, erect, painful to the touch.
Sexual desire excited: Nymphomania.

Respiratory Organs and Heart.
70. Burning in the chest.
Oppressed breathing, worse when talking and after eating.
Shortness of breath and suffocative attacks are caused by touching the larynx and are aggravated on moving the arms.
Periodical attacks of asthma (cannot lie down).
Hoarseness with a sensation of rawness and dryness in the larynx.
75. Contraction of the chest wakens him after midnight, with slow heavy wheezing breathing, compelling him to sit up with his chest bent forward.
Oppressive pain in the chest as if full of wind, relieved by eructations.
Stitches in the (left side of the) chest, with difficult breathing.
Pain as from soreness in the chest.

Pneumonia (hepatization of the inflamed lungs).
80. Palpitation of the heart, with fainting and anxiety.
Palpitation of the heart and choking from the slightest exertion.
Rheumatism of the heart.
Irregularity of the beats of the heart.
Constrictive sensation in the region of the heart.
85. Cough caused by pressure on the larynx, or by any covering of the throat; by a tickling in the pit of the throat and sternum; when falling asleep; from ulcers in the throat.
Cough, with rawness of the chest, difficult expectoration and pains in the throat, head and eyes.
Frequent attacks of short cough from tickling in the pit of the stomach, dry during the night; difficult sometimes watery salty mucus, which has to be swallowed again, is raised.
The cough is worse, during the day, after sleeping, from changes in the temperature, from alcoholic drinks, from acids and sour drinks.
Cough with hoarseness.—Diphtheria.

Back and Neck.

90. Pain in the small of back, with constipation, intermittent fever, palpitation of the heart or dyspnœa.
Pain in the os coccygis, when sitting down one feels as if sitting on something sharp.
Stiffness of the neck.

Extremities.

Upper. Lameness in the left shoulder.
Pain in the right shoulder-joint with headache.
95. Perspiration in the axillæ of strong smell (like garlic).
Pains in the wrist-joints as if sprained.
The hands go to sleep.
Trembling of the hands (in drunkards).
Tingling and pricking in the left hand.
100. Swelling of the hands.
Numbness on the tips of the fingers (morning).
Stinging in the tips of the fingers.
The hands are cold, as if dead.
Lower. Uneasiness in the lower limbs.
105. Trembling of the legs.
Stinging in the knees.
Sensation as if hot air were going through the knee-joints, which were shaky.

The (left) knee feels as if sprained.
Swelling of the knees.
110. Caries of the tibia.
Coldness of the feet.
Swelling of the feet, worse after walking (during pregnancy).
Tingling in the toes.
Cracked skin between and on the toes, deep rhagades like cuts across the toes.
115. Flat ulcers on the lower extremities, with blue or purple surroundings.
Gangrenous ulcers on the legs (toes).

Generalities.

Tearing, pricking, and pulsating pains.
Contractions of the muscles.
The left side is principally affected (paralysis), (throat), (ovaries).
120. Excessively cold and excessively warm weather causes great debility.
Inclination to lie down and aversion to move.

Sleep.

Sleeplessness, especially before midnight.
When falling asleep he is awakened by a tickling cough.
Restless sleep, with many dreams and frequent waking.
125. Sleeplessness in the evening with talkativeness.

Fever.

Pulse small and weak, but accelerated; unequal or intermittent, or alternately full and small.
Chill, with chattering of the teeth.
Chill ascending the back often on alternate days.
Chill and heat alternating and changing localities.
130. Heat, especially in the evening in the hands and feet.
Burning in the palms of the hands and soles of the feet at night.
Flushes of heat with great sensitiveness of the neck at night.
Internal sensation of heat, with cold feet.
Perspiration coloring the linen yellow red; cold; bloody.
135. *Intermittent fever*, the paroxysms come on every spring, or after the suppression of the fever in the previous fall by quinine; in the afternoon; are accompanied by violent pain in the small of the back and limbs, oppression of the chest, violent headache with a red face and cold feet; during the hot stage continuous talking; face yellow or ashy.

LACHNANTHES TINCTORIA.

Typhus fever, especially when the tongue is red or black, dry or in fissures especially on the tip, or when the tongue trembles when it is put out, or if, while endeavoring to put it out, the tip remains under the lower teeth or lip and cannot be put out.

Skin.

Itching.
Erysipelas.
Color of the skin bluish red (purple) or yellow (jaundice).
140. Ulcers with great sensitiveness to the touch, uneven bottom, ichorous, offensive discharge, or burning when touched, especially around the lower extremities; around the ulcer many small pimples or small ulcers on a purple skin.
Carbuncles, with purple-colored surroundings and many smaller boils around them.
Gangrenous ulcers.
Gangrenous blisters.
Purple spots.
145. Small wounds bleed a good deal. Ulcers bleed readily.
Cicatrices bleed readily.
Pain in old cicatrices.

Conditions.

Exacerbation in the evening.
Periodically (every spring, every fortnight,) returning attacks (sore throat), (intermittent).
150. All the symptoms are worse after sleep, especially after the siesta, or from taking acids, from alcoholic drinks, from the abuse of China and Mercury. After Lachesis, Lycopodium often follows well. Lachesis follows well after Arsenicum, Belladonna and Mercury.

LACHNANTHES TINCTORIA.

Mind and Disposition.

Restlessness, tosses about (during perspiration).
Great loquacity; afterwards, stupid and irritable.
Ill-humored and sleepy.
Great hilarity (evening).
5. Delirium, with circumscribed red cheeks (1 to 2 A. M.)

Head.

Giddiness in the head, with sensation of heat in the chest and around the heart, and perspiration.
Giddiness, with icy coldness of the forehead.
Dull headache and pressing in the forehead.
Head feels heavy.
10. Sensation as if the vertex were enlarged and were driven upward.
Headache pressing the eyes outward.
The head feels enlarged, and as if split open with a wedge from the outside to within; the body is icy cold; she cannot get warm also for a long time under a feather bed; the whole face becomes yellow; she has to whine with the headache; the head burns like fire, with much thirst; during the cold sensation the skin is moist and clammy.
Painful tearing in the forehead in the open air.
Tearing in the (right) temple, extending to the cheek.
15. Pricking headache (in the evening).
Sensation as if the head were standing on end; worse in the occiput.
Tearing in the vertex.
The scalp is very painful to the touch.
On the forehead elevated red pimples.
20. Wrinkles on the forehead, with longitudinal ridges from the interior corner of the eyebrows upwards.

Eyes.

Obscuration of sight; could not see in the evening; as if a cloud were before the eyes.
Pressing in the eyes as from dust; with secretion of white mucus.
Secretion of white mucus from the eyes (from the canthi).
Twitching of the right canthus.
25. Sensation of twitching in the upper eyelids, worse when closing them.
In the morning, violent lachrymation and burning of the eyes, with sensation of dryness.
The eyes feel heavy, as if they could not be kept open.
Eyes dry.
Eyes feel cold.
30. The eyebrows and upper eyelids are drawn upwards; he has his looks fixed.

Ears.

Singing in the ear when walking in the open air.
Tearing in the ears.
Crawling and itching in the ears.
Almost complete deafness (during fever).

Nose.

35. The nose bleeds profusely; the blood is pale.

Face.

Face swollen, with redness and blueness under the eyes.
Pale, sickly countenance; face and lips light blue; eyes dull, feel thick and cold.
Circumscribed redness of the face (1 to 8 A. M.), with violent delirium and brilliant eyes.
Redness of the face; yellow face.
40. Sensation as if something were crawling over the face.

Mouth and Throat.

Pain in all the teeth when drinking coffee or eating soup (from warm things).
All the teeth feel loose and too long; worse in bed.
Saliva of tough mucus.
Swelling and tension of the lips.
45. Lips red.
Sensation as if the mouth were sore and thick.
Great dryness in the throat, especially on awaking during the night, with much coughing.
Sore throat, with short cough.
When swallowing, itching (in a small spot) in the throat, left side.

Stomach and Abdomen.

50. Much thirst.
Hiccough in bed.
Sensation of qualmishness above the navel, when walking in the open air.
In the pit of the stomach, beating as from a pulse, as if a hammer were beating on an ulcerated spot.
Fulness in the pit of the stomach.
55. Rolling of wind in the abdomen (left side), hears it but does not feel it.
Fermentation and rumbling in the abdomen, and discharge of flatulency.
Sensation of heat through the abdomen.

Stool and Anus.
Frequent unsuccessful desire to evacuate.
With the evacuation, discharge of much flatulence.
60. Continuous stitch in the rectum.

Urinary Organs.
Pressure on the bladder while urinating.

Sexual Organs.
Men. Violent burning in the left half of the scrotum, drawing towards the right side.
Tingling and itching of the scrotum.
Perspiration and itching of the scrotum and penis.
65. *Women.* Catamenia too early, blood viscid, mixed with mucus.
During the catamenia, sensation of distention of the abdomen; it feels as if it were boiling.
Menstrual blood profuse, bright red.

Respiratory Organs and Heart.
Burning in the right side of the larynx.
Hoarseness (forenoon).
70. Cough dry, as if it came from the larynx; expectoration is streaked with blood, with severe pain in the chest (Pneumonia).
Sensation of fulness in the chest; is compelled to inhale deeply.
Stitches in the (left side of the) chest.
Stitches like knives in the right side of the chest.
Cough worse in bed and after sleeping.
75. Bubbling and boiling in the chest and the region of the heart; it rises to the head and he becomes giddy; he breaks out in a perspiration.
Sensation of heat in the region of the heart.
Stitches in the heart, with anxiety.
Frequent violent pulsations of the heart,—each beat is double, one hard and full, the other soft and small.
Trembling of the heart, with great debility
80. Feels hot and oppressed in the chest, with mild perspiration all over.

Back.
Stiffness and pain in the neck extending over the whole head down to the nose, and sensation as if the nostrils were pinched together.
Sensation of spraining in the neck when turning or moving the head backward.

Stiff neck; the head is drawn to one side (after Diphtheria, scarlet fever).
Sensation as if a piece of ice were lying on the back, between the shoulders, followed by a chill, with gooseflesh all over.
85. Sensation between the shoulder blades as if wet with cold perspiration, the skin being dry and cool.
Burning in the region of the left kidney, extending towards the right side.
Burning in the spine above the sacrum.
Burning in the sacrum.
Burning on the right shoulder-blade.

Extremities.

90. *Upper.* Tearing from the shoulder, extending to the finger-joints.
The thumb and index-finger feel as if sprained.
Tearing in the elbow-joints.
Tearing in the knuckles of the middle fingers of the right hand.
Burning of the palms of the hands and soles of the feet.
95. *Lower.* Tearing in the right ischium.
Small pimples around the left gluteus muscle, which discharge a watery fluid when scratched open.
Burning stinging in, above or below the left knee-pan.
Tearing in the left knee.
Tingling in both lower limbs and feet, worse in the heat.
100. Burning in the feet (soles of the feet).
Cramps in the feet (during the night).

Sleep.

Sleepiness, with yawning, the eyes feel so heavy that she cannot keep them open.
After waking and stretching, a shock followed by chilliness and gooseflesh all over.

Fever.

Continuous chilliness.
105. Sensation as if a piece of ice were lying on the back between the shoulders, then a shock, followed by coldness over the whole body with gooseflesh; these attacks recur on moving and go off after going to bed.
Feels hot, but the chills run all over her before the heat can develop itself.
Icy coldness of the body.

Flushes of heat, alternating with chilliness.
Evening fever, worse from 6 P. M. to midnight.
110. Fever with violent delirium, circumscribed redness of the cheeks and brilliant eyes (worse from 1 to 2 A. M.)
Fever with somnolency.
Perspiration after restless sleep (A. M.)
The skin is cold, damp and clammy during the coldness.
Icy cold perspiration, principally on the forehead.

Skin.

115. Sensation in the skin as if an eruption would appear.
The red pimples on the forehead suppurate.
Itching and burning in the skin all night; worse after scratching.

Conditions.

Sensation of great weakness, as if from loss of fluids.
Most symptoms are aggravated while lying down and are relieved by walking about.
120. Aggravation of most symptoms in the afternoon, and the fever is worse from 1 to 2 A. M.

LACTUCA VIROSA.

Mind and Disposition.

Anguish and internal uneasiness.
Sadness with exaggerated fancies.

Head.

Vertigo with heaviness of the lower limbs.
Giddiness with heaviness of the head, blackness before the eyes, and sensation as if the head were too large and expanded.
5. Difficulty of thinking.
Dulness of the head (early in the morning), dull pain in the whole head.
Pain in a small spot on the vertex.
Heaviness in the occiput with pressure (P. M.)
Painful spot near the vertex, the pain increases on touching it.

Eyes.

10. Biting in the eyes.
    Dim-sightedness, sight as through mist or gauze.
    Muscæ volitantes.
    The lids are covered with mucus.

Face.

Heat of the face, with trembling of the lips, and sensation as if they were swollen.
15. Twitching in the lips.

Mouth and Throat.

Tongue coated white.
The tip of the tongue feels burnt.
Increased flow of (acrid) saliva.
Tenacious mucus in the throat (early in the morning).

Stomach and Abdomen.

20. Increased appetite and thirst.
    Bitter taste in throat, as from bile.
    Pain in the stomach, with retraction of the pit of the stomach, worse on pressing on the part.
    Tightness in the pit of the stomach, with anguish in the precordial region.
    Icy coldness in the stomach and œsophagus.
25. Stitches in the pylorus.
    The pains in the stomach are relieved by sitting, bending, or by emission of fetid flatulence.
    Swelling of the liver with pressure or with tightness when pressing on it.
    Pinching in the umbilical region, increased by crossing the legs.
    Ascites, with induration of the liver and asthma.

Stool and Anus.

30. Dry, hard, knotty, difficult stool, with burning at the anus.
    Hæmorrhoidal tumors around the anus, with tenesmus of the rectum.

Urinary Organs.

Frequent micturition and increased secretion of urine, the urine is clear as water.
Burning at the orifice of the urethra.
Dragging pressing in the region of the bladder.

Sexual Organs.

35. Swelling of the lymphatic vessels in the penis, with painful erections during the morning slumber.

Respiratory Organs.

Roughness in the throat after reading aloud.
Cough from tickling in the throat, with a feeling of tightness in the chest.
Spasmodic, dry, hollow racking cough, as if the chest would fly to pieces.
Dry suffocative cough, with sensation of coldness in the stomach.
40. Difficult breathing with stitches in the left lobe of the lungs.
Frequent desire to take a deep breath, constant desire for air, with oppression of the chest.
Sensation as if the lower part of the chest were too tight.
Great oppression of the chest at night, waking him from sleep, and obliging him to sit up with anxious suddenness, feels as if he would suffocate, and suddenly he finds himself on his feet in the room.
Heaviness on the chest with tightness of breathing.
45. Feeling of fulness in the chest, sensation as if a heavy weight were oppressing the chest, obliging one to loosen the clothing.
Cannot bear anything to press on the chest, lest the breathing should become oppressed.
Hydrothorax.
Congestion of blood to the chest, with pressing and obliging one to breathe hurriedly.
Feeling of coldness in the chest.
50. Crampy, pressure in different parts of the chest.
Stitches in the chest.

Extremities.

Upper. Painful twitching in the hands.
Trembling of the hands.
Lower. Sensation in the legs as if the circulation were suspended, particularly when sitting.
55 Cold feet.

Sleep.

Irresistible drowsiness, in the day time.
Lethargic sleep.

Generalities.

Sharp, cramp-like twitchings in the neighborhood of the joints.

Indescribable feeling of lightness of the body.
60. Bruised feeling in all the limbs.

Fever.

Pulse slow, contracted, small.
Frequent coldness over the back and head, with heat in the face.
Chilliness in a warm room, with coldness of the hands and feet.
Dry heat of the upper part of the body, with icy coldness of the feet.
65. Profuse perspiration.

Skin.

Œdematous swelling of the whole body with asthmatic complaints.

Conditions.

Wants to sit erect.
Amelioration when taking exercise in the open air.

LAMIUM ALBUM.

Mind and Disposition.

Whining mood, inclination to weep, feels as if abandoned.

Sexual Organs.

Menses too early and too scanty.
Leucorrhœa profuse, painless, white mucus.

Back.

Bruised pain in the small of the back.

Extremities.

5. Blister on the heel from slight rubbing, afterwards bursting and changing to an ulcer with smarting and biting.

Skin.

Smarting and stinging in the ulcer (worse in the evening when lying), with redness and swelling around it, and smarting early in the morning in bed.

LAUROCERASUS.

Mind and Disposition.

Dulness of the senses; inability to collect one's ideas.
Insensibility and complete loss of sensation.
Weakness of mind and loss of memory; fear and anxiety about imaginary evils.
Loss of consciousness, with loss of speech and motion.
5. Intoxication.

Head.

Stupefaction, with vertigo.
Vertigo, with disposition to sleep.
Vertigo worse in the open air.
Stupefying pain in the whole head.
10. Sensation of coldness in the forehead and vertex, as if a cold wind were blowing on it, descending through the neck to the back; worse in the room, better in the open air.
Pulsation in the head, with heat or with coldness.
Sensation of looseness of the brain, as if it were falling into the forehead, when stooping, without pain.
The brain feels contracted and painful.
Stitches in the head.
15. Itching of the hairy scalp.

Eyes.

Pupils dilated, immovable.
Eyes open and staring; distorted eyes.
Objects appear larger.
Darkness before the eyes; obscuration of sight.

Ears.

20. Hardness of hearing.
Tingling in the ears.
Itching in the ears.

Nose.

The nose feels stopped up; no air passes through the nose —coryza with sore throat.

Face.

Sunken face, with livid gray-yellow complexion.
25. Distorted face.

Bloated face.
Twitching and convulsions of the facial muscles.
Titillation in the face, as if flies and spiders were crawling over the skin.
Eruption around the mouth.
30. Foam at the mouth.
Lock-jaw.

Mouth and Throat.

Dryness in the mouth.
Contraction of the œsophagus when drinking. Impeded deglutition.
Spasmodic contraction in the throat and œsophagus.
35. Dry and rough tongue.
White and dry tongue.
The tongue feels cold, or burnt and numb.
Swelling and stiffness of the left side of the tongue.
Loss of speech.
40. The drink he takes rolls audibly through the œsophagus and intestines.

Stomach and Abdomen.

Violent thirst, with dry mouth.
Entire loss of appetite, with clean tongue.
Nausea in the stomach and vomiting of the ingesta.
Hiccough.
45. Bitter eructations.
Violent pain in the stomach, with loss of speech.
Burning in the stomach and abdomen, or coldness.
Pain in the stomach like fainting.
Contractive feeling in the region of the stomach, and cutting pain in the abdomen.
50. Pinching about the umbilicus.
Sticking pains in the liver, with pressure.
Distention of the region of the liver, with pains, as from subcutaneous ulceration.
Induration of the liver.

Stool and Anus.

Constipation, stool hard, firm.
55. Ineffectual urging to stool, with emission of wind only.
Diarrhœa, with tenesmus.
Discharge of green liquid mucus.
Involuntary stools.
No stool or urine is discharged.
60. Constriction of the rectum.

Urinary Organs.

Suppression of urine; retention of urine as from paralysis of the bladder.
Involuntary secretion of urine.
The urine deposits a thick, reddish sediment.
Itching in the forepart of the urethra.

Sexual Organs.

65. *Men.* Gangrene of the penis.
Women. Menses too early and too profuse; blood thin, liquid.
Burning and stinging in and below the mammæ.

Respiratory Organs.

Scraping in the larynx, with increased secretion of mucus and hoarseness.
Roughness in the throat and trachea, with hoarseness and desire to cough.
65. Spasmodic constriction of the trachea.
Whizzing cough, with sensation as if the mucous membranes were too dry.
Cough, with copious jelly-like expectoration, mixed with bloody points.
Bloody cough.
Panting breathing.
70. Slow, feeble, almost imperceptible breathing.
Slow, moaning and rattling breathing.
Dyspnœa, with sensation as if the lungs would not be sufficiently expanded.
Spasmodic oppression of the chest.
Pressure on the chest as from a heavy load; pressure on the sternum.
75. Paralysis of the lungs.
Irregular beating of the heart, with slow pulse.
Stitches in the region of the heart.
Pain in every external part of the thorax on moving it.
Burning in the chest on taking an inspiration.

Back.

80. Painful stiffness in the small of the back.
Painful stiffness in the left side of the neck and nape of the neck.
Pressure in the nape of the neck, particularly in the open air, compelling him to bend the head forward.

Extremities.

Upper. Pressure on the right shoulder or in the joint.
In the right shoulder, pains as from lameness and stitches.
85. Stitch in both elbows.
Pain, as if sprained, in the right wrist-joint.
Distention of the veins on the hands.
Rough scaly skin between the fingers, with burning when touched by water.
Lower. Pain, as if sprained, in the left hip-joint.
90. Sticking in the left knee.
The feet go to sleep (when crossing the legs or sitting).
Ulcerated pains in the lower part of the heels.
Stiffness of the feet after rising from the seat.

Sleep.

Irresistible sleepiness, especially after dinner and in the evening.
95. Deep, snoring sleep.
Soporous condition.

Generalities.

Stinging and tearing in the limbs.
Painless paralysis of the limbs.
Want of energy of the vital powers and want of reaction.
100. Apoplexy, with paralysis.
Tetanus.
Epileptic convulsions, with foam before the tightly closed mouth.
Painlessness with the ailments.

Fever.

Pulse very irregular, sometimes small and slow, often imperceptible, again more rapid, seldom full and hard.
105. Chilliness and coldness in the afternoon and evening, which cannot be relieved by heat. Shuddering, with gooseflesh.
Chilliness and heat in alternation.
Want of natural heat.
Heat running down the back.
Perspiration during the heat, and continuing all night.
110. Perspiration after eating.

Conditions.

Aggravation in the evening.
Amelioration at night and in the open air.

LEDUM PALUSTRE.

Mind and Disposition.

Inclines to be out of humor and angry.
Vehement, angry mood; vehemence.
Dissatisfied; hates his fellow-beings.
Desire for solitude.

Head.

5. Vertigo, as from intoxication, especially when walking in the open air.
Vertigo, the head inclines backward.
Stupefying headache.
Raging, pulsating headache.
Pressing headache with distress when the head is covered.
10. A misstep causes the sensation of concussion of the brain.
Pimples and boils on the forehead (as in drunkards). Blood-boils on the forehead. The least covering is intolerable to the head.

Eyes.

Nightly agglutination of the eyes without inflammation or pain.
Violent suppuration on the eyes with discharge of fetid pus.
Lachrymation: the tears are acrid, and make the lower lids and cheeks sore.
15. Pupils dilated.

Ears.

Roaring in the ears as from wind.
Ringing and whizzing in the ears.
Hardness of hearing (right ear) as if the ear were obstructed by cotton.

Nose.

Burning (as from hot coals) in the nose.
20: Bleeding from the nose. The blood is pale.

Face.

Alternate paleness and redness of the face.
Bloated face.
Scaly, dry herpes in the face. burning in the open air.

Red tubercles also on the forehead, stinging when touched (as in drunkards).
25. Glandular swelling under the chin.

Mouth and Throat.

Stinging on the forepart of the tongue. Offensive breath.
Sore throat with fine stinging pain, worse when not swallowing.
Sensation as from a lump in the throat, when swallowing the pain is stinging.

Stomach and Abdomen.

Bitter taste in the mouth.
30. Nausea and qualmishness when spitting.
Pressure in the stomach after eating a small quantity.
Sensation of fulness in the upper part of the abdomen.
Colic every evening.
Colic as if diarrhœa would set in, from the umbilicus to the anus (with cold feet).
35. Ascites.

Stool and Anus.

Constipation; the stool is mixed with blood.
Diarrhœa, stool mixed with mucus and blood.

Urinary Organs.

Frequent discharges of small quantities of urine.
Frequent micturition of large quantities of urine.
40. Burning in the urethra, after urinating.
The stream of urine frequently stops during its flow.
Enuresis.

Sexual Organs.

Men. Inflammatory swelling of the penis; the urethra is almost closed.
Increased sexual desire.
45. *Women.* Menstruation too early and too profuse; the blood is bright red.

Respiratory Organs.

Spasmodic, double inspiration with sobbing, as one who had cried after having become angry.
Oppressed quick breathing; oppressed painful breathing.
Spasmodic constriction of the chest when walking and ascending.
Suffocative arrest of breathing and opisthotonos previous to coughing.

50. Violent, hollow, racking, spasmodic cough caused by tickling in the larynx, and suffocative oppression of breathing, with expectoration after midnight and in the morning, of fetid purulent matter, frequently of bright red, foaming blood.
Fetid breath.
Tingling in the trachea (bronchitis).
Burning soreness in the chest; soreness under the sternum.
Stitches in the chest.
55. Suppuration of the lungs.
An eruption like varicella on the chest (and upper arms).

Back and Neck.

Painful stiffness of the back and loins when rising from a seat.
Pain in the loins after sitting.
Sticking in the shoulder when lifting the arms.

Extremities.

60. *Upper.* Sticking in the shoulder-joint on lifting the arm.
Pressing pain in the shoulder and elbow-joints, worse on motion.
Rheumatic pain in the joints of the arms.
Tremor of the hands when seizing anything, and when moving the hands.
Fine stinging in the hands.
65. Itching rash on the wrist joint.
Gouty nodosities on the hand and finger-joints.
Perspiration in the palms of the hands.
Panaritium.
Lower. Laming, rheumatic pain in the hip-joint.
70. Pressure in the region of the right hip-joint, more violent during motion.
Rheumatic pains in the hip, knee and foot-joints.
Swelling, tension and stitches in the knee.
Swelling of the feet and up to the knee.
Tremor of the knees (and hands) when sitting or walking.
75. Hot swelling of the legs, with stinging, drawing pain.
Pain of the soles of the feet when walking, as if bruised.
The ball of the big toe feels soft, thick and painful when stepping.
Fine tearing in the toes of the (left) foot; podagra.

Generalities.

Gouty, rheumatic pains in the joints, aggravated by the heat of the bed and in the evening till midnight.

80. Tense, hard swelling of the affected joints.
Emaciation of the affected parts.
Painful (gouty) nodosities on the joints.

Sleep.

During the day sleepiness, as from intoxication.
Sleeplessness at night, with restlessness and phantastic illusions as soon as one closes the eyes.
85. Sleeplessness, with restlessness and tossing about.

Fever.

Pulse full and rapid.
Chilliness, with thirst and sensation as if cold water were poured over the parts.
Coldness and want of natural heat.
Morning and forenoon predominating chilliness with thirst.
90. General coldness with heat and redness of the face.
Heat without thirst more towards evening.
Burning in the hands and feet in the evening.
Heat and perspiration in alternation.
Perspiration all night, with inclination to uncover oneself.
95. Nightsweat, of putrid or sour smell.
Perspiration from the least exertion, principally on the forehead.
Perspiration causes itching.
Intermittent fever. Chilliness without subsequent heat, accompanied by thirst, especially a desire for cold water.
Heat all over without thirst; on waking up the body is covered with perspiration, accompanied by itching of the whole body.
100. Intermittent fevers with malignant rheumatic pains.

Skin.

Purple (bluish) spots over the body like petechiæ.
Dry, violent itching herpes, burning in the open air.
Blood-boils.
Œdematous swellings, also of the skin of the whole body.
105. Hot, tensive, hard swellings, with tearing pains.
Dryness of the skin and want of perspiration.

Conditions.

Cannot bear the heat of the bed, on account of the burning and heat of the limbs.
Heat aggravates.
Motion aggravates only the pains in the joints.
110. The rheumatic pains begin in the lower limbs and ascend.
Bad effects from alcoholic drinks.

LOBELIA INFLATA.

Desponding—sobbing like a child.
Apprehension of death and difficulty of breathing.

Head.

Vertigo with nausea.
Headache with slight giddiness.
5. Outward pressing in both temples.

Face.

Heat of the face.
Perspiration of the face with the nausea.
Chilly feeling in the left cheek extending to the ear.

Mouth and Throat.

Flow of clammy saliva in the mouth (with nausea).
10. Burning in the throat: dryness of the fauces, frequent spitting.
Tough mucus on the fauces, causing frequent hawking.
Dryness and prickling in the throat, not diminished by drinking.
Sensation of a lump in the pit of the throat, impeding deglutition.
Sensation in the œsophagus as if it contracted itself from below upwards.

Stomach and Abdomen.

15. Frequent flatulent eructations with flow of water in the mouth.
Frequent gulping up of a burning, sour fluid.
Acidity in the stomach with contractive feeling in the pit of the stomach.
Incessant, violent nausea, with shivering and shaking of the upper part of the body.
Hiccough, with abundant flow of saliva in the mouth.
20. Nausea, with profuse perspiration and copious vomiting.
Heartburn and running of water from the mouth.
Vomiting, with cold perspiration of the face.
Nausea and vomiting during pregnancy, with profuse running of water from the mouth.
Feeling of weakness of the stomach or in the pit of the stomach, extending through the whole chest.

25. Burning in the stomach.
    Feeling of weight in the stomach.
    Pain in the abdomen, worse after eating.

Stool and Anus.

Soft, whitish stool.
Discharge of black blood after stool.
30. Copious hemorrhages from the hæmorrhoidal vessels.

Urinary Organs.

Urine of a deep-red color, depositing a copious, red sediment.
Sticking pain in the region of the right kidney.

Sexual Organs.

Men. Smarting of the prepuce.
Sensation of weight in the genitals.
35. *Women.* During menstruation violent pain in the sacrum.

Respiratory Organs.

Sensation of a foreign body in the throat, impeding the breathing and swallowing.
Tightness of the breast, with heat in the forehead.
Dyspnœa and asthma, with sensation as of a lump in the pit of the throat, immediately above the sternum.
Burning feeling in the chest, passing upwards.

Back.

40. Rheumatic pain between the scapulæ.

Extremities.

Upper. Rheumatic feeling in the right shoulder-joint.
Rheumatic pain in the right elbow-joint.
Lower. Inflammatory rheumatism in the right knee.

Fever.

Pulse weak and small.
45. Intermittent fever. Thirst before the chill and through the whole fever; often only before the chill, not during the chill, but again during the heat.
Drinking increases the violence of the shaking chill and the coldness.
At the end of the heat, perspiration with sleep.

LUPULUS.

Head.

Vertigo, stupefaction.

Sleep.

Sopor. Great drowsiness.

Fever.

Pulse slow.
Profuse, greasy, clammy perspiration.

LYCOPODIUM.

Mind and Disposition.

Low-spirited, taciturn, melancholy; doubts about his salvation.
Desponding, grieving mood.
Weeping, sad mood; extremely sensitive.
Dread of men; desires to be alone, or aversion to solitude.
5. Extremely indifferent.
Headstrong, vehement, angry; irritable and nervous.

Head.

Stupefying headache, with heat in the temples and of the ears; dryness of the mouth and lips; worse from 4 to 8 P. M., when rising up, and on lying down.
Pressing headache on the vertex; worse from 4 to 8 P. M.; from stooping, lying down, exertion of the mind, and followed by great weakness.
Tearing in the forehead or in the right side of the head, extending down to the neck, with tearing in the face, eyes, and teeth; worse on raising oneself up, better on lying down and in the open air.
10. Tension in the head; worse at night when lying in bed, and on getting warm while walking in the open air; better when walking slowly in the open air, from cold, and when uncovering the head.

Stitches in the temples, mostly on the right side, from within to without; worse in the evening and at night when lying in bed, from heat and exertion of the mind; better from cold and in the open air

Congestion of blood to the head, especially in the morning when raising himself in bed.

Headache after breakfast.

Tearing, boring, and sensation of scraping on the external head, during the night.

15. Eruption of crusts on the back part of the head, moist, smelling fetid, easily bleeding, and burning; after scratching, more moisture and increase of the crusts.

The hair becomes gray early.

Baldness; the hair falls out, first on the vertex, later on the temples (after diseases of the abdominal viscera; after parturition), with violent burning, scalding, itching of the scalp, especially on getting warm from exercise during the day.

Eyes.

Stitches and soreness in the eyes in the evening, when looking at the light.

Inflammation of the eyes, with lachrymation during the day and agglutination during the night.

20. Photophobia.

Obscuration of sight, as from feathers before the eyes.

Perpendicular half sight.

Itching in the canthi.

Cold feeling in the eyes.

25. Styes on the eyelids near the internal canthus.

Dim, hot eyes. The eyes are wide open, insensible to light, fixed.

Dryness of the eyes, in the evening.

Sparks before the eyes, in the dark.

Ears.

Over-sensitiveness of hearing.

30. Music and sounds affect the ear painfully.

Roaring, humming and whizzing in the ears.

Sensation as if hot blood rushed into the ears. Congestion of blood to the ears.

Humid, suppurating scurfs on and behind the ears.

Ulceration and running of pus from the ears.

35. Hardness of hearing; the ears become closed with whizzing.

Singing in the ears, as from boiling water.

Nose.

Over-sensitiveness of the smell.
Bleeding from the nose, principally in the afternoon.
Scurf in the nose.
40. Nightly closing of the nostril by pus.
Dryness of the nose.
Obstruction about the root of the nose; can only breathe through the nose.
Dryness of the posterior nares.
Coryza, with acrid discharge, making the upper lips sore.
45. Violent coryza, with swelling of the nose.
Fan-like motion of the nostrils.

Face.

Paleness of the face, with deep furrows, especially towards evening.
Earthy, yellow complexion, with deep furrows, blue circles around the eyes, and blue lips.
Flushes of heat in the face.
50. Spasmodic twitching in the muscles of the face.
Eruption around the mouth.
A large ulcer on the vermilion border of the lower lip.
Soreness of the corners of the mouth.
Swelling of the upper lip.
55. Eruptions on the face, humid and suppurating.
The lower jaw hangs down.
Freckles.
Swelling of the submaxillary glands.

Mouth and Throat.

The teeth are excessively painful on touching them.
60. Yellow color of the teeth.
Toothache, with swelling of the cheek; relieved by the heat of the bed, and from warm applications.
Fistula dentalis.
The gums bleed violently on being touched.
Gum-boils.
65. Putrid smell from the mouth, especially in the morning when awaking.
Dryness of the mouth and tongue, without thirst.
Stiffness of the tongue and indistinct speech.
Vesicles on the tip of the tongue; they feel scalded and raw.
Soreness of the tongue.

70. Ulcers on and under the tongue.
    Convulsions of the tongue.
    The tongue is painful and swollen in different places (tubercles on the tongue).
    The saliva becomes dry on the palate and lips, and is converted into tough mucus.
    The posterior part of the mouth is covered by tough mucus.
75. Dry and bitter mouth (in the morning).
    Tongue dry; becomes black and cracked.
    Inflammation of the throat, with stitches on swallowing.
    Swelling and suppuration of the tonsils.
    The ulceration of the tonsils begins on the right side.
80. The pharynx feels contracted, nothing can be swallowed.
    Hawking up of bloody mucus.

Stomach and Abdomen.

Canine hunger.
Desire for sweet things.
Aversion to coffee and smoking, and to boiled, warm food.
85. Bitter taste or acidity in the mouth after a meal.
    Food tastes sour.
    Bitterness in the mouth with nausea in the morning.
    Nausea in the pharynx and stomach.
    Nausea in the morning and when riding in a carriage.
90. Vomiting of food and bile; of coagulated blood and matter.
    Vomiting between the chill and heat in intermittent fever.
    Heartburn.
    Hiccough frequently, periodically.
    Immediately after a (light) meal the abdomen is bloated, full, distended
95. Has a great appetite, but a small quantity of food fills him up and he feels bloated.
    After each meal pressure in the stomach with bitter taste in the mouth.
    Painful swelling and sensitiveness of the pit of the stomach to tight clothing and to contact.
    Cancer of the stomach.
    Tension in the hypochondria as from a hoop.
100. Inflammation and induration of the liver.
    Pressure and tension in the liver, especially on satisfying one's appetite.
    Indurations in the abdomen.
    Accumulation of flatulence—incarcerated flatulence, the flatulence cannot pass, and causes much pain.
    Gnawing, griping sensation in the region of the stomach.

105. Continuous rumbling in the abdomen.
 Hernia (right side).
 Palpitation of the heart during digestion.
 Full, distended abdomen with cold feet.
 Spasmodic contraction in the abdomen.

Stool and Anus.

110. Constipation. Hard stools with ineffectual desire to evacuate.
 Desire for stool followed by painful constriction of the rectum or anus.
 Small stool, with the sensation as if much remained behind, followed by excessive and painful accumulations of flatulence.
 Hemorrhage from the rectum, even after a soft stool.
 Feeling of fulness in the rectum continues after a copious stool.
115. Contractive pain in the perinæum, after scanty hard stool.
 Stitches in the rectum.
 Pale, putrid smelling stools.
 Diarrhœa (during pregnancy), with earthly color of the face.
 Itching and tension at the anus (in the evening in bed).
120. Itching eruption of the anus, painful to the touch.
 Painful closing of the anus.
 Protrusion of the varices.
 Distention of the varices of the rectum.

Urinary Organs.

 Frequent desire to urinate, with discharge of large quantities of pale urine.
125. Frequent micturition during the night, with scanty and rare discharges through the day.
 Dark urine with diminished discharge.
 Red, sandy sediment in the urine; greasy pellicle on the urine.
 Involuntary micturition.
 Discharge of blood from the bladder, painless.
130. Foamy urine
 Itching in the urethra during and after micturition.
 Stitches in the bladder.
 Stitches in the neck of the bladder and in the anus at the same time.
 Renal colic.

Sexual Organs.

135. *Men.* Sexual desire increased or suppressed.
 Impotence; penis small, cold, relaxed.

LYCOPODIUM. 375

     Feeble erections.
     Itching of the internal surface of the prepuce.
     Soreness between the scrotum and thigh.
140. Dropsical swelling of the genital organs.
     A quantity of yellowish humor behind the corona glandis.
     Falls asleep during an embrace.
     Discharge of prostatic juice without an erection.
     Excessive and exhausting pollutions.
145. *Women.* Menstruation too profuse and too long protracted.
     Suppression of the menses, also from fright.
     Before the menses, bloatedness of the abdomen, chilliness, low-spirited, desponding and melancholy.
     Dryness of the vagina.
     Burning in the vagina during coition.
150. Varices on the genitals.
     Leucorrhœa corroding, like milk, bloody, worse before the full moon.
     Disposition to miscarriages.
     Stinging in the nipples.
     Soreness of the nipples, or spreading scurf on them.
155. Hard, burning nodosity in the mammæ.

Respiratory Organs.

     Shortness of breathing in children, especially during sleep.
     Every exertion causes shortness of breathing.
     Oppressed breathing, worse when walking in the open air.
     Sensation as if there were too much mucus in the chest, with whizzing breathing in the day-time.
160. Rattling in the chest.
     Dry cough, day and night.
     Cough at night which affects the stomach.
     Cough, with expectoration through the day and without expectoration during the night.
     Titillating cough caused by deep breathing.
165. Cough, with copious purulent expectoration.
     Cough with gray, salty-tasting expectoration, or expectoration of blood.
     Hooping cough from irritation in the trachea as from fumes of sulphur, in the morning and during the day, with expectoration of fetid pus or of mucus streaked with blood.
     Morning cough, with green expectoration.
     Cough aggravated from 4 to 6 P. M., frequently on alternate days, from exertion, from stretching the arms out, stooping and lying down, when lying on the (left) side,

LYCOPODIUM.

       from eating and drinking cold things, in the wind, or in the warm room.
170. Hoarseness; voice feeble and husky.
       Roughness, soreness and tension in the chest.
       Cough with painfulness of the region of the stomach.
       Oppression of the chest, with shortness of breathing.
       Continuous pressure in the chest, it feels raw internally.
175. Stitches in the left side of the chest, also during an inspiration.
       (Typhoid and neglected) pneumonia. (Hepatization of the lungs.
       Paralysis of the lungs.
       Hydrothorax.
       Yellow, liver spots on the chest.
180. Itching on the chest.
       Palpitation of the heart, worse after eating.

Back and Neck.

       Pain and stiffness in the small of the back (at night).
       Stitches in the small of the back, especially when rising from a stooping position.
       Burning as of red-hot coals between the scapulæ.
185. Painful stiffness of the (left side) of the neck.
       Stiffness and swelling of one side of the neck.
       Swelling of the cervical glands.
       Large clusters of red pimples around the neck, with violent itching.
       Soreness of the neck.

Extremities.

190. *Upper.* Rheumatic tension in the right shoulder-joint.
       Pain in the bones of the arms at night.
       The arms and fingers go to sleep easily.
       Weakness of the arms when at work.
       Pain as from a sprain in the right wrist-joint.
195. Redness, inflammation and swelling of all the joints of the fingers.
       Twitching in the arms and shoulder.
       The skin of the hands is dry.
       Burning in the palms of the hands.
       Stiffness of the fingers from arthritic nodosities.
200. Itching pimples between the fingers. Panaritium.
       Lower. Nightly pains (tearing) in the legs.
       Rheumatic tension in the left hip.
       Pain as from a sprain in the hip.
       Swelling and stiffness of the knee.

LYCOPODIUM. 377

205. White-swelling of the knee.
Swelling of the knee, with perspiration.
Pain, as from contraction (cramps) in the calves when walking.
Swelling of the feet, around the ankles.
Swelling of the soles of the feet.
210. Pain of the soles when walking.
Cold, sweaty feet.
Profuse sweat on the feet, they become sore.
Stitches in the big toe of the right foot (in the evening).
Rhagades in the heel.
215. Cramp in the toes.
Stitches in the corns, with sore feeling.
Old ulcers on the lower legs, with tearing, itching and burning at night.

Generalities.

Drawing and tearing in the limbs, especially at night and during rest, or on alternate afternoons.
Numbness of the limbs, sensation as if circulation ceased.
220. Great emaciation, great internal debility.
Twitches through the body.
Contraction of some limbs.
Stiffness of all the joints.
The whole body feels bruised.
225. Involuntary, alternate extension and contraction of the muscles in different parts of the body.
Epileptic spasms, with screaming, foam at the mouth, loss of consciousness, throws the arms and limbs about, great anguish about the heart, and imagines he would have to die.
Faintishness at certain hours of the day.

Sleep.

Sleepiness during the day, but cannot go to sleep at night; his mind is too active
Restless sleep, with anxious dreams and frequent waking.
230. Loud coughing during sleep; screaming while asleep.
Sopor.
Starting when falling asleep.
Unable to find ease in any position.
Hunger at night when waking.
235. Unrefreshing sleep.

Fever.

Pulse only accelerated in the evening and afternoon.

Sensation as if the circulation stood still.
Chilliness in the afternoon from 4 to 8, with sensation as of numbness in the hands and feet.
Chilliness in the evening in bed, preventing sleep.
240. One-sided chilliness, mostly on the left side.
Chilliness followed by perspiration without heat after the chill.
Chills and heat alternating.
Want of natural heat.
Flushes of heat over the whole body, mostly towards evening, with frequent drinking of small quantities at a time; constipation and increased micturition.
245. Heat of one (left) foot with coldness of the other (right) foot.
Violent perspiration during the day from the least exertion.
Night and morning sweats, often with coldness of the face.
Night-sweats, clammy.
The perspiration is frequently cold, smelling sour, or offensive, or smelling like onions, or bloody.
250. Intermittent fever. Nausea and vomiting and then chilliness, followed by perspiration (without previous heat).
Chilliness in the evening, when in bed till midnight, this is followed by heat, in the morning sour-smelling perspiration.
Great heat and redness of the cheeks, alternating with chilliness.
Shaking chill 7 P. M., and great coldness as if lying in ice, with traction through the whole body, upon waking up from sleep, which is full of dreams, covered with perspiration, perspiration is followed by violent thirst.
Tertian fever, with sour vomiting (worse between chill and fever); the chills are followed by bloatedness of the face and hands.
255. Typhus fever (with threatening paralysis of the brain).

Skin.

Biting, itching when becoming warm through the day.
Humid, suppurating tetters, full of deep rhagades and covered with thick crusts.
Soreness of children, the sore places are humid.
Ulcers, at night, with tearing and itching pains, burning when touched. (Mercurial ulcers); bleeding and burning when dressing the otherwise painless ulcer.
260. Blood-boils (periodically).
Inflammation of the bones, with pains at night.

Softening of the bones.
Caries.
Fistulous ulcers, with hard, red-shining, everted edges, and inflammatory swelling of the affected parts.
265. Glandular swellings.
Chilblains.
Arthritic nodosities.
Freckles.
Liver spots (abdomen).
270. Dropsical swellings.

Conditions.

Great disposition to get cold.
Great desire for the open air or entire aversion to it.
Aggravation from 4 to 8 P. M., when everything is better, with the exception of the debility.
While at rest the debility is mostly felt, but there is also great aversion to exercise.
275. *Aggravation* on lying down, while sitting, when rising from a seat and when beginning to walk (the stiffness), after eating and having satisfied one's appetite, after eating oysters, from salt food, from cold food or drink, from wet (warm) poultices, from pressure of the clothes, from strong smells, while urinating.
Amelioration, on getting cold, from uncovering oneself, after rising from a seat and when continuing to walk, from warm food and drink.
It is not advisable to begin the treatment of a chronic disease with Lycopodium, it is better to give first another not antipsoric remedy.
Lachesis and Lycopodium follow well one after another.
Lycopodium follows well after Pulsatilla or Calcarea.

MAGNESIA CARBONICA.

Mind and Disposition.

Anxious, with perspiration all day.
Uneasiness, with trembling of the hands and absence of mind.
Sad mood, with indisposition to talk.

Anxious and warm through the whole body, especially in the head, while eating warm food.
5. Trembling, anguish and fear. as if some accident would happen, all day, going off after going to bed.

Head.

Vertigo, when kneeling or standing, as if everything were turning around.
Heaviness and dizziness in the head, early in the morning, when rising, going off after a walk.
Pressure in the forehead.
Pressing headache from mental exertion and when among many persons.
10. Violent darting headache after vexation (1 to 10 P. M.)
Lancinating headache early in the morning after rising.
Pulsating sensation in the forehead.
Congestion of blood to the head, especially when smoking.
Heat in the head and hands with redness of the face, alternating with paleness of the face.
15. Bruised sensation on the vertex.
Pain on the top of the head, as if the hair were pulled.
Dandruff on the scalp, itching during wet and rainy weather.
Falling off of the hair.

Eyes.

Inflammation of the eyes, with redness, burning, stinging and obscuration of sight, or dim-sightedness.
20. Swelling of the eyeball.
Agglutination of the eyes early in the morning.
Obscuration of the cornea.
Black motes before the eyes.
Obscuration of crystalline lens (cataract).
25. Dryness of the eyes.
Profuse lachrymation.

Ears.

Inflammation of the ears, with external redness and sensation of great soreness.
Great sensitiveness of the ear to noise.
Hardness of hearing with whizzing before the ears.
30. Whizzing, fluttering and buzzing in the right ear with hardness of hearing.

Nose.

Bleeding from the nose in the morning.
Vesicular eruption in the nose with pressing pain.

Dry coryza and obstruction of the nose, waking one at night.

Face.

Pale face, earthy, sickly complexion.
35. Alternate redness and paleness of the face.
Tension on the face, as if the white of an egg had dried on it.
Nightly tearing, digging and boring in the malar bone, insupportable during rest, and driving one from one place to another. Swelling of the malar bone, with pulsating pain.
Hard nodosities, bloatedness and swelling of the face.
Herpetic eruption around the (lower part of the) mouth.
40. Hard, little nodosities in both corners of the mouth.

Mouth and Throat.

Beating and stinging in the teeth after eating.
Toothache while riding in a carriage.
Toothache at night, compelling one to rise and walk about, the pain is insupportable while at rest.
Toothache, mostly burning, tearing, drawing, twitching, or great ulcerative pain, with twitching in the fingers and feet.
45. Toothache during pregnancy.
Ailments from cutting the wisdom teeth.
Looseness of the teeth, with swelling of the gums.
The toothache is aggravated from cold.
Burning vesicles on the gums, on the inside of the cheeks, tongue, lips, and palate, they bleed from the least contact.
50. Dryness of the mouth, especially at night and in the morning.
Stinging pain in the throat when talking and swallowing.
Burning in the throat and palate, with dryness and roughness, as if scraped by the beard of a barleycorn.
Frequent rising of mucus in the throat (morning) with roughness and dryness of the fauces.
Soft, fetid tubercles of the color of peas are hawked up.

Stomach and Abdomen.

55. Bitter taste in the mouth, the tongue coated white, the mouth and teeth are full of white, tough mucus, going off after rinsing the mouth.
Sour taste in the mouth.
Violent thirst for water, especially in the evening and at night.

Desire for acid drinks.
Sour eructations.
60. Nausea and vertigo while eating, followed by retching and vomiting of bitter, salty water.
Feeling of emptiness and qualmishness in the stomach, better after dinner.
Ulcerative pain in the stomach, with great sensitiveness to pressure.
Great heaviness in the bloated abdomen.
Colic, pressing, spasmodic—contractive pain.
65. In the region of the liver, hardness and stitches.
Colic followed by discharge of leucorrhœa.
Cutting and pinching in the aodomen.

Stool and Anus.
Constipation, frequent ineffectual urging to evacuate with small stool or only discharge of flatulence.
Diarrhœa painful, stools green and frothy.
70. Sour-smelling diarrhœa of children.
Ascarides and lumbrici.
Stitches in the anus and rectum, also with fruitless desire for stool.

Urine.
Secretion of urine increased, pale, watery or green.
Involuntary secretion of urine when walking or rising from the seat.
75. White sediment in the urine.
Burning and smarting during micturition.

Sexual Organs.
Men. Sexual desire diminished, erections wanting.
Discharge of prostatic fluid while passing flatulence.
Women. Pressing towards the pelvis, as if menstruation would come on, with cutting in the abdomen.
80. Menses too late or suppressed.
Menstrual blood thick, dark, like pitch.
During the menstruation, weakness, chilliness, headache, paleness of the face, pain in the small of the back, or spasmodic pressing pain in the abdomen with suppressed menstrual discharge.
Fluor albus, of acrid white mucus, preceded by colic.

Respiratory Organs.
Oppression of the chest with the sensation of constriction.
85. Sensation of soreness in the chest or in the left side of the chest, region of the heart.

Spasmodic cough from tickling in the larynx, with expectoration only in the morning and during the day of yellow, thin or tough mucus or of dark blood tasting salt.
The cough is worse in the evening till after midnight.

Back and Neck.

Stiffness in the neck.
Pain in the back and small of the back at night, as if broken.

Extremities.

90. *Upper.* Pain as from dislocation in the shoulder-joint when moving it.
Rheumatic pain in the shoulders (at night) with tingling down to the fingers; the pain prevents the least movement of the arm.
Heat of the fingers.
Red, inflammatory swelling of the fingers.
The skin of the hands becomes chapped.
95. Spreading blisters on the hands and fingers, with stinging.
Lower. Restlessness in the legs.
Drawing pains in the legs and feet.
Itching of the buttocks, with red spots after scratching.
Painful swelling in the bend of the knee.
100. Cramp in the calves (at night).
Burning spot on the tibia.
Blood-boils on the lower leg.

Generalities.

Epileptic attacks; while standing or walking he frequently falls down suddenly with consciousness.
Painfulness of the whole body.
105. Sensation of being tired, especially in the feet and when sitting.
A short walk tires much.
Restlessness in the limbs in the evening after sitting long.
Rheumatic pains in the limbs.

Sleep.

Sleepiness during the day.
110. Sleeplessness at night from oppression in the abdomen, or from anxious restlessness and internal heat, with aversion to being uncovered in the least.
Many and anxious dreams, with starts and crying out in the sleep.
Unrefreshing sleep, more tired in the morning than he was when lying down in the evening.

Fever.

Pulse slightly accelerated only during the night.
Chill and chilliness with external coldness in the evening, and after lying down, slowly going off.
115. Chill running down the back.
Heat mostly in the forenoon, frequently with perspiration on the head only.
Heat after the evening chill.
At night, anxious internal heat, with restlessness and aversion to being uncovered.
Perspiration with thirst, from midnight till morning.
120. Morning sweat.
Perspiration is greasy, coloring the linen yellow, smelling sour or putrid.

Skin.

Itching and great dryness of the skin.
Large, stinging nodosities under the skin.
Painful, small, red herpes, they scale off afterwards.
125. Spreading blisters.
Small blood boils (lower legs.)

Conditions.

Most symptoms come on at night and while at rest.
Symptoms coming on while sitting, disappear or are better while walking.

MAGNESIA MURIATICA.

Mind and Disposition.

Anxiousness in the room, relieved in the open air.
Fearful and inclined to weep.
Disinclination to talk, prefers solitude.

Head.

Vertigo in the morning on rising, during dinner, going off in the open air.
5. Stupefaction and dulness of the head.
Compressive sensation in the head, from both sides, with a hot feeling, and with beating in the forehead when pressing upon it.

Tearing and stitches in the temples, with great sensitiveness of the vertex, as if the hair were raised by pulling.
Heaviness in the head with reeling, as if one would fall down.
Sensation of numbness in the forehead, the head feels dull; worse in the morning when awaking and when lying; better from exercise in the open air and when wrapping the head up warm.
10. Congestion of blood to the head with painful undulation and whizzing as of boiling water on the sides upon which one rests.

Eyes.

Inflammation of the eyes, with violent burning and redness of the white of the eyes.
When looking into the light, lachrymation and burning of the eyes.
Nightly agglutination of the eyes.
Yellow color of the white of the eyes.

Ears.

15. Pulsation in the ears.
Hardness of hearing and deafness, as if something were lying before the ear.
Itching of old herpes behind the ears.

Nose.

Redness and swelling of the nose.
Swelling of the wings of the nose.
20. Sore pain and burning of the nostrils.
Scurf in the nostrils painful to the touch.
Ulcerated nostrils.
Distressing dryness of the nose.
At night the nose is obstructed.
25. Coryza with loss of smell and taste, and discharge of yellow fetid mucus.
Discharge of acrid, corrosive water from the nose.

Face.

Pale, yellowish complexion.
Severe cramp pains in the bones of the face.
Eruptions on the face.
30. Pimples on the forehead, itching in the evening.
Sensation of roughness on the inner side of the upper lip when touching it with the tongue.

Large water blisters on the margin of the vermilion border of the lower lip, itching, afterwards burning.
Chapped lips.

Mouth and Throat.

Toothache, almost insupportable if the food touches the teeth.
35. Sensation as if the upper cuspidati were elongated.
Painful swelling and easy bleeding of the gums.
Dryness of the mouth and throat without thirst.
The whole inner mouth feels as if it were scalded.
The surface of the tongue feels burnt, it burns like fire.
40. Rhagades in the tongue with violent burning.
Accumulation of water in the mouth.
Tongue coated white, early in the morning.
Dryness and roughness of the throat with hoarse voice.
Hawking up, with difficulty, of thick, tough mucus (sometimes mixed with blood).

Stomach and Abdomen.

45. Hunger, but does not know for what.
Violent thirst (3 A. M.).
Increased hunger followed by nausea.
Rising of the ingesta, while walking.
Violent hiccough, during and after dinner, which causes pain in the stomach.
50. Rising as of a ball from the stomach to the throat, relieved by eructation.
Nausea (in the morning after rising).
Nausea with faintness.
Tension, sensation of great soreness as if bruised in the abdomen, with external sensitiveness to the touch.
Throbbing in the pit of the stomach.
55. Distended abdomen, with constipation.
Painful induration in the abdomen, especially on the right side.
Pressing pain in the liver, when walking and touching it, worse when lying on the right side.
Tearing in the abdomen.
Tingling stitches in the abdominal muscles.
60. Colic (in the evening) in hysteric persons, extending to the thighs, followed by fluor albus.

Stool and Anus.

Constipation, stool hard, difficult and insufficient.
Knotty stool like sheep's dung.

Much pressure to stool with scanty evacuations or passage of flatus only.
Diarrhœa, discharges of mucus and blood.
65. The feces are covered with blood and mucus.

Urinary Organs.

Frequent desire to urinate day and night, with scanty discharge.
The urine can only be emitted by bearing down with the abdominal muscles.
The urine pale-yellow, followed by burning in the urethra.
Numbness in the urethra.

Sexual Organs.

70. *Men.* Itching on the genitals and on the scrotum, extending as far as the anus.
Frequent erections; early in the morning, with burning in the penis.
After an embrace burning pain in the back.
Women. Menses too early and too profuse.
Suppressed menses.
75. Menstrual blood black, clotted.
During menstruation paleness of the face, pain in the small of the back, debility.
Uterine spasms, extending into the thighs and followed by fluor albus.
Leucorrhœa, especially after exercise or preceded by uterine spasms.
Scirrhous indurations on the uterus.
80. Leucorrhœa immediately after stool.

Respiratory Organs.

Hoarseness, with roughness and dryness in the throat.
Hoarseness in the morning after rising.
Tingling in the larynx.
Dry cough evening and night, with burning and soreness in the chest.
85. Spasmodic cough at night, with tingling in the larynx.
Bloody expectoration brought on by sea-bathing.
Oppression in the pit of the stomach.
Sudden heaviness on the chest with oppression of breathing (while dining).
Tension and constriction of the chest.
90. Stitches in the heart, arresting the breath.
Palpitation of the heart while sitting, going off on motion.
Congestion of blood to the chest from bathing in the sea.

Back and Neck.

Pain as from bruises above and in the small of the back and both hips, with sensitiveness of the parts to the touch.
Contractive, spasmodic pain in the small of the back.
95. Stitches, tearing and burning in the small of the back.
Swelling of the glands on the neck.

Extremities.

Upper. Rheumatic pain in the shoulder-joint, extending down the arm to the hands, aggravated on motion.
The arms go to sleep when awaking in the morning.
Lower. Sensation of great fatigue in the legs, even while sitting.
100. Heaviness in the legs.
Twitching, tearing in the hips.
Restlessness and tension in the thighs.
Pressing pain in the knees.
Cramps in the calves at night.
105. Burning of the soles of the feet (in the evening).
Foot-sweat.
Tearing stitches in the loins.

Generalities.

Boring and spasmodic, contractive pains.
Paralytic drawing and tearing in the limbs.
110. Hysterical complaints and spasms.
Weakness as if it came from the stomach.
General sensation of soreness, with great sensitiveness to noise.

Sleep.

Sleepiness during the day with yawning.
Goes to sleep late and sleeplessness on account of nightly heat, with thirst and great restlessness of the body when closing the eyes.
115. Shocks through the body at night while waking.
Anxious, frightful dreams, with talking and crying out during sleep.
Nightmare.

Fever.

Face accelerated, with ebullitions while sitting.
Chill in the evening from 4 to 8, even near the warm stove.

120. Chill followed by heat in the evening till midnight.
Heat in the evening with perspiration only on the head.
Perspiration with thirst, from midnight till morning.
Morning sweat.

Skin.

Swelling of the glands.
125. Formication on the skin (face, chest and soles of the feet).
Blood-boils.

Conditions.

Liability to take cold.
Most of the symptoms appear while sitting, and at night, and are relieved on motion and by exercise.

MAGNESIA SULPHURICA.

Mind and Disposition.

Sad and weeping mood, with foreboding anxiety, as if some accident would happen.
Ill-humor, irritable.

Head.

Vertigo with heaviness of the head; with spontaneous closing of the eyes.
Dull or stupid feeling of the head, as if bandaged or screwed in.
5. Feeling of heaviness of the head with vertigo.
Stitches, stabbings in the head.
Boring in the vertex.
Sensation in the forehead on stooping as if something would fall forward.

Eyes.

Violent pains in the eyes, especially the right, as if it would start out of its socket.
10. Stinging in both eyes.
Dimness of the eyes with frequent drowsiness.
Burning of the eyes, especially at candle-light.
Lachrymation with photophobia.

Nose.

Bleeding of the nose (at night) with diminution of the headache.
15. Fluent coryza, with rough voice, pain in the chest and frequent flow of water from the nose.
Pain in the posterior nares as from air pressing through with violence, when coughing or talking.

Face.

Tearing in the right facial bones or in the left malar bone.
Burning of the lips in the evening, with dryness.

Mouth and Throat.

Toothache on entering the room from the cold air, aggravated by contact of food, and by cold and warm things.
20. Mouth and throat are very dry, as if numb.
Stinging in the fauces, more between than during the act of deglutition.
Frequent mucus in the throat, which can neither be swallowed nor hawked up.
Thirst early in the morning on rising, going off after breakfast.
Thirst in the evening, particularly during the menses.

Stomach and Abdomen.

25. Rising of water from the stomach, also with loathing and nausea.
Vomiting (in the afternoon), first of the ingesta, then of mucus.
Trembling of the stomach, with subsequent gulping up of water, which sometimes has a putrid taste.
Feeling of coldness in the stomach with inclination to vomit.
Sticking in the left hypochondriac region, particularly when sitting or in the evening.
30. Distention, fulness and hardness of the abdomen, even after a moderate meal.
Rumbling in the abdomen with emission of flatulence.
Itching of the left inguinal region, not removed by scratching.

Stool and Anus.

Alternation of hard and soft stools.
Liquid stools with tenesmus.
35. Diarrhœa preceded by rumbling in the abdomen.
Soft stools early after rising.
Discharge of ascarides at every evacuation.

Urinary Organs.

Increased emission of clear, greenish urine.
Nocturnal micturition (involuntary).

Sexual Organs.

40. *Men.* Frequent stinging about the penis when sitting or walking.
Erections without amorous fancies or sexual desire.
Women. During menses, great heaviness in the head; bruised pain in the small of the back; pain in the groins.
Discharge of blood between the menses.
Burning leucorrhœa particularly during motion.
45. Thick leucorrhœa, with bruised pain in the small of the back and thighs.

Respiratory Organs.

Deep hollow bass voice (as in catarrh).
Dry cough with burning from the larynx to the pit of the stomach.
Dry cough in the evening in bed, during which he falls asleep.
Loose cough with soreness in the mouth and throat.
50. Painful burning in the chest when coughing, as if a piece of the lungs would come out.
Oppression of the chest, with burning in the chest when walking.
Burning in the middle of the chest.
Burning under the upper part of the sternum.

Back and Neck.

Nightly pain in the small of the back and thighs.
55. Rheumatic pain between the shoulders.
Tension in the nape of the neck and between the shoulders, with stitches, particularly in the morning on rising, with great sensitiveness to the touch, relieved by walking.

Extremities.

Upper. Rheumatic pains in the left elbow, in the left wrist-joint.
Trembling of the hands.
Tingling in the fingers; going off by rubbing.
60. *Lower.* Rheumatic pain in the hip, in the left femur.
Cracking of the tarsal joint at every step.

Generalities.

Rheumatic pains in the limbs, particularly at night.
Great languor with staggering gait.
Languid weakness of the feet with trembling of the whole body.
65. Bruised feeling of the whole body.

Sleep.

Sleeplessness from violent headache, colic, pain in the small of the back which does not allow him to lie on his back.
Anxious dreams, with starting.

Fever.

Shuddering in the back, in the evening, from below upwards.
Chilliness with thirst, early in the morning after waking.
70. Chilliness in the evening, going off in bed.
Shaking chill with violent headache in the evening, 9 P. M., going off in bed, succeeded by thirst.
Chill from 9 P. M. till 10 A. M., followed by perspiration in the afternoon.
Alternation of heat and shuddering, with alternate redness and paleness of the face.
Heat and vertigo on raising the head in bed, accompanied with perspiration on the forehead and redness in the face.
75. Heat of the head with coldness of the rest of the body.
Cold feet all day, although otherwise he feels hot.

Skin.

Itching blotches, either hard or as from nettles with burning, after scratching.
Small red tetter (on the arms), with violent itching.

MANGANUM.

Mind and Disposition.
Out of humor, low-spirited and reflective.
Bitterness and long rancor.

Head.
Heaviness of the head, with the sensation as if it had become larger.
Burning, pressing headache, better in the open air.
5. Tension and stinging in the head in the open air, better in the room.
Congestion of blood to the head, as if the brain were to suppurate, better in the open air.
Sensation as if from concussion of the brain when moving.
Pressing, boring headache in the temples, extending towards the eyes and the forehead, going off on bending forward, but returning on sitting up, or on bending the head backward.
Stitches (like needles) and darts in the left side of the forehead.

Eyes.
10. Pressing in the eyes on using them and from candle-light.
Burning heat and dryness of the eyes.
Eyelids swollen and painful to the touch.
Agglutination of the eyes in the morning.
Short-sightedness.
15. Dim-sightedness with burning in the eyes.

Ears.
Otalgia.
Pains extend to and concentrate in the ear from other parts.
Stitches in the ear when talking, swallowing, laughing and walking.
Hardness of hearing (deafness) as if the ears were closed up; they open on blowing the nose, and are affected by the change of the weather.
20. Cracking in the ears on blowing the nose, on swallowing.
Whizzing and rushing in the ear.

Nose.
Violent dry coryza, with obstruction of the nose and no passage of air through it.

Painful crampy tearing between the root of the nose and the eyebrow.

Face.

Face pale, sunken.
25. Twitching stitches from the lower jaw to the temples, when laughing.
Drawing cramp in the muscles in the region of the left mastoid process, so that he had to incline his head to the right side.
Clear vesicles on the upper lip.
Dry, parched lips with shrivelled skin, without thirst.
Eruptions and ulcers at the corners of the mouth.
30. Cramp pain in the upper and lower jaw after eating.

Mouth and Throat.

Violent toothache, suddenly going from one place to another.
Smarting toothache, made insupportable when anything cold touches the tooth.
Smell from the mouth as if of clay or earth (early in the morning after rising).
Burning vesicles on the (left side of the) tongue.
35. Nodosities on the tongue.
Cutting soreness in the throat between the acts of deglutition.
When swallowing, dull stitches on both sides of the larynx, extending to the ear.
Dryness and scratching of the throat, with the sensation as if a leaf were closing up the trachea.
Chronic sore throat.
40. Dryness of the palate and lips.

Stomach and Abdomen.

Oily taste in the mouth.
Thirstlessness.
Aversion to food from a sensation of satiety.
Rising from the stomach, like heartburn.
45. Burning in the stomach rising up to the chest; sometimes with great restlessness.
Drawing in the region of the stomach with the sensation as if the pit of the stomach were enlarged, with nausea.
Pressure in the hypochondria.
Abdomen distended, bloated.
Pressing soreness in the upper part of the abdomen and in the pit of the stomach.

50. Warm contraction extending from the middle of the abdomen to the chest, with nausea.
Cutting in the region of the navel, when taking a long inspiration.
When walking, sensation as if the bowels were loose and shaking about.
Profuse secretion of flatulence.

Stool and Anus.

Constipation, stools rare, dry, difficult, knotty.
55. Yellow, granular stool, with tenesmus and constriction of the anus.
Loose and tenacious stools.
Contractive pain in the rectum when sitting.

Urinary Organs.

Frequent desire to urinate.
Sediment in the urine violet, earthy.
60. Darting in the urethra when emitting flatus.
Cutting in the middle of the urethra between the acts of micturition.

Sexual Organs.

Men. Sensation of weakness in the sexual organs, with burning and drawing in the spermatic cords, extending to the glans penis.
Itching on the corona glandis.
Stitches in the prepuce.
65. Itching in the interior of the scrotum, which cannot be relieved by pinching and rubbing.
Women. Menstrual discharge between the periods.
Menses too early and too scanty.
Pressure in the genital organs.

Respiratory Organs.

Roughness of speech early in the morning.
70. Roughness and hoarseness in the morning and in the open air.
Cough and hoarseness.
Dry cough brought on by loud reading and talking, with painful dryness, roughness and constriction of the larynx. (Bronchitis.)
In the morning, expectoration of yellowish-green lumps of mucus without cough.
Bloody expectoration from the chest.
75. Bruised pain in the chest.

Bruised pain in the upper chest when stooping, relieved by raising the head.
Breath hot and burning, with disagreeable heat in the chest.
Stitches in the chest and sternum, running up and down.
Beating in the chest.
80. Sudden shocks at the heart and in the left side of the chest from above downwards.

Back and Neck.

Pain in the small of the back on bending backwards.
Tearing in the whole spinal column, from above downwards.
Stiffness of the nape of the neck.
Red, swollen streak on the left side of the neck.

Extremities.

85. *Upper.* Pain as from a sprain in the shoulder-joint.
Rheumatic pains extending from the shoulders to the fingers.
Sensation of tension in the arm and carpal-joints.
Gnawing and boring in the humerus, as if in the marrow of the bone.
Tension in the elbow-joint as if too short.
90. Rhagades in the bends of the fingers.
Sensation of tension in the hands.
Lower. Twitching of the muscles in the legs from the least exertion.
Tension, drawing, stitches in the thigh.
Tension and stiffness in the legs.
95. Tearing in the knees.
Trembling and unsteadiness of the knees.
Inflammation and swelling of the ankle, with stitches extending to the lower leg.
Burning of the soles of the feet.
Sore rawness between the toes.

Generalities.

100. Rheumatic affections, generally in the limbs, and mostly in the joints, with red, shining swelling.
Drawing and tension in the limbs as from shortening of the tendons, especially on extending (stretching) them.
Inflammatory swellings and suppurations.
Weakness and trembling, especially of the joints.
Inflammation of the bones, with nightly, insupportable pains.
105. Every part of the body feels extremely sore when touched.

Sleep.

Much yawning.
Feels sleepy early in the evening.
Vivid, anxious dreams, which are well remembered.

Fever.

Pulse very uneven and irregular, sometimes rapid, sometimes slow, but constantly soft and weak.
110. Chilliness, generally in the evening, with icy cold hands and feet.
Chill with heat of the head and stinging pain in the forehead which continues after the chill.
Sudden flushes of heat in the face, on the chest, and over the back.
Profuse perspiration with short anxious breathing.
Night-sweats, itching, often only on the neck and on the lower legs.

Skin.

115. Inflammation of the bones, with insupportable digging pains at night.
Burning over the whole body; in the evening when rising from the bed.
Itching herpes.
The skin will not heal.
Rhagades in the bends of the joints, with soreness.
120. Inflammatory swellings and suppuration.

Conditions.

Most symptoms appear at night.
The symptoms which appear while in the room, disappear in the open air, and vice versa.
Many complaints change for the better or worse with the change of the weather.
Aggravation on stooping.
125. When touched ever so little, the parts feel intensely sore.

MARUM VERUM TEUCRIUM.

Mind and Disposition.

Indolence, aversion to all physical and mental exertion.
Irritability increased after eating (with pressure in the forehead).
Great sensitiveness and excitability.
Irresistible desire to sing.

Head.

5. Pressing pain in the forehead, over the eyes, worse on stooping.
The skin of the forehead feels sensitive to the touch.
The eyes look as if one had been weeping, with smarting in the canthi and redness of the conjunctiva.
Redness and puffiness of the upper eyelids.
Profuse smarting tears in the open air.

Ears.

10. Otalgia with lancinating pain.
A hissing sound in the ear when passing the hand over it, when talking, or when inhaling the air through the nose with force.
Dry herpes (with white dry scales) on the lobule of the (right) ear.

Nose.

Tingling (itching) in the nose.
Stinging, lancinating pain in the upper part of the nasal cavity.
15. Sensation in one nostril as if it were half stopped. Polypus.
Stoppage of both nostrils frequently through the day.
Frequent sneezing, with tingling in the nose, without coryza.
Coryza with stoppage of the nostrils.

Face.

Pale face.
20. Frequent sensation of flushes of heat, without redness.
On both sides of the under lip, two deep furrows with elevated edges.

Mouth and Throat.

Violent tearing in the roots and gums of the right lower incisors.

Smarting and scraping in the posterior fauces, and at the root of the tongue, especially on the left side.
Stinging or pressing pain in the throat, which hinders deglutition.
25. Much mucus in the mouth.
Smarting as from pepper, first on the left, later also on the right side of the root of the tongue.
After hawking up mucus, mouldy taste in the mouth.
Hunger in the morning and evening.
Feeling of hunger which prevents sleep.
30. Gulping up of bitter tasting food.
Sensation of emptiness and rumbling in the stomach.
Anxious oppression in the pit of the stomach.
Colic (cutting pain) after drinking (beer or water).
Frequent emission of silent, hot, hepatic-smelling flatulence.
35. Incarcerated flatulence.

Stool and Anus.

Swelling, itching and creeping at the anus as from ascarides, with restlessness at night and tossing about.
Creeping and violent stinging at the anus at night when in bed.
Creeping in the rectum after stool.

Urinary Organs.

Increased secretion of pale urine.

Genital Organs.

40. *Men.* Decreased sexual desire.

Respiratory Organs.

Short, dry cough from tickling in the upper part of the trachea, which is aggravated by coughing.
Sensation of oppression of the chest (without affecting the breathing).
Dryness in the trachea.

Extremities.

Upper. Rheumatic pain in the arms, especially in the bones and joints.
45. Burning in the tips of the fingers.
The finger-joints bend over easily.
Panaritium.
Lower. Rheumatic pains in the legs, especially in the bones and joints.
The toe-nails (of the right great toe) grow in and ulcerate.

Generalities.

50. Nervous, irritable, trembling sensation in the whole body. The limbs go to sleep.

Rheumatism in the limbs, especially in the bones and joints.

Sleep.

Restlessness at night, with tossing about, sleeplessness from excitability, especially before midnight; goes to sleep late.

Fever.

Chilliness and want of natural heat.

55. Chilliness after eating and when talking about unpleasant things.

Increased heat and exaltation in the evening, with great loquacity.

Skin.

Tearing in the bones.

Conditions.

Desire to take exercise in the open air, which does not fatigue.

At midday sensation of general debility.

MENYANTHES TRIFOLIATA.

Mind and Disposition.

Sad, weeping mood.
Taciturn and self-reflecting.
Anxiety about the heart, as if something evil were going to happen.

Head.

Continuous heaviness of the head.

5. Pressing or compressing headache, with the sensation when ascending as if a heavy weight pressed on the head, relieved by pressing the head with the hands.

Pressing pain from both sides of the head.
Dull headache in the room, with difficult flow of ideas; better in the open air.
External gnawing on the vertex.
Burning pain on the forehead.

Eyes.

10. The eyelids feel stiff as from tonic spasms.
    Pressing in the eyes.
    While reading, every thing becomes black before the eyes.

Ears.

Stitches in the ears.
Cracking in the ears when masticating.
15. Feeling of coldness in the ear.
    Running of the ears, especially after exanthemata.

Nose.

Tension in the root of the nose.
Nauseating smell before the nose as from rotten eggs.

Face.

Painless, visible twitching of the muscles of the face and of the eyelids.
20. Heat and redness of the face while sleeping. Heat in the face with cold feet.
    Pain and cracking in the articulation of the jaw when masticating.

Mouth and Throat.

Great dryness of the throat without thirst.
When yawning and coughing, paralytic feeling on the left side of the throat.
Dryness and roughness in the throat preventing deglutition.
25. Dryness of the palate, causing a stinging when swallowing.

Stomach and Abdomen.

Taste in the mouth bitter-sweet.
Frequent empty eructations.
After eating, painful dulness of the head.
Increased strong appetite preceded by heat in the stomach.
30. Constriction in the stomach.
    Continuous rumbling in the stomach as from emptiness.
    Sensation of coldness in the abdomen, especially when pressing with the hand on it, or in the morning when rising.
    Sensation of soreness of the abdominal walls.
    The abdomen is distended by flatulence.

Stool and Anus.

35. Constipation; hard stool with pinching pain in the abdomen.
    Bleeding, hæmorrhoidal tumors.

Urinary Organs.

Frequent desire to urinate, with scanty discharges.

Sexual Organs.

Men. Increased sexual desire without amorous fancies or erections.

Both testicles are drawn up, the right more than the left.

40. The spermatic cord is painful to the touch.

Respiratory Organs.

Rough, hoarse voice, the ears feel obstructed as if something had been stretched across.

Stitch in the anterior regions of the larynx, impeding deglutition.

Spasmodic contraction of the larynx; when an effort to inspire is made it causes a cough.

Constriction and stitches in both sides of the chest.

45. The stitches in the (right side of the) chest are worse during motion, and when breathing.

Stitches in the region of the heart.

Back and Neck.

Bruised pain in the small of the back, more on sitting quiet and when stooping.

Dull, boring stitch on the left shoulder-blade.

Feeling of heaviness and stiffness in the muscles of the neck and throat.

Extremities.

50. *Upper.* Tension and paralytic tearing in the arms, hands and fingers.

Spasmodic stiffness of the arms, the fingers are involuntarily clenched.

Painful jactitation of the muscles of the (right) upper arm and little finger.

Cramp-like pains in the muscles of the (left) lower arm, extending as far as the palm of the hand.

Lower. Bruised feeling of the thighs.

55. The (right) thigh and leg are spasmodically jerked upward, when sitting, relieved when standing or when drawing up the leg.

Generalities.

Painless twitching of the muscles in different parts (face, thigh), principally when at rest.

Great debility, especially when walking, often with chilliness.
Stinging, pinching pain (in the limbs: arthritic affections).

Fever.

Pulse. Slow during the cold stage and accelerated during the fever.
60. Chill predominates, icy coldness of the hands and feet and coldness in the abdomen.
Chill, which is relieved by the heat of the stove and only remains in the back.
Sensation of chilliness on the hands and lower legs.
Heat in the evening, mostly on the head, with cold feet.
Perspiration in the evening, as soon as he lies down, continuing all night.
65. Intermittent fevers, with sensation of coldness in the abdomen.

Conditions.

Chronic complaints from the abuse of cinchona and quinine.
Aggravation in the evening and during rest, while lying down, amelioration from motion, from pressing on the affected part.

MEPHITIS PUTORIUS.

Mind and Disposition.

Great talkativeness as if he were intoxicated.
Excited, with heat of the head.
Angry about trifles or about imaginary things.
The fancies are so vivid that he is unfitted for mental labor.

Head.

5. Numb and dull, with the sensation as if the head became enlarged, with ill-humor and nausea.
Vertigo when stooping; sudden vertigo while sitting.
Vertigo when turning in bed.
Headache while riding in a carriage.
Pain over the eyes.
10. Violent pain in the head, as if a fulness were pressing upwards.

Heaviness and heavy pressure in the back part of the head, as if fingers were pressing on it.

Eyes.
Pain in the eyes when turning them in certain directions.
Pain as if something had lodged in the eyes.
Pain in the eyes as from over-exertion.
15. Stitches in the eyes as from needles.
Heat and burning of the eyes.
Pressing on the lids with burning of the margins, as if a stye would form.
Inability to read fine print.
The letters become blurred, he is unable to discern them, they run together.
20. The weakness of sight is generally accompanied by headache and pain in the eyes.

Ears.
Erysipelas of the ear, with itching, heat, redness and blisters.

Nose.
Dry nose; bleeding from the nose.

Mouth and Throat.
Sudden jerks in the roots of the teeth.
Coppery taste in the mouth.

Stomach and Abdomen.
25. Nausea with emptiness in the stomach, and sensation as if the head were distended.
Pressure in the stomach, and colic.
Rheumatic pain in the region of the liver.

Stool and Anus.
Stools rare but soft.

Urinary Organs.
Frequent micturition with clear urine.
30. The urine is turbid in the morning, after evening fever.

Sexual Organs.
Men. Warmth of the genitals.
Itching of the scrotum.
Women. Soreness of the genitals and swelling of the labia.

Respiratory Organs.
When drinking or talking, liability to have something get into the larynx.

35. Cough with fluent coryza and soreness in the chest.
    Coughing from talking or reading aloud.
    Rattling cough every morning.
    Hooping-cough, worse at night and after lying down; with convulsions; with complete suffocative feeling, he cannot exhale; vomiting of all the food some hours after eating; bloated face.
    Pains in the chest (on the last left short rib) when touching and pressing on it; but especially when coughing and sneezing.

Back.

40. Stitches in the spinal column during motion.
    Pain in the back and all the limbs, with lameness.
    Tension and pain in the right side of the neck.

Extremities.

Upper. Rheumatic pains in the arms relieved on motion.
Restlessness in the left arm with insensibility.
45. Trembling of the arm when leaning on it.
    Twitching with the hands.
    Lower. Rheumatic pains from the hips down to the feet.
    Restlessness in the lower limbs as if they were to become insensible: the knee feels bruised.
    Stitches in the feet.
50. Cramp pain in the (left) foot.
    Arthritic pain in the heel.
    Pain in the big toe as if it were being pinched off.
    Corns with pain and burning.

Generalities.

Rheumatic pains.
55. Wandering pains, with much pressure to urinate and shocks.
    Sensation of lameness, especially with the pains.
    Fine, nervous vibrations, reaching to the interior of the bones, causing a good deal of anxiety.
    Inclination to stretch oneself, with disinclination to do any thing.

Sleep.

Frequent yawning with lachrymation.
60. Sleepiness during the day, even when in company.
    Wakens from sleep at night with congestion of blood to the lower legs.
    Nightmare.
    Vivid dreams which he well recollects.
    He wakens early and feels very well.

Fever.

65. Chilliness in the evening, with desire to urinate and colic, as if diarrhœa would set in.
Increased warmth, especially in the morning.
Warmth at night (genitals, head and lower legs).
Less chilliness than usual in cold weather, and no more aversion to cold washing.
Washing in ice-cold water causes a pleasant sensation.

Conditions.

70. Sensation of coldness, and restlessness predominates.
The cough is worse at night, and causes great distress when inhaling.

MERCURIUS VIVUS.

Mind and Disposition.

Anxiety, apprehension and restlessness, especially in the evening and at night, with fear of losing one's mind and understanding.
Disgust of life.
Great indifference to every thing.
Irritable, quarrelsome mood.
5. Continuous moaning and groaning.
Peevish, taciturn, and suspicious.
Hurried speech.
Desire to flee, with nightly anxiety and apprehensions.
Bad effects from fright, leaving one in a state of great anxiety and worse at night.
10. Home-sickness with nightly anxiety and perspiration.
Delirium; mental derangement of drunkards.

Head.

Fainting after sweetish rising in the throat, followed by sleep.
Vertigo when lying on the back, with headache, nausea every thing becomes black before the eyes.
Weakness of memory, forgets every thing.
15. Vertigo as if one were on a swing.
Dull and stupid feeling, with dizziness.
Vertigo on raising the head after stooping.

Burning in the head, especially in the left temple, worse at night when lying in bed, better on sitting up.
Compressive headache, the head feels as if it were in a vice with nausea; worse in the open air, from sleeping, eating and drinking; better in the room.
20. Inflammation of the brain with burning and pulsation in the forehead, with the sensation as if the head were in a hoop; worse at night, better after riding.
Sensation of subcutaneous ulceration in the whole head; worse at night when becoming warm in bed; better after rising, and while sitting still in a warm room.
Tearing in one (the left) side of the head and temple, extending from the neck, with insupportable heat and perspiration, worse at night and in the heat of the bed, relieved towards morning and while lying quiet.
Tension over the forehead as from a tape or hoop, worse at night in bed; better after rising and from laying the hand on it.
Headache as if the head would burst with fulness of the brain.
25. Congestion of blood to the head with heat in it.
Hydrocephalus.
Sensation of tension of the scalp.
The scalp is painful to the touch; worse when scratching, which is followed by bleeding.
Tearing and stinging in the bones of the skull. Stitches through the heart.
30. Itching on the hairy scalp, and forehead, and temples; worse from scratching, when it bleeds and becomes erysipelatous.
Dry, stinging, burning, fetid eruption like yellow crusts, on the forepart of the head and temples, when scratching inflammation and erysipelas.
Exostoses on the hairy scalp, with sensation of subcutaneous ulceration on touching them, most painful at night in bed.
Open fontanelles with dirty color of the face, restless sleep, and sour-smelling night-sweat.
Falling off of the hair, mostly on the sides of the head and on the temple; with humid eruptions on the head or after clammy perspirations of the head; with itching at night in bed; worse from scratching; with burning; with great tendency to perspiration.
35. Great chilliness with contractive, tearing pain of the scalp, extending from the forehead to the neck.

Fetid, sour-smelling, oily perspiration on the head and on the icy-cold forehead, with burning in the skin; worse at night in bed, better after rising.

Eyes.

Pain under the eyelids, as from a cutting body.
Stitches in the eyes.
Itching and heat in the eyes.
40. Inflammation of the eyes, with redness of the white of the eye, and great painfulness when looking into the bright light.
Violent lachrymation in the evening.
Blear-eyedness.
Pustules on the conjunctiva.
Ulcers on the cornea.
45. Scurfs around the eyes.
Swelling of the eyelids, they are covered on the edges with scurfs and ulcers.
The eyes are dim and without lustre.
Violent contraction of the eyelids, it is difficult to open them.
Periodical vanishing of sight.
50. Aversion to light and to look into the fire.
Mistiness before the eyes; amaurotic dimness before the left eye.
Black spots, flies, sparks and mistiness before the eyes.
Twitching of the lids.

Ears.

Inflammation of the internal and external ear (Otalgia), with stinging and tearing pain.
55. Soreness of the
Fungous excrescences in the ear.
Discharge of pus from the ear, with ulceration of the external ear.
Inflammatory swelling of the (right) parotid gland with stinging.
Pulsative roaring in the ears.
60. Hardness of hearing, all sounds vibrate violently in the ear, the ears feel obstructed, but open when swallowing or blowing the nose; or the obstruction is caused by an enlargement of the tonsils.
Buzzing, roaring, and ringing in the ears.

Nose.

Red, shining swelling of the nose with itching.
Greenish fetid pus is discharged from the nose.
Swelling of the nasal bones.
65. Blackish nose.
Scurfy nostrils, bleeding when cleansed.
Bleeding of the nose during sleep or when coughing.
Profuse fluent coryza, with profuse discharge of watery corrosive mucus.

Face.

Pale, yellow, earthy color of the face with dull eyes without lustre.
70. Heat and redness of the cheeks.
Swelling of one (right) side of the face with heat and toothache.
Yellow, dirty scurf in the face with discharge of fetid moisture, itching, bleeding after scratching.
Crusta lactea.
Tearing in the face.
75. Lips rough, black, dry, painful to the touch.
Cracks and rhagades in the lips and corners of the mouth.
Burning pimples with yellow crusts on the lips.
Pimples and eruptions on the chin.
Lockjaw with stinging pains and hard swelling of the submaxillary glands.

Mouth and Throat.

80. Almost complete immovability of the jaw, scarcely permitting one to open the mouth, with violent pain and inflammatory swelling of the lower jaw.
Caries of the jaw.
Looseness of the teeth, which are painful when touched by the tongue—they fall out.
Toothache aggravated from heat and cold (air), from eating, in the evening and at night, the heat of the bed makes it insupportable.
The nightly pulsating toothache extends to the ear.
85. Stitches in the teeth.
Itching, burning and redness of the gums.
Spongy, easily bleeding gums.
The gums recede from the teeth, they are painful to the touch, burning at night, and swollen.
The upper border of the gums looks indented, the indentations being white and ulcerated.

90. The swollen gums have white, elevated, ulcerated, pointed edges.
Bleeding of the gums when touching them ever so little.
Fetid smell from the mouth.
Inflammatory swelling of the inner mouth.
Burning ulcers on the inside of the cheeks.
95. Aphthæ of children: stomacace.
Ulceration of salivary glands.
Ptyalism, the saliva is often fetid and tenacious.
Tongue moist, soft, covered with mucus.
Tongue dry, hard, coated black.
100. Inflammation, swelling, induration and suppuration of the tongue.
Tongue swollen, soft, flabby, the edges become indented by the impression of the teeth.
Quick and stuttering speech.
Complete loss of speech and voice.
Accumulation of much tough mucus in the mouth.
105. Ranula.
Pain when swallowing as if a foreign body were swallowed down.
Burning in the throat as if from a hot vapor ascending from the stomach, with dryness in the throat when swallowing, and continuous desire to swallow, with accumulations of water in the mouth.
Redness and pain of the throat: erysipelatous inflammation of all the soft parts of the mouth and throat.
Inflammation and redness of the palate.
110. Angina especially with stinging pains aggravated by empty deglutition at night and in the cold air.
Continuous painful dryness of the throat; the mouth being full of water.
The fluid which is swallowed comes up through the nose.
Sticking pain in the tonsils when swallowing.
Ptyalism attends the sore throat.
115. Syphilitic ulcers in the mouth and throat.
Bitter, sweetish or putrid taste in the mouth.
Saltish taste on the lips.
The bread tastes sweet.

Stomach and Abdomen.

Canine hunger, even after eating.
120. Excessive hunger, but does not relish any thing he eats.
Has no appetite for dry food, likes liquid food.

Violent burning thirst, especially for beer and cold drinks, day and night.
Rising of air or acrid, bitter, putrid eructations.
Regurgitation of the ingesta, vomiting of food.
125. Nausea with sweet taste in the throat, vertigo, headache and heat.
At night restlessness with bitter, bilious vomiting.
Pressure in the stomach; it hangs down heavily, even after very light, easily digestible food.
Burning pain in the pit of the stomach.
Painfulness of the region of the stomach especially to the touch.
130. Great weakness of digestion with continuous hunger.
The stomach feels replete and constricted.
Swelling and induration of the liver.
The region of the liver is painfully sensative to contact.
Inflammation of the liver with stinging pains.
135. Distention of the abdomen with pressure and tension and painfulness to contact.
Cutting and pinching in the abdomen, especially after taking cold.
Cutting and tearing in the abdomen at night.
Stabbing in the abdomen as from knives.
Colic which only passes off in a recumbent position.
140. The intestines feel bruised if he lies on the right side.
Sensation of emptiness in the abdomen.
Colic, caused by the cool evening air, with diarrhœa.
Shaking sensation of the bowels on walking, they feel relaxed.
Inflammation of the peritoneum and of the intestines.
145. Inflammation, swelling and suppuration of the inguinal glands.
Buboes.

Stool and Anus.

Frequent ineffectual pressing to stool with tenesmus, worse at night.
Constipation, stool tenacious or crumbling, can only be discharged after violent straining.
Feces of small shape.
150. Stools undigested, black, tenacious (pitch-like), yellowish, white-gray, green, mucus, blood and mucus, undigested, smelling sour, excoriating the anus.
Chilliness between the diarrhœic stools.
During a diarrhœic stool nausea and eructations.

Discharges of bloody mucus accompanied by colic and tenesmus—dysentery.
Discharge of blood before, during and after a stool, if it is even hard.
155. Burning pain in the anus with a loose stool.
Discharge of mucus from the rectum.
After the stool prolapsus ani, or when pressing and straining to stool.
Discharge of ascarides and lumbrici.
Diarrhœa preceded by cool colic from evening air.
160. Rectum black, discharging blood.

Urinary Organs.

Frequent, violent desire to urinate, with scanty discharge in feeble stream.
Irresistible, sudden desire to urinate.
Involuntary emission of urine.
The quantity of urine emitted is larger than the quantity of fluid drank.
165. Urine dark-red, soon becoming turbid and fetid.
Urine smells sour and pungent.
The urine looks as if mixed with blood, with white flakes or as if containing pus; scanty, fiery red.
Hemorrhage from the urethra.
Burning and stinging in the urethra.
170. Thick greenish (or yellow) (gonorrhœic) discharge from the urethra, more at night.

Sexual Organs.

Men. Perspiration on the genitals when walking.
Soreness between the genitals and thighs.
Swelling of the lymphatic vessels along the penis.
Painful inflammation and swelling of the glans and prepuce.
175. Ulcers on the glans with cheesy bottom. (Chancres.)
Chancre ulcers on the prepuce and glans.
Hard swelling of the testicles with shining redness.
Lascivious excitement with painful nightly erections.
Nightly emissions of semen mixed with blood.
180. *Women.* Menstruation too profuse, with anxiety and colic.
Suppressed menstruation.
Congestion of blood to the uterus.
Sterility with too profuse menstruation; easy conception.
Swelling, heat and shining redness of the labia.
185. Inflammation of the ovaries and uterus.
Prolapsus vaginæ.
Fluor albus, purulent and acrid.

Hard swelling and suppuration of the mammæ with sore pains, ulcerated nipples. The infant rejects the milk.

Respiratory Organs.

Hoarseness with burning and tickling in the larynx.
190. Catarrh with cough, hoarseness, fluent coryza and sore throat.
Cough with hoarseness from tickling in the larynx.
Violent, racking dry cough, especially at night, as if it would burst the head and chest, sometimes with vomiturition.
Bloody expectoration.
Spasmodic cough (hooping cough); two paroxysms follow one another rapidly, from tickling in the larynx and the upper part of the chest, at night, without cough during the day, with expectoration of acrid yellowish mucus, which is sometimes mixed with coagulated blood, tasting putrid or salty.
195. The cough is aggravated in the night air, at night and when lying on the left side.
Dyspnœa (sensation of spasmodic contraction when coughing or sneezing).
Burning in the chest, extending to the throat.
Soreness and burning in the chest.
Stitches in the chest (right side, through from the shoulder-blade); inflammation of the lungs.
200. Sensation of dryness in the chest.
Palpitation of the heart.
Suppuration of the lungs after hemorrhages.

Back and Neck.

Bruised sensation of the shoulder-blades, back and small of the back.
Stinging pains in the small of the back, with the sensation of weakness.
205. Erysipelatous inflammation, extending from the back like a girdle around the abdomen (Zona).
Rheumatic stiffness and swelling of the neck.
Inflammation and swelling of the glands of the neck, with pressing pains and stitches.

Extremities.

Rheumatic pains in the shoulders and upper arms.
Twitching of the arms and fingers.
210. Red hot (arthritic) swelling from the elbow to the wrist.
Burning, scaly herpes on the forearms and hands.

Eruption like moist itch on the hands, with violent nightly itching.
Painful stiffness of the right wrist-joint.
Contraction of the fingers.
215. Painful and bleeding rhagades on the hands.
Swelling of the finger-joints.
Exfoliation of the finger-nails.
Lower. Tearing in the hip-joint and knee, worse at night or with pulsating pain, the suppuration beginning.
Rheumatic pains in the legs with stinging, especially in the hip-joint, femur and knee, worse at night, the affected parts feel cold.
220. Dropsical swelling of the legs.
Cold sweat on the feet.
Painful swelling of the metatarsal bones.

Generalities.

Great debility and weakness, with trembling and ebullitions from the least exertion.
Congestions to the head, chest and abdomen.
225. Rheumatic and arthritic pains, tearing and stinging, especially in the limbs and joints, worse at night, with profuse perspiration which gives no relief.
Stinging pains.
Contractions of some parts.
Inflammations ending in exudations and suppurations.
Rheumatic and catarrhal inflammations, with great tendency to perspiration.

Sleep.

230. Great sleepiness during the day.
Sleeplessness at night on account of anxiety, ebullitions and congestions.
Perspiration during sleep.

Fever.

Pulse irregular, generally full and fast, with violent beating in the arteries, at times weak, slow and tremulous.
Ebullitions with trembling from slight exertions.
235. Chilliness early in the morning when rising, but more so in the evening after lying down, as if cold water had been thrown over him, and not relieved by the heat of the stove.
Chilliness at night with frequent micturition.
Chilliness between the diarrhœic stools.
Internal chilliness with heat of the face.

Heat while in bed; as soon as one rises chilliness.
240. Heat after midnight with violent thirst for cold drinks.
Heat with anxiety and constriction of the chest, alternating with chilliness.
Perspiration, towards morning, with thirst and palpitation of the heart; from the least exertion, even when eating.
Perspiration in the evening before going to sleep.
Very debilitating night-sweats.
245. Perspiration has an offensive smell, or smells sour, and is cold, oily, clammy, and burns the skin.
The perspiration gives no relief, and accompanies all ailments.
Intermittent fever. Chilliness in the evening in bed, afterwards heat with violent thirst.
Chilliness and heat without thirst, towards morning thirst; during the perspiration, palpitation of the heart and nausea, the perspiration smells fetid or sour.

Skin.

Swelling and inflammation of the bones, with pains at night. (Rachitis.) (Caries.)
250. Skin dirty yellow, rough and dry. (Jaundice.)
Itching over the whole body, especially at night in bed, when getting warm.
Ulcers corroding and easily bleeding.
Itch—bleeding easily.
Itching eruptions, burning after scratching.
255. Herpes, burning when touched, humid with large scales on the edges.
Syphilitic ulcers and herpes.
Erysipelatous inflammation of external parts.
Suppurations.

Conditions.

Aggravation in the evening and at night; from the heat of the bed, before falling asleep, from the candle-light, during perspiration, when exercising.
260. Amelioration in the morning, when at rest, when lying down.

MERCURIUS SUBLIMATUS.

Mind and Disposition.

Anxiety, preventing sleep.
Weakness of the intellect; he stares at persons who talk to him, and does not understand them.

Head.

Vertigo, with coldness, cold perspiration; with deafness, when stooping.
Heaviness of the head.
5. Stitches in the forehead.
Swelling of the head and neck.

Eyes.

Burning and dryness of the eyes.
Inflammation of the eyes, the pain is pressing, burning, the pupils lose their roundness, are angular, the eyes feel too small.
The eye sparkling, very movable; pupils contracted, with red face.
10. Pupils contracted and insensible.
Objects appear smaller.
Double vision.

Ears.

Inflammation with stitches in the ear.
Discharge of fetid pus from the ear.

Nose.

15. Swelling and redness of the nose.
Fluent coryza, loss of smell.
Ozæna, discharge from the nose like glue, drying up in the posterior nares, perforation of the septum.

Face.

Face and cheeks swollen, hard, red, bloated.
Paleness of the distorted face.
20. Œdematous swelling of the face.
Yellow color of the face.
The face is covered with cold perspiration.

Mouth and Throat.

Swelling of the lips, mouth, tongue, and throat.
Swelling and turning up of the upper lip; dark-red, swollen lip.
25. The lips and tongue are whitish and contracted.
Tongue coated with thick white mucus, or dry and red; papillæ elevated like a strawberry; coated white and swollen, and stiff.
Looseness of the teeth; they pain, they fall out.
The gums swell, are covered with a false membrane, become gangrenous and bleed freely.
Mouth dry with unquenchable thirst.
30. Lymphatic exudations on the membranes in the mouth extending to the tonsils.
Ulcers (phagædenic) in the mouth, or the gums and throat, with fetid breath.
Burning in the mouth and gums.
Ptyalism with salty taste; bloody, yellowish, tough, acrid.
Painful burning in the mouth extending to the stomach.
35. Discharge of albuminous mucus from the mouth.
Swelling of the tongue with ptyalism.
Pricking in the throat as from needles.
Tonsils swollen and covered with ulcers.
Swelling of the throat, to suffocation, inability to swallow any fluid, with heat in the mouth, tongue and throat.
40. Pharynx dark red, painful to contact.
When he makes the effort to swallow, retching and vomiting.
Taste in the mouth, metallic or salty.

Stomach and Abdomen.

Burning, from the pit of the stomach to the mouth; in the stomach.
Swelling, distension of the pit of the stomach, not permitting the least touch.
45. Vomiting, of albuminous matter; of tough mucus; of blood; of stringy mucus, of green bitter substances like coffee grounds, with coagulated blood; of bile; of pus.
Stitches as if in the middle of the liver.
Bloated abdomen, very painful to the least touch.
Cutting below the navel.
Bruised pain in the abdomen.

Stool and Anus.

50. Diarrhœa, yellow, green, bilious, bloody, of mucus, of feces with mucus and dark clotted blood.

Burning in the rectum.

Painful, almost unsuccessful pressing, straining and tenesmus, with almost insupportable cutting pain in the abdomen, and discharge of small quantities of bloody mucus.

Tenesmus with dysenteric discharges, vomiting of bile, cramps in the calves, and stitches in the side.

Painful bloody discharges; with vomiting.

55. Dysentery.

Urinary Organs.

Tenesmus of the bladder; suppressed urine.

Increased discharge of urine.

The urine is only passed in drops, and with great pain.

Urine scanty, brown, with brick-dust sediment.

60. Itching in the forepart of the urethra.

Gonorrhœic discharges, first thin, then thicker, and then smarting pain when urinating, with stitches in the urethra.

Burning in the urethra, more before micturition.

Paraphymosis.

Sexual Organs.

Men. Violent erections during sleep.

65. Fine, painful stinging in the left testicle.

Women. Menses too early and too profuse.

Fluor albus, smelling sweetish, pale-yellow.

Respiratory Organs.

Hoarseness; aphonia.

Burning and stinging in the trachea, with loss of voice.

70. Respiration slow, interrupted, sighing.

Constriction of the chest, breathes with the pectoral muscles.

Oppression of the chest.

Stitches in the chest, through the thorax (right lower side).

Hæmoptysis.

Extremities.

75. Coldness in the extremities, they look purple, with small, spasmodic frequent pulse.

Upper. Rheumatic pains in the left shoulder and shoulder-blade.

The deltoid muscle feels relaxed.

The whole arm up to the shoulder is much swollen, red and covered with vesicles.
Lower. Stitches in the right hip-joint.
80. Sensation as if the legs had gone to sleep.
The muscles of the thigh and calf feel relaxed.
Cramps in the calves.
The feet are icy cold.

Generalities.

Drawing in the periosteum, with heat in the head.
85. Inflammation of the lymphatic vessels.
Twitches, convulsive contractions.
Convulsive twitchings of the muscles of the face, arms, and legs, and convulsions of the limbs.
Trembling.
Paralysis of the upper and lower extremities.

Sleep.

90. During sleep, violent hiccough.
Somnolence.
When trying to go to sleep violent starts.
Sleeplessness on account of vertigo; on account of anxiety.

Fever.

Pulse small, weak, intermitting, sometimes trembling.
95. Chilliness from the least movement and in the open air, generally with colic.
Chilliness in the evening, especially on the head.
Chilliness at night in bed.
External heat with yellowness of the skin.
Burning and stinging heat in the skin.
100. Heat when stooping, and coldness when rising.
Night-sweat.
Towards morning the perspiration becomes fetid.
Cold perspiration, often only on the forehead.
The whole skin is covered with cold perspiration, with anxiety.

Skin.

105. Painful drawing in the periosteum, as if a chill would set in.
Inflammation of the periosteum (lower jaw).
Necrosis of the upper jaw.
Burning and redness of the skin, with the formation of small vesicles.
Swelling of the glands (neck, buboes.)
110. Gray color of the nails.

Conditions.

Aggravation in the evening and at night.

MERCURIUS PROTO-IODATUS.

Mind and Disposition.

Destructiveness, moodiness, depression of spirits.

Head.

Dizziness when reading, and when rising from a chair.
Occasional shooting pains in the temples; sharp stitches in the temples.
The head feels dull and compressed, as if a heavy weight were pressing it down on the pillow.
5. The head feels full and heavy.
Throbbing pain in the (fore) head.
Dull headache on awaking in the morning.
Sharp pain on the vertex.
Sensation as if the skull were cracking.
10. Violent pain in the right side of the head (over the right temple).

Eyes.

Severe pain and soreness of right orbit (on rising in the morning).
Black clouds float before his eyes, when lying on his left side.

Ears.

Sharp, throbbing, boring pain, from within outward, deep in the (left) ear.

Nose.

Pain at the root of the nose (shooting pain).
15. A great deal of mucus in the nose.
A great deal of mucus descends through the posterior nares into the throat.
The right side of the septum and right nostril are very sore and much swollen.

Face.

Dull bruised pain in the right malar bone, radiating into the forehead and right side of the head, a small spot pulsates and burns like fire.
Sharp stitches through the head and face.
20. Soreness of all the bones of the face.
Stinging in the left cheek.

Mouth and Throat.

The teeth feel too long; cannot eat.
Mouth, teeth and lips dry and sticky, the back part of the tongue is heavily coated.
Fine bright and red eruption on the roof of the mouth.
25. Tongue coated; yellowish white; dirty yellow; light brown.
Small, red, raised elevations on the tongue.
Coating on the back part of the tongue (thick, dirty yellow).
Coating bright yellow, the tips and edges are red.
Burning in the throat when swallowing the saliva.
30. Dryness of the mouth and throat with frequent empty swallowing.
Dryness of the mouth and throat.
Pharynx, tonsils and uvula are red and congested.
Throat dry and burning with pain when swallowing.
Excessive secretion of mucus in the throat, difficult to dislodge, and which causes retching.
35. The mucous patches on the tonsils and walls of the pharynx are easily detached.
Accumulation of mucus in the throat in the morning.

Stomach and Abdomen.

Thirst excessive, for acids or sour drinks.
Nausea, with suffocation about the heart and dizziness.
Weak, empty feeling at the stomach, with nausea.
40. Nausea with sensation of disgust at the sight of food.
Burning at the stomach, with pain as from a blow.
Hardness of the abdomen.
Heat at the umbilicus, as if from a hot coal, worse when inspiring.
Small stool, of very tough feces, almost of the consistency of putty, requiring great straining for their evacuations.
45. Stitching pain in the region of the liver relieved by pressing the hand against it.
Pain in the left hypochondrium, with dizziness on awakening in the morning.

Urinary Organs.

Urine copious and of a dark red color.

Sexual Organs.

Men. Sharp, shooting stitches in the end of the penis, through the glans.
Copious seminal emissions, preceded by lewd dreams.

50. Dreams that he must urinate; this was followed by an emission.
Seminal emission, of which he knew nothing till morning

Respiratory Organs.

Sharp pain in the chest, behind the sternum.
Stitches through the (right side of the) chest.
Slight hacking cough when inspiring.
55. Stitching pain in the heart.

Back.

Throbbing pain between the shoulders.
Severe pain as if bruised over the entire scapular region.
Throbbing pain on the right scapula.

Extremities.

Upper. Numbness and wearied feeling in the right arm, aggravated by writing.
60. Lameness and stiffness of the right shoulder.
Rheumatic, laming pain in the right arm, aggravated by writing.
Soreness and lameness of the left shoulder and arm at night when lying on the left side.
Soreness and pain of the right arm; worse from pressure, rubbing and passive motion.
Sharp pain in the right shoulder, obliging him to cease writing.
65. Heavy feeling of the right arm.
Lame numbness of the left shoulder and left arm.
Rheumatic pain in the right hand, at night, in bed.
Lower. Weariness in the legs, with dull pains and tingling.
Heavy laming pains in the calves of both legs, with pain in the left knee-joint.
70. Pain in the sole of the left foot (causing faintness), with feeling of faintness through the whole body.

Generalities.

Sticking pains: both scapulæ, right temple, right side of the chest, left ear, along the outer borders of both hands and both little fingers.
Heaviness of the limbs, with laziness and drowsiness.
He feels languid and sleepy.
Excessive tired feeling of all the limbs, especially when lying on the left side, relieved by lying on the right side.

Sleep.

75. Sleeplessness without restlessness; before 1 A. M.
Frightful dreams; nightmare.

Fever.

Pulse weak, irregular and laboring.
Chills with trembling all over the body.

Skin.

Troublesome itching over the whole body, not relieved by scratching.
80. Persistent itching spots over the whole body, following each other in rapid succession.

Conditions.

While in church she felt as if she would faint.
The stools during the day-time are copious, soft and of a dark or light yellowish brown color; at night they are scanty, hard and black.
Steady pressure sometimes relieves the pain.
Aggravation; in the evening, at night until 1 A. M., or after dinner until 4 P. M.; during rest; during passive motion; by writing.
85. *Amelioration;* from active motion; while exercising.

MERCURIUS SULPHURICUS (TURPETHUM.)

Mind and Disposition.

Low-spirited; with chilliness and yawning.
Ill-humor after eating.

Head.

Sensation of giddiness while standing, after headache.
Fulness in the head with occasional stitches.
5. Soreness and heaviness through the head (after breakfast and when walking about).

Ears.

Burning in the ears and in the face, after a chill.
Swelling of the parotid gland.

Nose.

Fluent coryza with sneezing.
Swelling and soreness of the tip of the nose.
10. Itching of the nose.

Face.

Pale, anxious looking countenance.
Burning heat of the face and ears after the chill.

Mouth and Throat.

Gums black and ulcerated.
The mouth is clammy and full of mucus in the morning.
15. Burning, smarting, stinging pain on the tip of the tongue (left side, in the evening).
Soreness, as if scalded on the tip of the tongue.
The tongue is coated white heavily, yellowish at the root of the tongue, the enlarged papillæ stand up like red points, with flat taste in the mouth and a reduced pulse.
Heat and sensation of constriction in the throat.
Dryness of the tongue and throat.
20. Burning in the mouth and throat.
Ptyalism.

Stomach and Abdomen.

Vomiting and diarrhœa.
Coldness or burning in the abdomen.

Stool and Anus.

After drinking coffee, pain in the abdomen as if diarrhœa would set in.
25. Stools soft and earlier in the morning than usual.
Sudden and violent pressing to stool while walking, compelling him to stand still, causing an anxious perspiration; later the stools are forcibly gushing out in a hot burning stream of yellow water; followed by great debility, hiccough and belching.
After the diarrhœic stools sensation of fulness as from congestions to the legs, especially the feet, they feel numb when standing.

Urinary Organs.

Diminished secretion of urine, does not micturate frequently but has constant pressure; urine dark, becoming turbid with a scum on it.
Increased secretion of urine, without a sediment.

Sexual Organs.

30. Gonorrhœa and syphilitic diseases, with great congestions to the parts.

Swelling of the testicles.

Respiratory Organs.

Roughness in the throat, and hoarseness.
Sensation of heat in the larynx.
Increased expectoration of mucus from the larynx and trachea.
35. Pain in the chest prevents him from breathing.
Pain in the right side of the chest, extending to the scapula, can scarcely breathe, worse from 4 to 5 P. M.
Pressure on the chest.
Dyspnœa; in children: Hydrothorax.

Extremities.

Upper. Numbness in the left forearm and hand, later numbness in the right hand.
40. Hands icy cold with blue nails.
Stiffness in the arms.
Lower. Pain in the knees and lameness, especially when walking.
Foot-sweat with soreness at the ends of the nails.
Ulcers on the ankles.

Generalities.

45. Most of the pains feel as if a dull stick pressed on the parts and were moving in diverse curved lines, feels as if this pain were in the bones.
Debility with sleepiness.
Rheumatic pains.

Sleep.

Frequent yawning and great sleepiness in the afternoon.
Sleeplessness after midnight.
50. Awakens with headache in the morning.

Fever.

Chilliness running up the back, with yawning and depression of spirits, followed by dull pain in the forehead, burning in the face and ears and slight fever.
Chilliness, restlessness and heaviness in the upper part of the abdomen, frequent yawning and diminished secretion of urine (in the afternoon).

Chill with nausea from 10 A. M. till 2 P. M.
Chill every other day.
55. The whole body feels cold externally.
Icy coldness of the hands.
Painful burning over the whole body, especially in the face but not on the feet, with violent thirst.

Skin.

Induration of the glands.
Psoriasis: Lepra.

Conditions.

60. In the sunshine sneezing.
The dyspnœa and chest symptoms are worse in the afternoon.
In hydrothorax it has proved a successful remedy where the dyspnœa and swollen extremities had yielded to no other remedy.

MERCURIALIS PERENNIS.

Head.

Giddiness on descending the stairs.
Head confused as if inflated.
The scalp feels tense and numb, is moved with difficulty.
Burning on the vertex.

Eyes.

5. Eyelids feel heavy and dry, it is difficult to move them.
Weakness of the upper eyelids.
Trembling of the upper eyelids.
Dilated pupils with great sensitiveness of the eyes to the light.

Nose.

The breath from the nose is cold.
10. Crawling and burning of the nose.

Face.

Feeling of coldness in the face.
Feeling of tension in the face and head.
Great redness of the cheeks.
Lips dry and parched, with increased thirst.

Mouth and Throat.

15. Dryness of the mouth, it is difficult to move the tongue and impedes chewing.

Burning in the mouth and tongue.

The tongue feels heavy and dry, numb, insensible, with loss of taste.

Burning, stitching blisters on the tongue, inside of the lips and cheeks; they form very painful spreading ulcers.

Burning dryness in the throat.

Stomach and Abdomen.

20. Chilly feeling or burning in the stomach.

Fever.

Cold over the whole body, with hot flush in the face; must be warmly covered, then sleeps and perspires.

Cold over the whole body, emanating from the right side, particularly from the right arm, shuddering, great debility, sleepiness.

Gooseflesh on the cold right arm, extending over the whole body; after midnight an offensive perspiration on both sides, particularly on the arms.

On going to bed in the evening chill, during the night and towards morning heat with intense thirst; perspiration in the morning.

MEZEREUM.

Mind and Disposition.

Restlessness when alone and longing for company.

Hypochondriac mood, with low spirits and weeping.

Indifference about every thing and everybody around him.

Aversion to talk, it seems to him to be hard work to utter one word.

5. Disposed to reproach others or to quarrel.

Irresolute.

Unable to recollect, the mind is easily confused.

Head.

Head feels dull or as if intoxicated.

Headache with chilliness, worse in the open air.

10. Headache in the temples, and sides of the head after an exertion and from talking much.

Violent headache and great sensitiveness to the least contact after a slight anger.

The head is covered with a thick leather-like crust, under which thick and white pus collects here and there, and the hair is glued together.

On the head great elevated white scabs, under which ichor collects in great quantity, and which begins to be offensive and breed vermin.

The scabs on the head look chalky and extend to the eyebrows and the nape of the neck.

15. Burning, biting itching on the scalp, principally on the vertex; when scratching the locality changes but the itching becomes worse; this is followed by very sore boils and humid eruptions, worse at night and when lying down.

Pain in the bones of the scalp (on both sides) with swelling and caries, great sensitiveness to contact, cold, motion, worse in the evening.

Numbness of the scalp, with drawing pain in it, generally only on one side; worse from cold, contact and in the evening.

Ameliorated by heat.

Dandruff, white, dry.

Eyes.

20. Inclination to wink with the eyes.

Dryness in the eyes, with pressure in them; the eyes feel too large.

Twitching of the muscles around the eyes.

Lachrymation, with smarting in the eyes.

Staring at one spot.

Ears.

25. Itching behind the ears, scratching causes small elevations, they are scratched off and feel sore.

The ears feel as if they were too open, and as if air were pouring into them, or as if the tympanum were exposed to the cold air, with a desire to bore with the fingers into the ear.

Otalgia.

Nose.

Twitching (visible) on the root of the nose.

Fluent coryza, soreness of the nose, scabs in the nose, and soreness and burning of the upper lip.
30. The sense of smell is diminished, with dryness of the nose.

Face.

Gray, earthy complexion.
Frequent, troublesome twitching of the muscles in the middle of the right cheek.
Dull cramp pain and benumbing pressure in the right malar bone, extending to the temples.
Swelling of the lower lip, with rhagades.
35. The child scratches the face constantly; it becomes covered with blood.
Face and forehead hot and red, with great restlessness and peevishness.
In the night the child scratches its face, so that the bed is covered with blood in the morning; and the face is covered with a scab, which the child keeps constantly tearing off anew, and on the spots thus left raw, large fat pustules form.
The ichor from the scratched face excoriates other parts.
A honey-like scab around the mouth.
40. The skin of the face is of a deep inflammatory redness, the eruption is humid and fat.

Mouth and Throat.

Stinging toothache, which extends to the malar bones and temples.
The teeth feel dull, and elongated.
Boring, stinging in decayed teeth, extending to the malar bone.
The teeth decay suddenly.
45. The teeth pain when touched by the tongue.
Burning in the mouth and throat.
Burning of the pharynx and œsophagus.
Constriction of the pharynx, the food presses on the part during deglutition.

Stomach and Abdomen.

Beer tastes bitter and causes vomiting.
50. Increased appetite noon and evening.
Sensation of nausea in the throat.
Sensation as if the posterior part of the throat were full of mucus, the same after hawking.
Unusual longing for ham fat.
Burning in the stomach, mouth and throat, relieved by eating (swallowing the food).

55. Dull pain in the region of the spleen.
Many short, fetid, flatulent discharges, especially before the stool.

Stool and Anus.

Constipation, stool dark brown, in knots, very hard balls, with great straining but not painful.
Stools soft, brown, smelling sour.
Soft stool in the evening, fermented stool, not fully digested, smelling very offensive or sour.
60. Excessive diarrhœa (small stools) with intolerable colic.
Brown feces, containing some white glistening bodies.
Chill before and after the stool.
During the stool, prolapsus ani with constriction of the anus, which makes it very difficult to replace it.
Before and after the stool, creeping in the rectum as from ascarides.
65. Stitch in the rectum upwards (in the afternoon).

Urinary Organs.

Decreased secretion of urine.
In the morning and forenoon, frequent discharges of large quantities of pale urine.
The urine becomes flaky and has a red sediment.
Hæmaturia.
70. Sticking in the kidney, and pain as if torn.
After micturition, itching at the prepuce.

Sexual Organs.

Men. Discharge of mucus from the urethra.
Heat and swelling of the penis.
Violent erections and increased sexual desire.
75. Painless swelling of the scrotum.
Swelling of the testicles.
Women. Menses too frequent and lasting too long.
Leucorrhœa, resembling albumen, malignant, corroding.

Respiratory Organs.

Dyspnœa, as if the chest were contracted, and as if there were adhesion of the lungs.
80. Sensation of constriction of the (muscles of the) chest.
Desire to draw a long breath.
The chest feels too tight on stooping.
Burning and dryness in the trachea, with hoarseness.
Soreness and burning in the bones of the thorax.
85. Stitches in the (right side of the) chest, worse from drawing a long breath.

Spasmodic, violent hooping-cough, caused by an irritation in the larynx, extending to the chest, expectoration in the morning, of a yellow, albuminous, tough mucus, tasting salt.

The cough is worse in the evening, till midnight; or day and night, with tension over the thorax; when eating or drinking any thing hot (has to cough till the food is vomited up); from drinking beer.

Back.

Rheumatic pains in the muscles of the shoulder-blade; they feel tense and swollen, and prevent motion.

Extremities.

Upper. The right arm feels sprained on top of the shoulder.
90. The right hand cold (while writing), the left warm (in a warm room).

Cold hands.

Trembling of the right hand.

The tips of the fingers are powerless, cannot hold any thing.

The hands (and feet) go to sleep continually.

95. *Lower.* The right hip-joint feels sprained on walking.

Twitching of the whole right leg.

Pain in the hip, the leg is shortened.

The whole chin is covered with elevated white scabs.

Cracking in the right knee, when rising in the morning.

100. The legs and feet go to sleep.

Stitches in the toes, of the right foot.

Pain in the periosteum of the long bones, especially the tibia, worse at night in bed, and then the least touch is intolerable.

Generalities.

Tension in the muscles.

Twitching in the muscles.

105. Burning of the internal parts, with external chilliness.

Sensitiveness to the cold air.

Sensitiveness to washing with cold water in the morning.

Sleep.

Great inclination to sleep from debility.

Sleep disturbed by violent pain in the face.

110. Awakens after midnight, from vivid dreams and with nightmare.

Fever.

Pulse full and hard; in the evening accelerated; intermitting at times.
Chill predominates even in the warm room.
Chill with thirst and desire for heat.
Chill from the upper arms, extending to the back and legs.
115. Heat in bed, mostly in the head.
Perspiration during sleep, following the chill, without previous heat.
Intermittent fever; chill over the whole body, accompanied by asthmatic contraction and tightness of the chest, in front and back.
During the cold stage, a peculiar thirst; dryness in the back part of the mouth, with accumulation of saliva in the fore part without any desire to drink.
During the cold stage, drowsiness in the warm room.

Skin.

120. Inflammation and swelling of the bones, rachitis, caries.
Itching in the evening when in bed, aggravated and changed to burning by touch or by scratching.
Sensitiveness to touch.
Ulcers: with an areola, sensitive and easily bleeding (when removing the linen, which sticks to the ulcer), painful at night, the pus tends to form an adherent scab, under which a quantity of pus collects, burning and stinging with inflammation.
Vesicles around the ulcers, itching violently and burning like fire.
125. Desquamation of the whole body.
Suppuration after inflammations.

Conditions.

Aggravation in the evening, at night, from contact, and motion.
One side of the body is generally affected. Bad consequences from the abuse of mercury.
Amelioration when walking in the open air.

MILLEFOLIUM.

Mind and Disposition.
Very excited, with pain in the pit of the stomach.
Sighing and groaning of children.

Head.
Vertigo when moving slowly, walking, but not when taking violent exercise, with nausea when stooping, not when lying down.
Sensation as if all the blood ascended to the head.
5. Violent headache, with twitching of the eyelids and muscles of the forehead.

Eyes.
Glistening eyes.
Agglutination of the eyes in the morning.
Lachrymation and discharges from the eyes.

Face.
Redness of the face without internal heat.

Nose.
10. Bleeding from the nose.

Mouth and Throat.
Ulcers on the gums.
Stomacace.
Tongue swollen and coated.
Elongation of the palate.
15. Ulcers in the throat.

Stomach and Abdomen.
Painful gnawing and digging in the stomach as from hunger.
Burning in the stomach, extending to the chest.
Violent pain in the pit of the stomach (during retrogressive small-pox).
Vomiting when coughing.
20. Nausea with vertigo.
Pain in the region of the liver.
Congestions to the portal system.
Colic during menstruation.
Ascites.
25. Incarcerated hernia.

28

Frequent emission of fetid flatulence.
Violent colic, with bloody diarrhœa (during pregnancy).
Dysentery.

Stool and Anus.

Hemorrhages from the rectum, caused by too violent exertion.
30. Mucous diarrhœa.
Profuse bleeding from the hæmorrhoidal tumors.

Urinary Organs.

Hæmaturia.
Involuntary micturition (Incontinence of urine).

Sexual Organs.

Men. Swelling of the penis or testicles.
35. The semen is not discharged during an embrace.
Sycotic excrescences.
Women. Hemorrhage from the uterus from too violent exertions.
Menses too profuse.
Suppressed menstruation with epileptic attacks.
40. Barrenness, with too profuse menstruation.
Suppressed lochia with violent fever, suppressed secretion of milk, or convulsions; convulsive motion of all the limbs and violent pain.
Lochia too profuse.
Sore nipples.

Respiratory Organs.

Very difficult breathing, with tetanic spasms.
45. Oppression of the chest, with bloody expectoration.
Hæmoptysis (after falling from a height, in the afternoon, in connection with hæmorrhoidal symptoms).
Violent palpitation of the heart and spitting of blood.

Extremities.

Upper. Pricking and numbness of the left arm.
Heat of the hands.
50. *Lower.* The feet go to sleep; first the left foot, later the right, disappearing on walking.
Heat of the feet.

Generalities.

Rheumatic and arthritic complaints.
Convulsions and fainting attacks of infants.
Hysterical spasms.

55. Paralysis and contraction of the limbs.
    Tetanus.
    Convulsions after parturition.
    Epileptic spasms from suppressed menstruation.
    Hemorrhages from various organs.

Sleep.

60. Violent yawning without being tired.
    Goes to sleep late, and does not feel refreshed in the morning.

Fever.

Pulse accelerated and contracted.
Chilliness with pain in the kidneys.
Colliquative perspirations.

Skin.

65. Suppressed itch, and from it fever.
    Painless varices of pregnant women.
    Fistulous ulcers.
    Ulceration of internal organs.
    Cancerous ulcers.
70. Wounds—after the operation for the stone of the bladd
    Bruises, bleeding from the wounds.
    Bad effects from a fall (from a height) and sprains.

Conditions.

Especially suitable for aged persons, children and for women.
Coffee causes congestion to the head.

MOSCHUS.

Mind and Disposition.

Great anxiety with palpitation of the heart.
Hypochondriacal anxiety and ill humor.

Head.

Vertigo as soon as the head is moved.
Stupifying, compressing headache, mostly in the forehead,
   with nausea in the evening, worse when moving the
   head and in the room, better in the open air.
5. Tension in the back part of the head and neck with nausea,
   worse in the evening, when sitting in the room, and
   when becoming cold, better in the open air, and when
   getting warm.

Headache with nausea, compelling one to lie down.
Congestion of blood to the head, heaviness of the head.
Compressing headache, especially right over the root of the nose.

Eyes.

Pressing, itching and pimples on the eyes.
10. The eyes are turned upwards, fixed and glistening.
Attacks of sudden blindness.

Ears.

Detonation in the (right) ears like the report of a cannon, accompanied with the discharge of a few drops of blood.
Hardness of hearing.

Nose.

Bleeding from the nose.
15. Crawling in the point of the nose.

Face.

Earthy, pale complexion.
Pale face, with perspiration.
Redness of the right cheek without heat, with paleness of the left, which feels hot.
Heat in the face without redness, and with dimness of sight.
20. Tension in the facial muscles, as if too short.
Peeling off of the lips.
Movement of the lower jaw, as if he were chewing.

Mouth.

Great dryness in the mouth.

Stomach and Abdomen.

Sudden nausea, as from the pit of the stomach; the umbilicus being drawn in.
25. Sensation of fulness and oppression in the pit of the stomach, with qualmishness, worse from eating.
Hysterical abdominal spasms.
Sensation as if every thing in the abdomen were constricted, compelling one to move about, cannot do any work, or remain quiet anywhere.
Incarcerated flatulence.

Stool and Anus.

Stools soft, smell sweetish.
30. Involuntary loose stools during sleep.
Stitches in the anus, extending to the bladder.

Urinary Organs.
Copious watery urine.

Sexual Organs.
Men. Violent sexual excitement.
Involuntary emissions, painful, without erections.
35. Erections with desire to urinate.
Impotence occasioned by a cold.
Women. Violent sexual desire.
Menses too early and too profuse.
Pressing and drawing in the genitals, as if the menses would appear.

Respiratory Organs.
40. Constriction of the trachea, as from the vapors of sulphur.
Suffocative spasmodic constrictions of the chest, especially as soon as he becomes cold.
Soreness of the thorax under the arms, when pressing on it.
Hysterical spasms of the chest.

Extremities.
Lower. Sensation of coldness on the tibia.
45. Restlessness in the lower extremities, he has to move them all the time.

Generalities.
Fainting and weakness, especially at night in bed, or in the open air, or with hysterical persons.
Convulsions—tetanic spasms.
Hysterical complaints.
Hypochondriacal complaints, originating in the sexual system.

Sleep.
50. Sleepiness in day-time.
Cannot lie at night in one position, because the parts on which one lies feel as if dislocated and sprained.
Sleeplessness from over-excitability; of hysterical persons.

Fever.
Pulse full and accelerated, with ebullitions.
Weak pulse, faintings from anæmia.
55. Chill and chilliness, which extends itself over the whole body, from the scalp.
Sensation as if cold air were blowing on him, especially on uncovered parts.
External coldness, with internal heat.
One cheek is pale and hot, the other is red and cold.

Burning heat in the evening, in bed, frequently only on the right side, with restlessness and inclination to uncover oneself.
60. The one hand is burning hot and pale, the other is cold and red.
Clammy perspiration in the morning, smelling of musk.

Skin.
Herpes with excessive burning.

Conditions.
Aggravation in the cold air.
Amelioration on getting warm, or being in the warm air.

MUREX PURPUREA.

Mind and Disposition.
Weakness of memory, and difficulty of connecting words.

Head.
Headache in the morning on waking, going off after rising.

Ears.
Cramp pains behind the ears.

Nose.
Coldness of the nose all day.

Face.
5. Burning of the right cheek towards evening, and of the left cheek early in the morning.

Urinary Organs.
Frequent desire to urinate, urine colorless.
Urine smells almost like Valerian, forms a white sediment; after urinating, discharge of mucus.
Discharge of some blood in urinating.

Sexual Organs.
Women. Violent excitement in the sexual organs, and excessive desire for an embrace; excited by the least contact of the parts.
10. Feeling of dryness and constriction of the uterus.
Beating in the uterus.

Sore pain in the uterus, as if cut by a sharp instrument.
Violent pain in the right side of the uterus, extending through the abdomen to the chest.
Feeling of heaviness in the vagina during the colic.
15. Feeling of heaviness and enlargement of the labia majora.
Menstruation too profuse—hemorrhages.
During the profuse menstruation, sensation of constriction at the uterus.
Bloody leucorrhœa, during stool.
Violent pains, acute stitches in the mammæ.
20. Leucorrhœa; watery, greenish, thick, bloody.

Respiratory Organs.

Altered voice; hoarseness.
Wheezing in the chest, when breathing in the evening.
Pain in the chest as if bruised.
Palpitation of the heart, and throbbing in the carotids.

Extremities.

25. *Upper.* Pain in the forearm below the elbow.
Heat in the hands.
Lower. Pain (burning, as if sore) in the loins.
Pains in the hips and loins when lying in bed.
Great weakness and weariness in the lower limbs.
30. Weariness and contused sensation in the thighs.

MURIATIC ACID.

Mind and Disposition.

Sad, taciturn, with anxious apprehension.
Sadness, peevishness.
Irritable, disposed to anger and chagrin.

Head.

Vertigo, with tottering gait.
5. Headache, as if the brain were torn or demolished.
Feeling as if the brain were loose.
Tearing and stitches in the head, coming on in periodical shocks.
Heaviness in the back part of the head, with obscure sight, aggravated by the effort to see.

Headache from walking in the open air, especially in the cold wind.
10. Headache, aggravated from rising up in bed, and from moving the eyes, ameliorated by moving the body.

Eyes.

Itching, smarting in the corners of the eye.
Itching in the eyes.
Stitches out of the eyes.
Swelling and redness of the eyelids.
15. Perpendicular half-sightedness.

Ears.

Otalgia, with pressing pain.
Beating in the ear.
Hardness of hearing deafness.
Very sensitive to noise and over acuteness of hearing.
20. Tingling, humming and whizzing in the ear.

Nose.

Continuous bleeding from the nose.
Sore nostrils with stinging pain.
Obstruction of the nose.
Coryza, with thick yellow or watery, corrosive discharge.

Face.

25. Heat in the face, and glowing redness of the cheeks when walking in the open air, without thirst.
Pimples forming scabs on the face, forehead and temples.
Bloated lower lip, it feels heavy and burns.
Burning of the lips.
Pimples around the lips forming a scurf.
30. Freckles.

Mouth and Throat.

Toothache (pulsating), aggravated from cold drinks, better from heat.
Tingling in the teeth.
Scorbutic gums, swollen, easily bleeding and ulcerating.
Great dryness in the mouth.
35. The tongue feels heavy as if it were lead, which prevents him from talking; feels as if paralyzed.
Deep ulcers (with black base) and vesicles on the tongue.
Sensation in the mouth as if it were glued up with insipid mucus; much saliva in the mouth.
The tongue becomes sore and bluish.
The tongue dwindles (shrinks), (atrophy of the tongue).

40. Rawness and smarting of the feces.
   Dry throat with burning in the chest.
   Every thing tastes sweet.
   Acrid and putrid taste in the mouth, like rotten eggs, with ptyalism.

Stomach and Abdomen.

Excessive hunger and thirst.
45. Aversion to meat.
   Hiccough (before and after dinner).
   Bitter, or putrid eructations.
   Vomiting of the ingesta.
   Sensation of emptiness in the stomach.
50. Pressing and tension in the hypochondria.
   Fulness and distension of the abdomen, from small quantities of food.

Stool and Anus.

Stool is discharged with difficulty, as from inactivity of the intestines.
Diarrhœa, with smarting and burning in the rectum and anus.
Involuntary discharge of thin, watery stool while urinating.
55. Discharge of blood with the stool.
   Prolapsus ani, while urinating.
   Hæmorrhoidal tumors, swollen, blue, with burning soreness.

Urinary Organs.

Frequent micturition with profuse discharge.
Profuse discharge of watery urine.
60. Slow emission of urine; weakness of the bladder.
   Involuntary discharge of urine.

Genital Organs.

Men. Feeling of weakness in the genital organs, penis relaxed (impotence).
Soreness in the margin of the prepuce.
Itching of the scrotum, not relieved by scratching.
65. *Women.* Menses too early and too profuse.
   Pressing on the genitals as if the menses would appear.
   During the menses sad and taciturn.

Respiratory Organs.

Breathing deep and groaning; moaning.
Oppression across the chest (evening).
70. Stitches in the chest, and on the heart, when taking a long breath and on violent motion.
   Tension and pain on the sternum.

Hoarseness, with sore feeling in the chest.
Violent palpitation of the heart, which is felt in the face (at night).

Back.

Pressing pain in the back, as from a sprain, or as if he had stooped long.

Extremities.

75. *Upper.* Heaviness of the arms, especially the fore-arms.
Scabby eruption on the back of the hands and fingers.
Numbness, coldness and deadness of the fingers at night.
Swelling and burning of the tips of the fingers.
Lower. Wavering gait from weakness of the thighs.
80. Swelling, redness and burning of the tips of the toes.
Putrid ulcers on the lower extremities.

Generalities.

Rheumatic pains in the extremities during rest, better from motion.
Great debility as soon as he sits down, his eyes close; the lower jaw hangs down, he slides down in the bed.
Great sensitiveness to damp weather.

Sleep.

85. Great sleepiness during the day, going off as soon as one moves about.
Sleeplessness before midnight, tossing about and delirium, he slides down in the bed.
Wakens early in the morning with a chill.

Fever.

Pulse weak and slow, frequently intermitting every third beat.
Chilliness predominates.
90. Chill in the evening, with coldness in the back, with external warmth and burning in the face.
Shuddering over the whole body, with hot cheeks and cold hands.
Chill and heat without thirst.
Internal heat with desire to uncover oneself, and restlessness in the body.
Burning heat, especially in the palms of the hands and soles of the feet.
95. Perspiration during the first sleep, till midnight, especially on the head and back.
Night and morning sweat.

In the evening, in the bed, the perspiration is first cold on the feet.

Typhus fever, the lower jaw hangs down, atrophy of the tongue, involuntary watery stools when passing urine, great debility, with sliding down in the bed, loud moaning.

Skin.

Scurfy eruptions, itching when getting warm in bed.
100. Blood-boils, pricking on being touched.
Painful putrid ulcers (lower legs), with burning at their circumference.
Fetid odor of the ulcers; also, they are covered with a scurf.
Black pocks.
Dropsical swellings.
105. Painfulness and drawing in the periosteum, as in intermittent fever.

NATRUM CARBONICUM.

Mind and Disposition.

Restlessness, with attacks of anxiety, especially during a thunder-storm.
Aversion to man and society.
Hypochondriacal mood, tired of life.
Mind much agitated, every event (music) causes trembling.
5. Out of humor, peevish, irritable, angry.

Head.

Vertigo from drinking wine and from mental exertion.
Inability to think and to perform any mental labor; the head feels stupefied if he tries to exert himself.
Difficulty in comprehending what one hears or reads and in connecting ideas.
Dulness of the head, when at rest or when in the sun.
10. Headache from the sun or when turning the head rapidly.
Tension and obstruction in the head, as if the forehead would burst.
Stupefying, pressing headache in the forehead, with nausea, eructations and dimness of sight, in the evening; worse in the room.

Stitches in the head and out of the eyes.
Pulsating headache in the vertex every morning.
15. Congestion of blood to the head, with heat in it.
Tearing pain in the forehead, returning at certain hours of the day.

Eyes.

Heaviness of the upper eyelids.
Stitches in the eyes from within outwards.
Inflammatory swelling of the eyelids (right upper lid).
20. Aversion to light.
Ulcers on the cornea.
Cannot read small print.
Black spots (before the eyes when writing) or dazzling flashes before the eyes.
Sensation as of feathers before the eyes.
25. Dim eyes; has to wipe them constantly.

Ears.

Otalgia, with sharp-piercing stitches in the ears.
Hard hearing, as if the ears were closed up.
Over-sensitiveness of hearing, sensitiveness to noise.

Nose.

Red nose with white pimples on it.
30. Peeling off of the dorsum and tip of the nose; painful when touched.
Ulcerated nostrils, high up in the nose.
Coryza with cough, from the least current of air, only going off by sweat.
Obstruction of the nose; hard, fetid clots come out of one nostril.
Thick, yellow or green discharge from the nose.
35. Coryza on alternate days.

Face.

Bloated face.
Burning heat and redness of the face.
Swelling of the cheeks, with redness.
Pale face with blue rings around the eyes, swollen eyelids.
40. Freckles in the face.
Yellow blotches on the forehead and upper lip.
Humid, herpetic eruptions and ulcers on the nose, around the mouth, on the lips.
Swelling of the upper lip.
Burning rhagades in the lower lip.

Mouth and Throat.

45. Flat ulcers and blisters inside of the mouth, burning and painful when touched.
    Digging, boring toothache, especially during or after eating sweatmeats or fruit.
    Great sensitiveness of the lower teeth.
    Nightly pressing toothache, with swelling of the lower lips and of the gums.
    Stuttering on account of heaviness of the tongue.
50. Burning about the tip of the tongue, as if it were cracked.
    Throat and œsophagus feel rough, scraped and dry.
    Accumulation of mucus in the throat.
    Much nasal mucus passes through the posterior nares.

Stomach and Abdomen.

Incessant thirst: great desire for cold water a few hours after dinner.
55. Increased and ravenous hunger in the forenoon, from sensation of emptiness in the stomach.
    Empty eructations (after eating).
    Aversion to milk, and diarrhœa from it.
    Very weak digestion; after eating, hypochondriacal humor.
    The food tastes bitter.
60. After every meal pressure in the stomach.
    Sensitiveness of the pit of the stomach to the touch, and when talking.
    Continuous qualmishness and nausea.
    Colic, with constriction around the stomach.
    Stitches in the left hypochondrium; also after drinking very cold water.
65. Stitches in the region of the liver and spleen (chronic inflammation of the liver).
    Hard, bloated, swollen abdomen.
    Tumors on the abdomen, as if the intestines were distended by wind here and there.
    Colic, with contraction of the navel and hardness of the integuments of the abdomen.
    Accumulation of flatulence, incarcerated flatulence, and loud rumbling of the flatulence.
70. Passes much flatus, smelling sour or fetid.

Stool and Anus.

Frequent ineffectual urging to stool, or too scanty, inefficient evacuations.

Soft or watery discharges, with violent sudden pressure and tenesmus.
Diarrhœa; stools yellow, or with colic, after taking cold.
The stool is watery and is discharged in a gush.
75. Stools bloody.
Burning and cutting in the anus and rectum during and after stool.
Itching and creeping at the anus.
With the stools discharge of tape-worm.

Urinary Organs.

Frequent strong desire to urinate, with profuse discharge.
80. Involuntary micturition at night (wetting the bed).
Urine dark-yellow, smelling fetid or sour, depositing a mucous sediment.
Burning in the urethra during and after micturition.

Sexual Organs.

Men. Increased sexual desire. (Priapism.)
Continuous painful erections.
85. Inflammation, swelling, and easy excoriation of the prepuce and glans penis.
Heaviness and drawing in the testicles.
The testicles feel bruised.
Discharge of prostatic fluid after micturition and after a difficult stool.

Respiratory Organs.

Dyspnœa and shortness of breathing, occasioned by tension of the chest.
90. When breathing, tension in the chest.
Stitches in the chest.
Hoarseness, with roughness of the chest, coryza, chilliness, and scraping, painful cough.
Violent dry cough, when entering a warm room, while coming from the cold air.
Cough, with expectoration of salty, purulent, greenish pus.
95. Short cough, with rattling in the chest.
Chilliness in one (left) side of the thorax.
Violent, anxious palpitation of the heart, when ascending, and at night when lying on the left side.
Painful cracking in the region of the heart.

Back.

Stitches in the small of the back, when sitting.
100. Tingling (formication) in the back.
Stiffness of the neck.

NATRUM CARBONICUM. 447

Cracking in the cervical vertebra when moving the head.
Swelling of the glands of the neck.
Goitre; pain, pressing.

Extremities.

105. *Upper.* Rheumatic pain of the shoulder, arms and elbows, with weakness of the arms.
Twitches and twitching sensation in the arms and fingers on taking hold of any thing.
Cutting pain in the hands.
Trembling of the hands (morning).
Burning-itching and burning blisters on the fingers.
110. Contraction of the fingers.
The skin of the hands is dry, cracked and chapped.
Warts or herpes on the hands.
Swelling of the hands (in the afternoon).
Lower. Heaviness of the legs and feet, with tension in them when sitting or walking.
115. Tension in the bend of the knee; the muscles are shortened.
Cramps and tension in the calves, as if too short.
Blotches (as in lepra) on the legs.
The lower legs are swollen, inflamed, red and covered with ulcers.
Cutting pain and cramps in the feet.
120. Swelling of the feet and soles of the feet, with stinging in them when walking or stepping on them.
Easy dislocation and spraining of the ankle; the ankle is so weak that it gives way; the foot bends under when stepping on it.
Cold feet.
Black, ulcerated pustule on the heel.
Ulcer on the heel, arising from spreading blisters.
125. Smarting and soreness between the toes.
Swelling, tearing and soreness in the (big) toes, preventing sleep.
Blisters on the points of the toes, as if scalded.
Boring, drawing and stinging in the corns.

Generalities.

Involuntary twitching in the muscles and limbs.
130. Tingling, stinging in the muscles.
Contractions of the muscles (hands, bend of the knee, neck).
The whole body is relaxed and limber.
Great emaciation, with pale face, dilated pupils and dark urine.
Great liability to take cold; aversion to the open air.

135. Great debility; a short walk fatigues much; playing on the piano causes trembling.

Sleep.

Irresistible sleepiness during the day; difficulty of going to sleep late in the night and difficulty of waking in the morning.
Unrefreshing sleep, disturbed by vivid, voluptuous, disconnected dreams, violent erections and seminal emissions.
During the night, great restlessness, ebullitions, palpitation of the heart and nightmare.
During sleep, starts and twitches.

Fever.

140. Pulse accelerated mostly at night, with ebullitions.
Coldness and chilliness the whole day, more so in the forenoon, with cold hands and feet with hot head, or the reverse, hot hands and feet with cold cheeks.
Heat with great debility and sleep.
Heat with perspiration over the whole body.
Violent, anxious perspiration from every slight exertion.
145. Burning hot perspiration on the forehead when the hat presses him.
Night-sweats, with alternate dryness of the skin.
Perspiration while eating.
Cold, anxious perspiration, with trembling from the pains.

Skin.

Swelling and induration of the glands.
150. Herpes, in yellow rings, or suppurating.
Ulcers, with swelling and inflammatory redness of the affected parts.
Formication under the skin.
Skin, dry, rough and chapped.
Red, hard blotches.
155. Warts painful to the touch.
Cutting pain, burning and stinging in wounded parts.

Conditions.

Most symptoms appear while sitting, and go off on motion, pressing and rubbing.
Aggravation; in the forenoon; during a thunder-storm; after the slightest exertion; in the rays of the sun (headache); before eating; from talking.

NATRUM MURIATICUM.

Mind and Disposition.

Melancholy, dejected, sad, weeping, aggravated by consolations from others, with palpitation of the heart.
Apprehension for the future.
Hypochondriacal, tired of life.
Joyless, indifferent, taciturn.
5. Great tendency to start.
Hurriedness.
Passionate vehemence; gets angry at trifles.
Difficulty of thinking; absence of mind, weak memory.

Head.

Vertigo, when rising in bed in the morning, or when rising from bed and walking.
10. Emptiness of the head, with anguish.
Weariness in the head.
Vertigo, periodically appearing, with nausea, eructations, colic and trembling of the limbs.
Pressing headache, from both sides, as if the head were in a vice, in the morning; better when lying down.
Beating and pulsation in the head, mostly in the forehead, with nausea and vomiting; worse in the morning and when moving, better when lying with the head high; relieved by perspiration.
15. Rheumatic (tearing) pain in the head, from the root of the nose extending to the forehead, with nausea, vomiting, vanishing of sight; worse in the morning when waking from sleep, from mental exertion and motion; better when sitting still or when lying down.
Heaviness in the back part of the head; it draws the eyes together; worse in the morning; from warmth and motion; better when sitting, lying, or perspiring.
Violent headache, as if the head would burst.
Sensation of congestion of blood to the head; the head feels heavy.
Stitches through the head, extending to the neck and chest.
20. Heat in the head, with redness of the face, nausea and vomiting.

Periodical headaches during, after or before the menses.
Falling off of the hair as soon as it is touched, more on the forepart of the head, the temple, the whiskers, and on the genitals, especially during child-bed; with great sensitiveness of the scalp; with greasy, shining face, frequent headaches in the morning and from cold air.
Liability to take cold in the head.
Great sensitiveness of the scalp to the touch, especially on the temple, forehead and the borders of the hair; worse in the warm room, better in the open air.
25. Sensation as if the scalp were constricted; worse from talking and in the open air, better when sitting or lying.
The headache ceases on one side of the head; it continues more violent on the other side.
Burning on the vertex.

Eyes.

Itching in the eyes.
Stinging-smarting and burning of the eyes.
30. Spasmodic contraction of the eyelids (evening).
Red, ulcerating eyelids.
Inflammation of the eyes, with ulcerated eyelids and glutinous mucus in the (external) canthi.
Acrid tears in the eyes (morning).
Obscuration of sight when stooping and walking, when reading and writing.
35. The letters run one into another when reading.
Double vision.
One half of the object is visible, the other half is dark.
Black points or streaks of light before the eyes.
Fiery, zigzag appearance around all things.

Ears.

40. Stitches in the ears.
Pulsation and beating in the ear.
Swelling, burning and heat of the ears.
Hardness of hearing.
Discharge of pus from the ears.
45. Humming, ringing, and singing in the ears.
Painful cracking in the ear when masticating.
Itching behind the ears.

Nose.

One-sided (left side) inflammation and swelling, and swelling of the nose with painfulness to the touch.
The nose feels numb on one side.

50. Soreness in the nose, with swelling of the interior wings.
Scabs and scurf in the nose.
Loss of smell (and taste).
Bleeding of the nose (when coughing at night), (when stooping).

Face.

Face shining, as from grease.
55. Complexion yellowish, pale, livid.
Redness of one (the left) cheek (afternoon, night).
Heat in the face.
Swollen face.
Itching and eruptions on the face (crusta lactea).
60. Pain in the cheek-bones, as if bruised when masticating.
Lips dry, cracked, with rhagades, or sore and ulcerated, with burning-smarting eruptions and scabs, easily bleeding.
Fever-blisters on the lips.
Herpetic eruption around the mouth.
Swelling of the upper lip.
65. Ulcer on the (left) cheek.
Blood-blisters on the inside of the upper lip.
Eruptions and ulcers on the chin.
Tingling and numbness of the lips.
Swelling of the submaxillary glands.

Mouth and Throat.

70. Teeth very sensitive to the air and contact.
Pain (drawing, tearing) in the teeth, extending to the ears and throat, after eating and at night, with swelling of the cheek.
Decayed teeth feel lose, burn, sting and pulsate.
Fistula dentalis.
Gums very sensitive to warm and cold things, swollen, inflamed, putrid, easily bleeding.
75. In the mouth and on the tongue blisters and ulcers, with smarting-burning pain when touched by the food.
Hæmoptysis.
Heaviness of the tongue, with difficulty of speech.
Numbness and stiffness of one side of the tongue.
Sensation as of a hair on the tongue.
80. Dryness of the mouth, lips, and especially of the tongue.
Ptyalism.
Burning at the tip of the tongue.
Swelling; sensation of constriction and stitches in the throat.

Long-continued sore throat, with the sensation as if she had to swallow over a lump.
85. Hawking up of mucus in the morning.

Stomach and Abdomen.

Loss of taste (and smell).
The water tastes putrid.
Putrid or sour taste while fasting.
Bitter taste in the mouth.
90. Continuous thirst (with nausea).
Excessive appetite.
Longing for bitter food and drink.
During meals perspiration in the face.
After eating, empty eructations, nausea, acidity in the mouth, sleepiness, heartburn, palpitation of the heart.
95. Soreness, as if bruised in the pit of the stomach, when pressing on it, with swelling.
In the region of the liver, stitches and tension (chronic inflammation of the liver).
In the region of the spleen, stitches and pressure.
Swelling of the abdomen.
Colic with nausea, relieved by discharge of flatulence.
100. Red spots on the pit of the stomach.
Burning in the intestines.
Nausea in the morning; vomiting, first of food, later of bile.
Rumbling in the abdomen.

Stool and Anus.

Constipation; stools difficult to discharge, hard, dry, crumbling, like sheep's dung.
105. Evacuations difficult, with stitches in the rectum.
Diarrhœa like water, with colic.
Involuntary stools.
Passes blood with the stool.
Alternate constipation and papescent stools.
110. During and after stool, burning in the anus and rectum.
Smarting and pulsations in the rectum.
Hæmorrhoidal tumors with stinging pain.
Soreness at the anus and around it when walking.
Tetter at the anus.

Urinary Organs.

115. Frequent and strong desire to urinate (day and night), with profuse discharge.
Involuntary micturition, when coughing, walking and laughing.

Pale urine with brick-dust sediment.
Discharge of mucus from the urethra.
During micturition stitches in the bladder, smarting, burning in the urethra; smarting and soreness in the vulva.
120. After micturition spasmodic contraction in the abdomen; burning, drawing and cutting in the urethra, and a discharge of thin, glutinous substance.
Urine dark, like coffee, or black.

Sexual Organs.

Men. Excessive irritability of the sexual instinct or impotence.
After an embrace, seminal emissions.
Itching, soreness and herpes between the scrotum and the thighs.
125. Itching and stinging on the glans penis and on the scrotum.
Women. Pressing and bearing down in the genitals.
Menstruation too early and too profuse, or too late and too scanty.
Suppressed menstruation: difficulty in the appearance of the first menses.
During the menstruation, melancholy, colic.
130. Before, during and after the menstruation, headache.
Itching on the genitals.
Aversion to an embrace.
Sterility, with too early and too profuse menstruation.
Fluor albus, acrid, greenish; increased discharge when walking; with yellow complexion.

Respiratory Organs.

135. Hoarseness, with dryness in the larynx.
Accumulation of mucus in the larynx (in the morning).
Dry cough, from tickling in the throat or in the pit of the stomach, day and night, especially when walking and drawing a long breath.
Morning cough.
Hooping-cough, caused by tickling in the throat or pit of the stomach, with expectoration (only in the morning) of yellow or blood-streaked mucus, with violent pain in the head, as if the forehead would burst, or with shocks; beating and hammering in the head; involuntary micturition; stitches in the liver.
140. The cough is worse in the evening after lying down.
Dry cough with rattling in the chest.
Cough, with expectoration of bloody mucus.

Shortness of breathing on walking fast; relieved when exercising the arms and in the open air.
Sensation and pain in the chest, as from tension.
145. Stitches in the chest and sides, with shortness of breathing, especially when taking a long inspiration.
Violent palpitation of the heart from every exertion, and especially when lying on the left side.
Fluttering motion of the heart.
Irregular, intermitting beats of the heart.

Back and Neck.

In the small of the back pain, as if bruised, as if lame; stitches, cutting, pulsation.
150. Tension and drawing in the back.
Over-sensitiveness of the spine.
Stitches in the neck and back part of the head.
Painful stiffness of the neck.
Scabs in the axilla; painful soreness of the cervical glands when coughing.
155. The pain in the back is relieved by lying on something hard.

Extremities.

Upper. Sensation of lameness and of a sprain in the shoulder-joint.
Cramp in the arms, hands, finger and thumb.
Weakness and paralytic heaviness of the arms.
Stitches in the muscles and joints of the hands and fingers.
160. Involuntary movement of the hands.
Tingling in the hands (and feet), especially on the joints and tips of the fingers (and toes).
Brown spots on the hands.
The finger-joints move with difficulty.
Dry, cracked skin of the hands, especially around the nails.
165. Warts in the palms of the hands.
Perspiration of the hands.
Trembling of the hands when writing.
Swelling of the right hand.
Hang-nails.
170. Pain in the hip, as if sprained, with stitches.
Restlessness in the legs, compelling one to move them constantly.
Sensation as if the legs were paralyzed, especially the ankles.
Twitching of the muscles of the thighs.
Tension in the bends of the limbs, and sensation as if the tendons were shortened; painful contraction of the hamstrings.

175. Pain as if the knees and ankles were sprained.
 Weakness in the knees and calves.
 Cramps in the lower legs and calves.
 Great heaviness of the legs and feet.
 Burning of the feet.
180. Swelling of the feet.
 Cold feet.
 Sensation in the tarsal joint as if bruised when walking and when touching it.
 Suppressed perspiration of the feet.
 Redness of the big toe, with tearing and stinging on walking or standing.
185. Sensation as if the limb had gone to sleep (feet, fingers).
 Corns, with boring, stinging pains.

Generalities.

Great weakness and relaxation of all bodily and physical powers from the least exertion.
Disinclination to move and walk after rising, with great heaviness and indolence in the morning.
The limbs feel weak and as if they were bruised, especially in the morning after rising.
190. Hysterical debility; the debility is greatest in the morning in bed.
 Great emaciation.
 Stiffness of the joints; they crack on moving them.
 Shortening, contraction of the muscles.
 Twitching in the muscles and limbs.
195. Pulsations in the whole body from the least exertion.
 Restlessness in the limbs; they have to be moved constantly.
 Paralysis.

Sleep.

Sleepiness during the day with sleeplessness at night; is unable to go to sleep.
In the morning he feels unrefreshed.
200. Sleep with vivid, frightful dreams; dreams of burning thirst; starts and talks in the sleep and tosses about.
 Wakens with fright, violent headache and perspiration; with erethism of the blood; violent throbbing in the arteries.

Fever.

Pulse very irregular, frequently intermitting, especially when lying on the left side.
Pulse at one time rapid and weak, at another full and slow.
The pulsations shake the whole body.

205. Chill predominates; chilliness internally, as from want of natural heat, with icy coldness of the hands and feet (evening).
Continuous chilliness from morning till noon.
Flushes of heat with violent headache, chilliness over the back and perspiration in the axilla and soles of the feet.
Continuous heat in the afternoon, with violent headache and unconsciousness; they are gradually relieved during the perspiration which follows.
During the heat generally violent thirst.
210. Violent perspiration, relieving the painful symptoms present during the fever.
Much perspiration during the day, and inclination to perspire from the least exertion.
Debilitating, somewhat sour-smelling perspiration.
Night and morning sweat.
Intermittent fever. Chilliness with great thirst; afterwards great heat with violent thirst and excessive headache; at last profuse perspiration.
215. Chilliness, with increasing headache in the forehead every day at 9 A. M. until noon; afterwards heat with gradually appearing perspiration and thirst, the headache decreasing afterwards gradually.
In the forenoon chilliness for three hours, with blue nails and chattering of teeth; this is followed by heat, lasting as long, accompanied by obscuration of sight, stitches in the head, much thirst, pains in the back, followed by perspiration.
Chilliness at 10 A. M., commencing at the feet, followed by heat with headache and, later, perspiration.
Anticipating chilliness in the morning, with external coldness, great thirst, violent headache, stupefaction; afterwards slight heat, with some perspiration, faintishness, and weakness of the eyes.
Intermittent fevers after the abuse of Chininum sulph., or with yellow complexion, great debility, drawing pain in the limbs, headache (worse during the hot stage), pressure in the stomach, loss of appetite, excessive thirst, fever-blisters on the lips.

Skin.

220. Nettle-rash after violent exercise (itching).
Itching and pricking in the skin.
Large red blotches, itching violently.

Rash over the whole body, with stinging sensation in the skin.
Pain and redness of an old cicatrix.
225. Varices.
Blood-boils.
Herpes (in the bend of the knee).
Warts in the palms of the hands.

Conditions.

Bad effects from anger (mortification caused by offence).
230. Bad effects from acid food and bread.
The nightly pains cause dyspnœa and a one-sided paralysis.
Most of the complaints appear or are renewed while lying down, especially at night, or in the morning, and are relieved when sitting up.
Aggravation at 10 A. M.; every exertion increases the circulation; on looking fixedly at an object; from talking (the weakness), when writing or reading.
Amelioration while fasting, while lying on the back or on the right side, after lying down.
235. Natrum mur. is an antidote to Argentum nitricum (especially if it has been applied locally), and to Chininum sulph.
It follows well and is well preceded by Apis mel.; to which it also stands in an antidotal relation.

NATRUM NITRICUM.

Ears.

Otalgia; the pain seems to be in the tympanum, in the evening; with warmth in the ear, coldness of the right concha, burning heat of the left, which extends beyond the temple.

Stomach and Abdomen.

Sourish taste; sourish eructations.
Distended abdomen, with a feeling of heaviness in it, followed by emission of a quantity of wind and eructations.
Flatulence, with pressure in the pit of the stomach and under the sternum.
5. Painful retraction of the abdominal muscles towards the spinal column.

Stool and Anus.

Constipation; the stool is discharged with difficulty, slow, and with the sensation after the stool as if the feces were still remaining.

NATRUM SULPHURICUM.

Mind and Disposition.

Sadness; inclined to weep.
Lively music disposes one to weep.

Head.

Vertigo after a meal; the heat extends from the abdomen to the head; relieved after the forehead becomes moist.
Heaviness in the head, with bleeding of the nose.
5. Periodical attacks in the right side of the forehead.
Pain, as if the forehead would burst, after a meal.
Jerks in the head, tossing it to the right side (forenoon).
Feeling of looseness of the brain, as if it were falling to the left temple (in the forenoon on stooping).
Sensitiveness of the scalp; the hair is painful on combing it.

Eyes.

10. Burning in the eyes, with discharge of burning water, with dimness of sight.
Burning and dryness of the eyes.
Dimness of sight, from weakness of the eyes.

Ears.

Pressing in the ears as if the tympanum were pressed out.

Nose.

Itching of the wings of the nose, inducing rubbing.
15. Bleeding of the nose during the menses (in the afternoon).

Face.

Pale complexion.
Itching of the face.
Vesicles on the lower lip.
Dryness of the upper lip, the skin peels off.
20. Pimples on the chin, they burn when touching them.

Mouth and Throat.

The gums burn like fire.
Feeling of numbness and roughness in the mouth.
Dryness, with redness of the gums and thirst.
Burning of the tongue; it feels as if covered with blisters.
25. The tongue is covered with mucus; slimy taste in the mouth.
Burning blisters on the tip of the tongue.
Burning of the palate as if sore and raw (during the menses).
Blisters on the palate, with great sensitiveness; relieved by cold.
Frequent constriction of the throat when walking.
30. Inflammation of the tonsils and uvula, with painful deglutition, and urging to swallow saliva.
Dryness of the throat, extending to the œsophagus.
Accumulation of mucus in the throat, particularly at night; with hawking up of salt mucus in the morning.

Stomach and Abdomen.

Great thirst for cold things; worse after exercise and in the forenoon.
After eating, perspiration in the face.
35. Gulping up of sour water.
Hiccough in the evening; after eating bread and butter.
Vomiting of sour mucus, or of saltish sour water (preceded by giddiness).
Qualmishness before eating.
Boring in the stomach, as if it would be perforated, or burning and pinching, in the morning after rising; better after breakfast.
40. Beating in the stomach, with nausea.
Stitches in the region of the liver, while walking in the open air.
Great sensitiveness of the region of the liver while walking.
Stitches in the left hypochondrium while walking in the open air.
Colic, griping in the abdomen; worse before breakfast; relieved in the afternoon by the emission of flatulence.
45. Painful digging in the abdomen during the menses, in the evening, followed by thirst.
Contractive pain in the abdomen, extending to the chest, with tightness of breath, and subsequent diarrhœa.
Pain, as if bruised, in the abdomen and small of the back.

Pinching in the abdomen, with the sensation as if the bowels were distended.

Pinching in the whole abdomen, with rumbling, shifting and subsequent diarrhœa.

50. Flatulent colic; accumulation and difficult emission of flatulence.

Incarceration of flatulence.

Emission of fetid flatulence (in the morning, after meals, and with the loose stools).

Stitch from the (left) groin to the axilla.

Stool and Anus.

Stool hard, with pressure; streaked with blood.

55. Looseness of the bowels.

Half-liquid stools, with tenesmus.

Diarrhœa, preceded by pain in the groins and hypogastrium.

Yellow liquid stools after rising from bed in the morning.

During stool profuse emission of flatulence.

60. Constant uneasiness in the bowels and urging to stool. (Chronic diarrhœa; tuberculosis abdominalis.)

After stool, burning at the anus.

Itching of the anus.

Urinary Organs.

Copious micturition, with brick-dust sediment.

Burning during or after micturition, or with pain in the small of the back on retaining the urine.

65. Gonorrhœa.

Sexual Organs.

Men. Itching of the glans or penis, obliging one to rub.

Itching of the scrotum, with burning after scratching.

Itching of the perineum and mons veneris.

Excited sexual desire (evening); erections (morning).

70. *Women.* Retarded, scanty menses, with colic.

Profuse menstruation, particularly when walking in the afternoon.

Menstrual blood acrid, corrosive and flowing profusely the first days; the last days (flowing longer than usual) discharge of lumps of coagulated blood.

Leucorrhœa.

Respiratory Organs.

Dry cough (in the morning, after rising from bed). At night, with soreness of the chest and roughness of the throat; has to sit up and hold the chest with both hands.

75. Loose cough, with expectoration; shortness of breathing; stitches in the left side of the chest.

Stitches in the left side of the chest, when sitting, when yawning, during an inspiration.

Back and Neck.

Pain in the small of the back, all night; has to lie on the right side; the back feels bruised when turning on it.

Pain as if stabbed between the shoulders.

Stitches in the nape of the neck (at night).

Extremities.

80. *Upper.* Twitchings of the hands (and feet), during sleep (more so after midnight).

Trembling of the hands on waking, and also when writing.

Loss of strength of the (left) hand, is unable to hold any thing heavy.

Tingling, ulcerative pain under the nail.

Panaritium.

85. Tingling in the tips of the fingers.

Lower. Pain in the hips, in the morning on rising, and all day, particularly on making certain motions (on stooping), more violent when rising from a seat or on moving about in bed.

Stabbing pain in the left hip (after a fall).

The pain in the hip is better in certain positions, but compels one to move again after a short time, causing intense suffering.

Legs and thighs feel weary and exhausted.

90. In the heels, lancinating pain, tearing and ulcerating pain.

Itching on or between the toes, in the evening on undressing.

Sleep.

Drowsiness in the forenoon, especially when reading or writing.

Starting as if in a fright, soon after falling asleep.

Anxious, frightful dreams disturb the sleep.

Fever.

95. Internal coldness, with yawning and stretching.

Coldness and shuddering with thirst.

Waking at night with chilliness, shaking and chattering of teeth, with anguish and thirst.

Chilliness, with warmth of the forehead and hands.

Dry heat in the afternoon.

100. Perspiration in the morning.

Conditions.

When lying long in one position, the restless desire to move compels a change which is very painful, and it is very difficult to find a new position which gives relief.

Aggravation of many symptoms in the morning, and amelioration after breakfast and in the open air.

NICCOLUM.

Mind and Disposition.

Low-spirited; fears something evil will happen.
Vexed and very angry from the least contradiction.

Head.

Dulness, does not comprehend the conversation, and is unable to relate properly in conversation.
Vertigo; in the morning; when rising after stooping, in the evening, when awaking with nausea and desire to vomit.
5. Fulness and heaviness in the head, compelling to rub the forehead with the hand.
Heaviness in the forehead in the morning, as if she had not slept sufficiently.
Heat and heaviness in the forehead (afternoon).
Headache all day, in the forenoon with vomiting of bile.
Heat in the head, compelling him to seek the open air, with thirst (afternoon).
10. Pressure on the vertex as from a hand.
The headache is worse in the room, after walking in the open air.
Stitches in the head (when stooping).
Tearing in the head and the left eye in paroxysms.
Periodical (every fortnight) headache.

Eyes.

15. Heat and redness of the eyes, with pressing in them.
The eyes are swollen, and cannot be opened in the morning.
Agglutination of the eyes in the morning.
The eyelids are red and swollen, with lachrymation and swelling of the meibomian glands.
Cold water causes redness of the eyes with tension.

20. Dryness and heat of the eyes (in the evening).
    Burning and pressing in the eyes (in the evening).
    Violent twitching in the eye, with lachrymation and difficulty of vision.
    The vision is very much impaired, especially in the evening.
    Objects appear too large; the light appears double; is surrounded by the colors of the rainbow.
25. Objects look blue (before the right eye).
    Cloud before the eyes (morning).
    Stitches in the edge of the eyelids like electric sparks, worse on touching them.

Ears.

Stinging in the ears.
Sudden deafness, with roaring and humming in the ears.

Nose.

30. Dryness of the nose.
    The nose is stopped up (right side) at night.
    Coryza, fluent during the day, and dry during the night.
    Stinging, tearing and soreness at the root of the nose.
    Redness and swelling at the tip of the nose, with burning.

Face.

35. The right side of the face is red and hot.
    Redness of the face, with burning and itching like erysipelas.
    Swelling of the right side of the face, with sore throat.
    The pain in the swollen face wakens him at night, it is relieved by cold.
    The skin of the face is chapped.
40. Twitching of the upper lip at intervals.

Mouth and Throat.

When the molar teeth (decayed) are sucked, a sour fetid water is drawn from them.
All the teeth feel loose and elongated.
Toothache, with tearing in the right ear.
Accumulation of thick mucus in the throat, with stinging pain.
45. Stitches in the throat (uvula) on swallowing.
    The whole throat feels sore as if ulcerated, on swallowing, worse in the morning, the (right side of the) neck is very sensitive, painful to pressure.
    The sore throat is worse in the evening, when talking and yawning.

Stiffness of the tongue, it is difficult to talk.
Bitter taste in the mouth in the morning.
50. The breath is offensive, of which he himself is not aware.

Stomach and Abdomen.

Aversion to meat.
Violent thirst day and night.
Hiccough (at night).
Bitter and sour eructations.
55. Nausea (morning).
Sensation of emptiness in the stomach, without hunger.
Sensation of great fulness in the stomach after eating.
Pressure in the stomach, relieved by eructations.
Painful sensation of constriction of the stomach.
60. Stitches in the stomach and pit of the stomach.
In the pit of the stomach, violent pain, like stabs with a knife.
Stitches in the stomach, extending to the back.
Burning in the stomach.
Pinching around the navel.
65. Painless rumbling in the abdomen.
Tension of the abdomen, and discharge of flatulence (during the menses).
Violent stitches, as with knives in the hypochondria.

Stool and Anus.

Constipation; ineffectual urging to go to stool, stool very hard and only discharged with great effort, has to press hard to discharge the soft stool.
Diarrhœa, with yellow mucus; expulsion with great force and with much flatulence.
70. Diarrhœa after drinking milk, and tenesmus.
During stool, burning and stitches in the rectum and anus.
After stool, itching, burning and stitches at the anus.

Urinary Organs.

Increased secretion of urine.
Burning at the orifice of the urethra, during micturition.
75. After micturition, discharge of thin leucorrhœa.

Sexual Organs.

Men. Erections (after dinner).
Itching on a small spot of the scrotum, scratching does not relieve it.
Women. Menses too late and too scanty.
During the menses, bloated abdomen, colic, pain in the small of the back, great debility, burning of the eyes.

80. Leucorrhœa, watery, especially after micturition.

Respiratory Organs.

Roughness in the throat, relieved by coughing.
Hoarseness, day and night; every year at the same time.
Cough from tickling in the trachea: in the evening, after lying down.
Dry, scraping cough, from tickling in the trachea, with sleeplessness from midnight till 4 A. M.
85. At night violent cough, compelling one to sit up and to hold the head.
Expectoration of white mucus.
When coughing, dyspnœa and pressure on the chest.
Stitches in the chest (left side) when breathing.
Pressure and heaviness on the chest.

Back and Neck.

90. Cracking in the neck when moving the head (forward or backward).
Pain in the neck, as from a sprain.
Stitches in the small of the back (afternoon).
Pain in the small of the back during a soft stool.
Itching and pimples in the small of the back.

Extremities.

95. *Upper.* Pain in the shoulders, as if sprained.
Itching on the shoulders; scratching does not relieve.
Rheumatic pains in the elbows, extending to the hands.
The hands feel heavy, tremble, feel bruised.
Rheumatic pains in the fingers.
100. *Lower.* Itching herpes on the hips.
Stitches in the right patella.
Rheumatic pains from the knees downward.
The feet feel heavy, tremble and are weak.
Stitches in the heel of the left foot.
105. Itching on the left heel.

Generalities.

Great restlessness; worse at night; is compelled to change the position continually; with vomiting and colic after suppressed menstruation.
Great debility, especially in the evening.
Heaviness in the hands and feet, relieved by motion.

Sleep.

Sleeplessness from over-wakefulness.

110. Feels refreshed in the morning, without having slept.
Restless sleep.
At 3 A. M., restlessness and heat; every thing feels sore, compelling one to rise and to walk about to obtain relief from it.
Awakens after midnight with colic.

Fever.

The chill is preceded or begins with yawning and sleepiness.
115. Chill, with chattering and shaking, followed by profuse general perspiration (in the evening in bed).
Heat in the evening, followed by chill.
Continuous chill, with moist palms of the hands.
Heat, restlessness and vomiting at night (must rise).
Anxious heat with violent thirst.
120. Dry heat with thirst, every afternoon at 3 o'clock.
Heat with perspiration and thirst, followed by chill.
Morning sweat.

Skin.

Itching; over the whole body, but mostly on the neck, as from fleas; not relieved by scratching, but followed by small vesicles.

NITRUM.

Mind and Disposition.

Despondency, out of humor, uneasy.
Timidity and apprehension (of death).

Head.

Headache, causing the eyelids to close; worse when the head is allowed to hang down (stooping).
Stupefying heaviness of the head in the morning, as after free indulgence in intoxicating drink.
5. Pain, as from constriction in the back part of the head; all the parts feel stiff, compelling one to bend the head backward, and relieved by tying up the hair.
Constricting headache, which concentrates in the tip of the nose.
Stinging pain in the head.

Pressing headache, aggravated by coffee and relieved by riding in the open air.
Headache after eating veal.
10. Great painful sensitiveness of the scalp.

Eyes.

Burning in the eyes, with lachrymation and aversion to light, especially in the morning, after washing in cold water.
In the evening, rainbow-colored circles around the light.
Every thing appears black before the eyes (after smelling Camphor).

Ears.

Tingling in the ears.
15. Deafness from paralysis of the auditory nerves.
Stitches in the ears at night; worse when lying on the ear.
Tension, sticking and tearing behind the (right) ear.
Inflammation and swelling of the right lobe, with violent burning and jerking.

Nose.

The tip of the nose is inflamed with stinging pains.
20. Swelling of the internal nose.
Ulcers in the nose (covered by a scurf).
Bleeding of the nose; the blood is acrid and sharp, like vinegar.
The nasal bones are painful, especially to the touch.

Face.

Color of the face pale.
25. Redness of the cheeks, with tension in them, while the headache becomes worse.
The pain like contraction in the eyes, forehead and face concentrates in the tip of the nose.
Pain in the bones of the face.

Mouth and Throat.

Stitches in hollow teeth, when touching them.
Pulsating toothache at night; worse from cold things.
30. Stinging or tearing toothache, with tearing in the head.
Inflammatory swelling of the gums; they bleed easily.
Fetid odor from the mouth.
Burning blister at the tip of the tongue.
The tongue is coated with white mucus.
35. Inflammation of the throat, with stinging pain during deglutition.

Pain in the throat, as if it were going to close at night, with dyspnœa.
Impeded deglutition from tension and cutting in the larynx.

Stomach and Abdomen.

Violent thirst, with want of appetite.
The appetite is strongest in the evening.
40. Nausea, especially at night.
Vomiting of mucus with blood.
Pressure in the pit of the stomach, with gnawing and faintish weakness.
Burning in the stomach or sensation of coldness (inflammation of the stomach).
Contractive, spasmodic colic, especially after eating veal.
45. Incarcerated flatulency, especially in the evening.

Stool and Anus.

Constipation; stool hard and only discharged by violent pressing.
Soft stools, with colic.
Stools watery, bloody.

Urinary Organs.

Frequent micturition, with discharge of large quantities of pale urine with reddish clouds.

Sexual Organs.

50. *Women.* Menstruation too early and too profuse, with black blood.
Before and during the menstruation violent colic and pain in the small of the back.
Leucorrhœa thin, stiffening the linen, discharged with violent pains in the small of the back.

Respiratory Organs.

Hoarseness, with roughness and scraping in the larynx.
Cough, which awakens one at 3 A. M., with violent stupefying headache.
55. Cough in the open air, when ascending, when arresting the breathing.
Cough, with cutting pain in the chest; with stitches in the chest and expectoration of clear blood.
Suppuration of the lungs, with profuse (colliquative) perspiration.
Dyspnœa, not allowing to lie with the head low.
Constrictive pain in the chest, as if the lungs were constricted from the back.

60. Stitches in the chest on drawing a long breath, while lying and coughing, with great anxiety and dyspnœa. (Inflammation of the lungs.)

Violent palpitation of the heart, especially at night when lying.

Back and Neck.

Stitches in and between the shoulder-blades, which impede the breathing; worse at night while lying on the back, better while lying on the right side.

Violent pain in the small of the back at night, or in the morning on waking, and when stooping.

Violent pain in the neck, extending to the shoulders, as if one were drawing the hair backwards with great violence.

Extremities.

65. *Upper.* Rheumatic pains in the shoulders at night.

Rheumatic pains and stitches in the joints of the shoulder, of the elbow, hands and fingers, especially at night, with the sensation as if the hands and fingers were swollen and too large.

Numbness and tingling in the arms and hands.

Stiffness and tension in the finger-joints.

Lower. Rheumatic pains in the legs.

70. Great debility and paralytic weakness in the lower legs after a short walk.

Numbness and tingling in the feet.

The toes are contracted.

Generalities.

The affected parts feel numb, as if they were made of wood.

Great debility, with sensation of heat in the face and hot forehead (morning).

75. Rheumatic pains and stitches in the limbs and joints.

The debility is worse while sitting than when moving about moderately.

Inflammation of internal organs.

Sleep.

Sleepiness during the day.

Restless sleep at night; nightmare.

Fever.

80. Pulse full, hard and rapid.

Pulse slow in the morning, rapid in the afternoon and evening.

Chilliness and coldness in the afternoon and evening; aggravated from every exertion and ceasing when lying down.
Chill, followed by perspiration without previous heat.
Chill in the evening, with pain.
85. Coldness in the afternoon, with thirst.
Heat at night, without thirst and without perspiration following.
Very debilitating perspiration from the least exertion.
Night-sweat most profuse on the lower extremities.
Morning-sweat most profuse on the chest.

Skin.

90. Pricking in the skin like needles, followed by burning, especially in the face.
Burning vesicles filled with a yellow fluid; they burst when scratched and relieve the burning.
Sudden hydropical swelling.

Conditions.

Aggravation after midnight, afternoon and evening; from smelling camphor; from eating veal.
The conditions which are aggravated during the day are relieved in the evening, after lying down.

NITRIC ACID.

Mind and Disposition.

Sadness, despondency.
Anxiety about his disease, with fear of death.
Excessive nervousness, great excitability, especially after the abuse of mercury.
Taciturn, disinclined to communicate any thing.
5. Irritable disposition.
Vexed at trifles.
Attacks of rage, despair, with cursing and maledictions.

Head.

Vertigo, especially in the morning, obliging one to lie down.
Great weakness of memory, with aversion to mental exertion.
10. Headache in the morning on awaking.
Headache, with nausea and vomiting.

NITRIC ACID.

Stitches in the head, compelling one to lie down and disturbing the sleep.
Congestion of blood to the head, with much heat in it.
Pressing headache from without to within, with tension extending to the eyes, with nausea; aggravated by noise, relieved on lying down or when riding in a carriage.
15. Great sensitiveness of the head to the rattling of wagons, especially over the paved streets, and against stepping hard.
Humid, stinging-itching eruption on the vertex and on the temples, extending down to the whiskers, bleeding very easily on scratching it, and feeling very sore when lying on it.
Inflammatory swellings on the scalp, suppurating or becoming carious; most painful from external pressure or when lying on them.
Great sensitiveness of the head to touch and pressure, even to the pressure of the hat; worse in the evening and on the places on which one lies.
The hair falls off, with humid eruptions, paining as if splinters were thrust in it, or when touched; also on the genitals, after the abuse of mercury; with nervous headaches, great debility and emaciation.
20. Pain in the bones of the skull, with the sensation as if they were constricted by a tape; worse in the evening and at night; better from cold air and while riding in a carriage.

Eyes.

Eyes dull and sunken.
Pressure and stinging in the eyes.
Inflammation of the eyes, especially after suppressed syphilis or after the abuse of mercury.
Spots on the cornea.
25. Paralysis of the upper eyelids.
Black spots flying before the eyes.
Double vision; short-sightedness.
Fistula lachrymalis.

Ears.

Stitches in the (right) ear.
30. Suppuration of the ears; discharge of pus from the ears.
Hardness of hearing, especially from induration and swelling of the tonsils (after the abuse of mercury).
Cracking in the ears when masticating.
Beating and humming in the ears.
Echo in the ears of one's own speech.

35. Caries of the mastoid process.
    Steatoma at the lobe.

Nose.

Stitch in the nose, as from splinters, when touching it.
The tip of the nose is red and covered with scurfy vesicles.
Itching herpes on the wings of the nose.
40. Bleeding of the face; when weeping; in the morning the blood is black, clotted.
Disagreeable smell in the nose on inhaling air.
Fetid, yellow discharge from the nose; fetid smell from the nose.
Condylomatous excrescences on the nose.
Soreness, burning and scurf in the nose.
45. Unsuccessful attempt to sneeze.
The nose is dry and stuffed up; complete obstruction of the nose; water is dropping out.
Dry coryza, with dryness of the throat and nose; the wings of the nose are inflamed and swollen.
Fluent coryza, with obstruction of the nose; the mucus is only discharged through the posterior nares.
Coryza, with dry cough, headache, hoarseness and stitches in the throat.

Face.

50. Pale face with sunken eyes.
Yellow complexion or yellowness around the eyes, with red cheeks.
Dark yellow, almost brown, complexion.
Bloatedness around the eyes on waking early.
Swelling of the cheeks.
55. Pimples on the face, forehead and temples.
Black pores in the face.
Scurfy pustules on the face with large red areola.
Swelling of the lips.
Lips cracked.
60. Ulceration of the corners of the mouth and of the lips.
Ulcers in the red part of the lips.
Blood-boils on the chin.
Painful swelling of the submaxillary glands.

Mouth and Throat.

Pulsating or stinging pain in the teeth, mostly in the evening, in bed, or during the night.
65. The teeth become yellow or loose.
Pain in hollow teeth.

The teeth feel elongated.
Gums white, swollen, bleeding.
Stomacace.
70. Ulcers in the mouth and fauces, with pricking pains.
Putrid, cadaverous smell from the mouth.
Great dryness in the mouth, with thirst.
Ptyalism; also with ulcers on the fauces, or in attacks of fever.
Mercurial and syphilitic ulcers in the mouth and fauces, with pricking pain.
75. Inflammation of the throat; with pricking pains also after the abuse of mercury, or with burning and soreness.
Painful soreness of the soft palate, the tongue and inside gums, with stinging pain and ulceration of the corners of the mouth.
Great dryness and heat in the throat.
The tongue is very sensitive; even mild food causes a smarting sensation.
White, dry tongue, in the morning.
80. The tongue is coated green (with ptyalism).

Stomach and Abdomen

Violent thirst: in suppuration of the lungs, in the morning violent thirst.
Bitter taste after eating.
Sour taste, with burning in the throat.
Longing for fat, herring, chalk, lime, earth.
85. Aversion to meat, to bread, and when eating it, sour taste and vomiting.
During and after eating, perspiration.
Milk is not digested.
After eating, fulness in the stomach, debility, and, from the least exertion, heat, perspiration and palpitation of the heart.
Bitter and sour vomiting, with much eructation.
90. Pain in the cardiac orifice on swallowing food.
Stitches in the pit of the stomach.
Colic from cold.
Cutting and pinching in the abdomen, especially in the morning in bed.
On touching the abdomen, stinging pain, soreness.
95. Incarcerated flatulency in the upper part of the abdomen, and especially morning and evening.
Inguinal hernia also of children.
Swelling and suppuration of the inguinal glands.

Stool and Anus.

Constipation; stool dry, difficult, irregular.
Diarrhœa; discharges putrid or of mucus, fetid and undigested.
100. Dysenteric, bloody stools, with tenesmus.
Before the stool colic; after the stool nervousness and debility.
Itching and burning or stinging at the anus and rectum.
Humid moisture at the anus.
Varices of the anus, swollen, burning and bleeding after every evacuation.

Urinary Organs.

105. Incontinence of urine.
Frequent desire to urinate, with a scanty discharge of dark-brown, bad-smelling urine.
The urine is cold when it passes.
The urine has an intolerably offensive, strong smell, or smells like horse urine.
While urinating, smarting and burning in the urethra.
110. Discharges from the urethra of mucus, or of bloody mucus, or of pus.
Ulcers in the urethra.

Sexual Organs.

Men. Itching at the genitals.
Swelling, inflammation and phymosis of the prepuce.
Chancre-like ulcers on the prepuce and on the corona glandis, with pricking, stinging pains.
115. Sycotic condylomata.
Red, scurfy spots on the corona glandis.
Deep ulcer on the glans, with elevated, lead-colored, extremely sensitive edges.
Inflammatory swelling of the testicles, with painful drawing in the spermatic cords, extending into the abdomen.
Small, itching vesicles on the prepuce, bursting soon and forming a scurf.
120. Painful spasmodic erections at night, or entire want of sexual desire and erections.
Great falling off of the hair of the genital organs.
Women. Soreness in the genitals.
Ulcers in the vagina, burning and itching.
Menses too early, or suppressed menstruation.

125. During the menses colic and pressing and bearing down on the genitals.
Leucorrhœa; acrid, offensive, like brown water.

Respiratory Organs.

Scratching and stinging in the larynx, with hoarseness, especially when talking for a long time.
Hoarseness, with coryza, cough, and stinging pain in the throat.
Bronchitis.
130. Violent, shaking, barking cough, caused by tickling in the larynx and pit of the stomach, with expectoration during the day of blood mixed with clots, or of yellow, acrid pus, tasting bitter, sour or salt, and of offensive smell.
Dry, barking cough in the evening, after lying down.
Phthisis pulmonalis (after Kali carb).
When coughing, stitches in the small of the back.
Shortness of breath; panting breathing during work.
135. Dyspnœa, palpitation of the heart and anguish when going up stairs.
Cramp-like contractive pain in the chest.
Stitches in the chest; right side and scapula.
Soreness in the chest when breathing and coughing.
Congestion to the chest, with anxiety, heat and palpitation of the heart.
140. Nodosities in the mammæ, or atrophy of the mammæ.

Back and Neck.

Stitches in and between the shoulder-blades, with stiffness of the neck.
Pain in the back and small of the back from cold.
Swelling of the glands on the neck and of the axilla.

Extremities.

Upper. Rheumatic pains in the arms, especially in the fore-arms and fingers.
150. Weakness and trembling of the fore-arms and fingers.
Cold hands.
Chilblains on the hands and fingers.
Herpes between the fingers.
Swelling of the fingers, especially the joints, with stinging pain.
155. White spots on the finger-nails.
Lower. Sensation as if the hip were sprained with limping.
Rheumatic pains in the legs and feet.

Restlessness in the limbs in the evening.
Pain in the patella, impeding walking; stiffness and stitches in the knee.
160. Violent cramp in the calf at night and when walking after sitting.
Foot-sweat very offensive, or suppressed.
Chilblains on the toes.

Generalities.

Pricking pains, as from splinters, especially from contact.
Rheumatic pains in the limbs (from taking cold).
165. Cracking in the joints.
Hysteria.
Epileptic attacks.
Great debility, with heaviness and trembling of the limbs, especially in the morning.
Syphilis (secondary).
170. Sycotic condylomata; and sycosis.

Sleep.

Sleepiness during the day from debility, with vertigo.
During the sleep, pain and starts.
Difficulty of going to sleep in the evening; and in the morning one wakens too early or too late, and with great difficulty.

Fever.

Pulse very irregular: one normal beat is often followed by two small rapid beats,—the fourth entirely intermits; alternate hard, rapid and small beats.
175. Chilliness mostly in the afternoon and evening, and after lying down.
Chilliness, with internal heat at the same time.
Chilliness in the morning in bed, after previous heat.
Continuous chilliness.
Heat, especially on the hands and face.
180. Flushes of heat with perspiration on the hands.
At night, internal, dry heat, with inclination to uncover oneself.
Heat, with perspiration and debility after eating.
Perspiration every night, or on alternate nights; the most profuse on the side on which one lies.
Perspiration smelling offensive or sour, or like horse urine.
185. *Intermittent fever.* Chilliness in the afternoon (an hour and a half, while in the open air), followed by dry heat when in bed, accompanied by all sorts of fancies while in a

state of half waking, without sleep; sleep and perspiration only come on towards morning.

Chilliness in the afternoon, for an hour; then heat over the whole body, for a quarter of an hour; afterwards profuse perspiration for two hours over the whole body; there is no thirst either in the cold or in the hot stage.

Skin.

Dryness of the skin.
Itching nettle-rash, in the open air, even in the face.
Black pores.
190. Brown-red spots and dark freckles on the skin.
Painful chilblains and corns.
Frostbitten, inflamed, itching limbs, from a slight degree of cold, with cracked skin.
Large blood-boils.
Violently bleeding ulcers or wounds, with stinging pain, as from splinters, or with burning, especially when they are touched.
195. Ulcers, with bloody, ichorous matter.
Mercurial ulcers.
Carious ulcers.
Cicatrices pain on the change of weather.
Inflammation, swelling and suppuration of the glands.
200. Painfulness and inflammation of the bones.—Caries.

Conditions.

Especially suitable, after alkalies, for lean persons with dark complexion, black hair and eyes.
Pains on change of temperature and of the weather.
Great inclination to take cold.
The pains are felt during sleep.
205. *Aggravation* in the evening and at night, on waking, on rising from a seat; from touching the parts.
Amelioration from eructations; while riding in a carriage.

NUX JUGLANS.

Mind and Disposition.

Indisposition and aversion to converse.
Inattention when reading and disinclination to work.

Head.

Excitement as if intoxicated, with the sensation as if one were flying.
Headache above the eyes, especially the left; worse on motion.
5. Burning heat in the head in the evening, with icy-cold extremities.

Mouth and Throat.

Painful swelling and abscess on the gums (on an upper left incisor).
Tongue coated with white mucus in the morning on waking.
Accumulation of mucus in the throat with hawking.

Stomach and Abdomen.

Thirstlessness while eating and aversion to wine.
10. Frequent loud eructations.
Fulness and bloatedness of the stomach, which prevent one from eating while one has a good appetite, better from eructations.
Fulness, bloatedness, tension and heaviness in the abdomen, with frequent desire to go to stool, relieved by eructations and discharge of flatulence.
Tympanitic hardness of the abdomen.

Stool and Anus.

Itching at the anus in the evening in bed, with stitches, compelling one to walk about.

Urinary Organs.

15. Continuous desire to urinate and frequent micturition day and night, with very profuse discharge.

Sexual Organs.

Men. Ulcer with hard, high edges, white bottom and easily bleeding, and suppurating profusely between the glans penis and prepuce.
Women. Menstruation too early and too profuse; discharge of a large quantity of black clots.

Respiratory Organs.

Itching on the sternum.
Aphonia or great hoarseness.

Back.

20. Violent stitches in the small of the back, causing one to tremble.

Extremities.

Lower. Pain in the hips or knees, impeding walking.

Fever.

Pulse full and frequent in the evening.
Frequent and sudden attacks of flushes of heat.
Burning hot face in the evening, with cold extremities.
25. Alternation of cold and heat in short attacks during the day.

Skin.

Painful, large blood-boils on the shoulder and in the region of the liver.
Glandular swellings (scrofulous swellings).
Pustules as in eczema, with burning-itching, red, cracked skin, discharging a greenish fluid stiffening the linen.
Syphilitic. scrofulous and mercurial ulcers and herpes.

Conditions.

30. Aggravation in the evening and at night.
Amelioration after passing the stool and flatulence.

NUX MOSCHATA.

Mind and Disposition.

Changeable disposition; hysteria with suddenly changing disposition, great drowsiness and disposition to faint.
Very irresolute, changes his intention continually.
Absence of mind; vanishing of thoughts in reading, disposition to go to sleep.
Dulness of senses, thoughtlessness, with slowly returning consciousness.
5. Great inclination to laugh at every thing, especially in the open air.
Slowness of ideas; loss of memory.
Idiocy; craziness.
Delirium with violent vertigo, strange gestures, improper talk, with loud tone and voice and total sleeplessness.

Head.

Vertigo and giddiness as from intoxication, with delirium, or craziness, or insensibility.
10. Reeling (while walking in the open air) with staggering, gradual rigidity and insensibility.
Fainting, with palpitation of the heart, followed by sleep.
Sensation of looseness of the brain, and when shaking or moving the head as if the brain were striking against the skull, with sleepiness after a meal; worse from cold, better from warmth and heat.
Sensitiveness of the head as from soreness, especially sensitive to the slightest touch, in a draft of air (wind); worse in the cold and from lying down, better from hard pressure and from external heat.
Pulsating, pressing pain on a small spot over the left eye.
15. Painless pulsation in the head with fear to go to sleep.
The headache generally appears after eating, especially after breakfast or after overloading the stomach.

Eyes.

Sensation of dryness and dryness of the eyes, can move the eyelids only with difficulty.
Tension around the eyes and in the lids.
Sensation of fulness in the eyes with contracted pupils.
20. Illusions of visions; objects appear too distant.
Weakness of sight.

Ears.

Otalgia with stinging pain (right ear).
Pain in the eustachian tube as from a rough body (on change of weather) previous to the setting in of wind and rain.

Nose.

Sneezing; early in the morning.
25. Stoppage, especially of the left nostril.

Face.

Heat in the face with slight redness of the cheeks.
Blue margins around the eyes (with pale face).
Sensation of swelling of the left cheek, with pricking as from electric sparks.
Freckles in the face.

Mouth and Throat.

30. Toothache of pregnant women.

Stinging and tearing in the teeth, extending to the ears and temples, with stitches in the teeth when sucking them, and aggravation from contact and cold air.
Sticking pain in the teeth, relieved by the application of warmth.
The teeth feel dull, as if covered with lime.
Toothache from damp, cold evening air; the teeth feel as if they were grasped by the forceps, with pain in the neck.
35. The gums bleed readily.
Shocks in the molar teeth from drinking cold water.
Toothache from washing, from cold, from damp cold air.
Dryness and sensation of dryness in the mouth without thirst.
Dryness and sensation of dryness of the tongue, extending to the mouth and throat.
40. The tongue is coated white (with mucus).
Paralysis of the tongue.
Aphthæ.
Great dryness in the throat without thirst.
Difficulty of deglutition as from paralysis of the throat.
45. The breath has a very offensive smell.

Stomach and Abdomen.

Taste in the mouth like chalk, pappy; or as if he had eaten strongly salted food.
Appetite increased; thirst diminished.
After eating, debility; scraping eructations.
Weakness of digestion (especially in old persons).
50. Nausea and vomiting during pregnancy.
Nausea while riding in a carriage.
Fulness in the stomach, with oppressed breathing.
Colic pain in the abdomen, immediately after eating and worse after drinking only during the day, with dry mouth and thirstlessness.
Sensation of heat and burning in the stomach.
55. Cutting in the abdomen and screwing pain around the navel, as from worms, with sleepiness.
Abdomen distended from flatulence, preventing sleep.
Swelling of the liver; heaviness in the region of the liver; swelling of the spleen.

Stool and Anus.

Slow, difficult soft stool.
Diarrhœa from debility or from cold; predisposition to diarrhœa.

60. Diarrhœic stools, like scraped eggs, with loss of appetite in children.
Summer complaint—summer diarrhœa.
Diarrhœa with loss of appetite and great sleepiness in children.
Diarrhœa of undigested food, with fainting.
Putrid, bloody diarrhœa in typhus fever.

Urinary Organs.

65. Painful strangury.
Burning and cutting while urinating.
The urine smells like violets.
Renal colic.

Sexual Organs.

Men. Debility of the sexual system; desire with relaxed organs.
70. Discharge of prostatic fluid.
Women. Irregular menstruation, sometimes too early, then again too late.
The menstrual blood is dark and thick.
Before menstruation pain in the small of the back, debility, pressure in the stomach, water-brash and pain in the liver.
During a hemorrhage from the uterus or menstruation, pressure in the abdomen, drawing down into the legs from the navel.
75. Spasmodic, false labor-pains.
Threatening miscarriage.
Pain of the uterus from the pessary.

Respiratory Organs.

Altered voice; hoarseness; sudden from walking against the wind.
Cough with great soreness in the larynx or the chest.
80. Dry cough with oppressed breathing from taking cold by standing in the water.
Cough with or without expectoration when becoming warm in bed in the evening or when becoming warm from working.
Hæmoptysis.
Cough during pregnancy.
Shortness of breathing after eating.
85. Oppression of the chest, originating in the pit of the stomach.
Sensation of constriction of the chest.

Fulness and sensation of a heavy weight pressing on the chest.
Palpitation of the heart with attacks of fainting (followed by sleep).

Back and Neck.

Sensation of great weakness in the small of the back (and knees).
90. Drawing in the muscles of the neck from the draft of moist air.
Pain in the back or small of the back as if broken and bruised.
Pain in the small of the back when riding in a carriage.
Tabes dorsalis.

Extremities.

Upper. Cold hands as if frozen, with buzzing in the hands on entering a room.
95. *Lower.* Pain in the (right) knee as if sprained, especially when moving and going up-stairs.
Weakness of the knees (and small of the back).

Generalities.

Great soreness of all the parts on which one lies.
Rheumatic pains (from cold damp air).
Wandering pains, only attacking a small spot and lasting but a short time, returning frequently.
100. Hysterical paroxysms.
Inclination to faint.
Convulsions (of children).
Great debility from the least exertion, compelling one to lie down with sleepiness.
Apoplexy.

Sleep.

105. Great sleepiness with all complaints.
Irresistible drowsiness; deep sopor.

Fever.

Pulse accelerated.
Chill whenever uncovering oneself and chilliness in the open, especially wet, cold air, with very pale face; at once relieved in the warm room.
Sensation of coldness of the feet with heat of the hands.
110. Chilliness in the evening with great drowsiness.
Chilliness and drowsiness predominate.

Heat in the face and hands in the morning, with hypochondriac mood and thirstlessness and dryness of the mouth and throat.

Perspiration scanty, but at times red like blood.

Intermittent fever. Double tertian intermittent fevers, with sleepiness, white tongue, rattling breathing, bloody expectoration and very little thirst only during the hot stage.

115. Intermittent fever with sleepiness, and during the heat great dryness of the mouth and throat with thirstlessness.

Skin.

Dry, cold skin and not disposed to perspire.
The skin is very sensitive to cold moist air.
Bluish spots on the skin.

Conditions.

All the ailments are accompanied by drowsiness and sleepiness; and inclination to faint.

120. Especially suitable for women and children.

Aggravation from cold, wet air or in cold, wet weather; while lying on the painful side; from cold food; from spirituous liquors; when riding in a carriage; from water and washing; from changes of the weather; in windy (stormy) weather.

Amelioration in the room; from warm air; in dry weather; from wrapping up warmly.

NUX VOMICA.

Mind and Disposition.

Anger, with habitual malicious, spiteful disposition.
Fiery, excited temperament.
Inclined to find fault and scold; morose; stubborn.
Over-sensitiveness to external impressions, noise, smells; light and music are unbearable and affect him much; anxiety and restlessness in the evening.

5. Anxiety with irritability and inclination to commit suicide; but is afraid to die.

Hypochondriac humor of persons of sedentary habits, and of those who dissipate at night, with abdominal sufferings and constipation.

Delirium tremens with over-sensitiveness, nervous excitability and malicious vehemence.

The time passes too slow.

After anger, chilliness alternating with heat, vomiting of bile and thirst.

10. Great laziness and aversion to occupy oneself.

Head.

Reeling vertigo in the morning and after dinner; with vanishing of sight and loss of hearing.

Cloudiness as from intoxication in the head.

Intoxication from the drunkenness on the previous day, with vanishing of sight and hearing; worse after dinner and in the sun.

Congestion of blood to the head, with burning in it and with heat and redness of the bloated face; worse in the morning, on moving the head and when walking in the open air.

15. Burning in the forehead in the morning on waking and after eating; worse from mental exertion and when exercising in the open air; better when at rest and in the warm room.

Stunning headache in the morning, after eating, and in the sunshine.

Pressing headache in the forehead, with sour vomiting; worse in the morning in bed, better when leaning the head against something or when lying on the back.

Pressing pain on the vertex, as if a nail were driven into it.

Pressing headache, as if the skull were pressed asunder.

20. Sensation as from a bruise in the back part of the head.

Rheumatic headache with nausea and acid vomiting.

Tension in the forehead as if it were pressed in at night and in the morning, worse on exposing the head to the cold air.

Bruised sensation of the brain, generally one (right) sided, better when lying on the painless side.

The brain seems to shake when walking or running in the open air; better when wrapping the head up in the warm room and when at rest.

25. Pressing in the head, as if something heavy were sinking down in the forehead or head.

Periodical headache in the forehead, sore as from ulceration, with constipation.

Semi-lateral headaches from excessive use of coffee.

The scalp is sensitively painful, on the least touch, to the wind, and is relieved by warmly covering the head.

Fetid perspiration of one half of the head and face, which is cold to the touch, relieving the pain, and with anxiety and dread from uncovering the head.

30. Liability to take cold on the head mostly from dry wind, draft of air.

The head symptoms are worse in the morning, in the open air, and from mental exertion and from motion; and better after rising in the morning and during the day, in the warm room, and from sitting quiet or when lying down.

Eyes.

Inflammation of the sclerotica, with stitches and aversion to the light of the sun.

Painless, circumscribed red spots, like extravasation of blood, in the white of the eye.

Exudation of blood from the eyes.

35. Yellowness of (especially of the lower part of) the eyeball.

In the morning the light of day is insupportable.

Streaks like lightning before the eyes.

Burning and smarting in the eyes as from salt.

Twitching of the eyelids.

40. Anxious staring look.

Ears.

Otalgia with tearing-stinging pains.

Tension in the ears when he raises his face.

Painful sharp shocks and stitches in the ears, especially in the morning in bed.

Pain in the ear on swallowing, as if it were pressed outward.

45. Strong reverberation of sounds in the ear.

The pains in the ear are worse after entering the room and in bed.

Nose.

Sensitiveness and inflammatory redness of the internal nose.

Bleeding from the nose in the morning.

Smell before the nose like old cheese or brimstone.

50. Coryza; fluent during the day, worse in the warm room, better in the cold air; dry coryza during the evening and night.

Dry coryza with stoppage of the nose (in infants).

Acrid discharge from the obstructed nose.

Face.

Pale, yellowish and earthy color of the face.
Yellowness around the mouth and nose, or around the eyes.
55. Swelling of one cheek, with faceache and pain in the cheek-bone.
Red, swollen face; burning redness of the face with heat.
Twitching of the muscles of the face, in the evening when lying down.
Painful pealing off of the lips.
Crusts on the lips.
60. Trismus.
Corroding ulcers in the corners of the mouth.
Periodical prosopalgia nervosa, worse at night.
Pimples in the face from the excessive use of spirituous liquors.
Swelling of the submaxillary glands; with stinging on swallowing.

Mouth and Throat.

65. Tearing in the teeth extending to the head through the bones of the face, renewed from cold drink, relieved by warmth.
Stinging in decayed teeth; burning-stinging in one whole row of teeth.
Looseness of the teeth.
The gums swollen, white, putrid, bleeding.
Toothache from taking cold.
70. The toothache is caused or aggravated by wine, coffee, cold air and mental exertion, and is relieved by heat.
Bad odor from the mouth.
Stomacace.
Aphthæ (of children).
Inflammatory swelling of the roof of the mouth, throat and gums, with difficulty of deglutition.
75. Sensation as of a plug in the throat.
Sensation of soreness in the throat on inhaling cold air.
When swallowing, stitches in the throat and sensation as if it were too narrow or constricted.
Inflammatory swelling and stitches in the palate.
Heavy white coating on the tongue.
80. The tongue is black and dark-red and cracked on the edges.
Heaviness of the tongue with difficulty of speech.
Fetid ulcers in the mouth and throat.

Stomach and Abdomen.

Hunger with aversion to food, especially to bread, coffee and tobacco.
Ravenous hunger after drinking beer.
85. Thirst, in the morning, with aversion to water and beer.
Longing for brandy and chalk.
Tastelessness of all food.
Sour taste, especially in the morning or after eating and drinking.
Putrid taste (in the morning).
90. After dinner (some hours after) pressure in the stomach, dulness of the head and hypochondriacal mood.
Bitter, sour eructations.
Violent hiccough.
Nausea, especially in the morning and after dinner.
Empty vomiturition; straining to vomit (in drunkards).
95. Periodical attacks of vomiting; of food, of sour-smelling mucus, of dark, clotted blood; and during pregnancy.
Bloatedness, and pressure in the stomach and pit of the stomach, as from a stone, especially after eating.
Colic and pressure in the stomach, extending to the shoulders, in the morning, fasting and after eating.
Constrictive colic generally, with water-brash.
Colic of brandy and coffee drinkers.
100. Pressure and tension in the pit of the stomach, with tension opposite, between the shoulder-blades.
Cannot bear his clothes tight around the hypochondria.
Pressure and stinging in the region of the liver. Inflammation and induration of the liver.
Labor-like spasms in the abdomen and in the uterus, extending into the legs.
Pressing in the abdomen towards the genitals.
105. Painful soreness of the abdominal muscles when moving, pressing on them, coughing or laughing.
Periodical (colic) pains in the abdomen, especially after eating and drinking.
Disordered stomach after over-eating.
Hernia; incarcerated hernia.

Stool and Anus.

Constipation; stool insufficient, black, hard, often streaked with blood, as from inactivity of the intestines; with ineffectual efforts to go to stool (in infants).
110. Stools like pitch, with blood.

Dysenteric stools, with cutting at the navel, pressing and straining on the rectum, and discharge of bloody mucus with feces.
Frequent small mucous discharges, with pressing and straining.
Painful, spasmodically closed anus.
Painful blind hæmorrhoidal tumors.

Urinary Organs.

115. Strangury; painful, ineffectual urging to urinate.
Pressure to urinate at night, with discharge of a few drops of red, bloody, burning urine.
Hæmatorrhœa.
During and after micturition, discharge of viscid, purulent mucus from the bladder.

Genital Organs.

Men. Increased secretion of smegma behind the corona glandis.
120. Inflammation and swelling of the testicles, with stinging and spasmodic contraction, extending to the spermatic cords, the testicles being hard and drawn up.
Easily excited, strong sexual desire, with painful erections.
Hydrocele.
Women. Menses too early and too profuse, with dark, black blood.
During and after menstruation, appearance of new and aggravation of old ailments.
125. Congestion to and bearing down of the uterus. Inflammation of the uterus and the external parts.
Prolapsus uteri.
False and inefficient labor-pains, with frequent pressure to urinate and to pass stool.
After-pains too violent and of too long duration.

Respiratory Organs.

Suffocative attacks after midnight from spasmodic constriction of the larynx.
130. Dyspnœa; asthma from spasmodic constriction of the lower part of the thorax.
Catarrhal hoarseness, from scraping in the throat, with viscous mucus in the larynx and on the chest.
Itching in the larynx.
Acute bronchitis.
Cough from exertion,—reading or mental exertion,—or thereby aggravated.

135. Dry cough, with pain in the head, as if it would burst, or with great soreness in the upper part of the abdomen.
Dry cough; worse at night or early in the morning.
The cough is dry in the evening and at night; expectoration during the day.
Hooping-cough, caused by a tickling in the throat and larynx, with expectoration during the day of yellow, gray, cold mucus, mostly tasting sour or sweet, and last of bright-red blood.
The cough is aggravated after midnight and in the morning, from exertion, from cold air, when lying on the back, from eating and drinking, from smoking tobacco, from becoming cold, from acids.
140. Heavy, pressing pain in the chest, as from a heavy load.
Sensation as if something were torn loose in the chest.
Congestion to the chest, with heat and burning in it.
Anxious palpitation of the heart.

Back and Neck.

Tension between the shoulder-blades.
145. Burning, pressing and stitches between the shoulder-blades.
Pain, as if bruised in the small of the back and back, so violent that he cannot move.
Sensation in the small of the back as if lame (also after difficult parturition).
Heaviness and stiffness in the neck.

Extremities.

Upper. Paralysis of the arm, with violent jerks in it, as if the blood would start out of the veins.
150. Soreness in the shoulder-joint.
Drawing in the arms, extending from the shoulder to the fingers, with sensation as if the arm were asleep; loss of motion of the arm, especially at night.
The hands go to sleep and feel dead.
Cold, sweaty hands, with cold nose.
The veins on the hands and arms are prominent, enlarged.
155. *Lower.* Numbness, stiffness and tension in the legs.
Sensation of paralysis of the legs, with the sensation of a painful stripe down on the inside of the thigh; numbness and paralysis of the legs.
Staggering walk and weakness of the legs.
Painful swelling of the knee-joint.
Numbness and deadness of the lower legs.
160. When he walks he drags the feet; he cannot lift them up.

Dryness and cracking in the knee-joint, when walking.
Cramp in the calves at night.

Generalities.

Great debility of the nervous system, with over-sensitiveness of all the senses.
Periodical attacks of indisposition.
165. Sensation of heaviness of the body, alternating with sensation of lightness.
Stitches in jerks through the whole body.
Feeling of soreness all over the body in the morning, in bed.
Great inclination to lie down or to sit, with aversion to move about and to the open air.
Rheumatic pains, especially during windy (stormy) weather.
170. Disposition to take cold and great sensitiveness to draft of air, and aversion to the open air.
Paralysis, with coldness of the paralyzed parts.
Convulsions and spasms; epileptic attacks.
Attacks of fainting (in the morning; after eating).
Gastric and bilious complaints, especially of pregnant women.
175. Inflammation of internal organs: congestion.
Very suitable for thin, slender persons.

Sleep.

Goes to sleep late from crowding of thoughts on him.
Goes to sleep late; wakens at 3 A. M. and lies awake till break of day, when he falls into a dull sleep full of dreams, from which he is hard to rouse and wakens late, feeling tired.
The morning sleep aggravates all the complaints.
180. Great drowsiness during the day and after eating.

Fever.

Pulse full, hard, accelerated, especially during the heat.
Pulse small and rapid; every fourth or fifth beat intermits.
Chilliness and coldness, which cannot be relieved by external heat.
Chilliness with shuddering, in the evening and during the night in bed till morning; aggravated from every movement and from drinking.
185. Chilliness with hot face.
Chilliness and heat alternating.
Chilliness and shuddering during exercise in the open cold air.
After the chill he sleeps till the hot stage sets in.

General internal, burning heat.
190. Heat during the night, without thirst.
Heat, with aversion to be uncovered, and from it at once chilliness.
Heat, which is aggravated from the least exertion or motion, even in the open air.
Heat precedes the chill.
Heat of single parts while others are chilly.
195. Heat is ascending from the throat.
Perspiration after midnight and during the morning.
Perspiration smells sour or offensive.
Perspiration only on one (right) side of the body, or only on the upper part of the body.
Cold, clammy perspiration in the face.
200. Perspiration which relieves the pain in the limbs.
Intermittent fever. Chill in the evening; then one hour's sleep, which is followed by heat, with headache, tingling in the ears and nausea.
Violent chill with shaking, increased by drinking; afterwards heat, which is followed by perspiration.
Chilliness after the perspiration, and then perspiration again.
Anticipating morning fever; first moderate chilliness, with blue nails without thirst,—then thirst and long-lasting violent fever and heat, with stitches in the temples, followed by light perspiration.
205. Chill without thirst, followed by violent heat with thirst, headache, vertigo, redness of the face, vomiting, red urine, pain in the chest, followed by partial perspiration.
Intermittent fevers, with the prevalence of gastric and bilious symptoms or with constipation.
Congestive intermittent fevers, with vertigo, anguish, chills, delirium, accompanied by vivid visions and distention of the stomach; with stitches in the sides and abdomen.
Intermittent fever, characterized by a sense of paralysis and want of strength in the limbs in the beginning of the fever.

Conditions.

Every mental exertion causes or aggravates the symptoms.
210. Bad effects from coffee, tobacco, and spirituous liquors; from over-exertion of the mind, sedentary habits and loss of sleep; over-eating.
Aggravation from motion and slight touch, but strong pressure relieves.

Most symptoms are most severe on waking in the morning and after eating.

The ailments which appear in the open air and from motion are relieved in the room and when at rest; but the reverse also takes place occasionally.

Is an antidote to almost all narcotic, drastic and vegetable remedies, especially against citrate of magnesia, and often suitable to begin the treatment of cases after drugging.

OCIMUM CANUM.

Urinary Organs.

Turbid urine, depositing a white and albuminous sediment.
Urine of a saffron color.
Crampy pain in the kidneys.
Renal colic, with violent vomiting; moans and cries, wrings the hands; after the attack, red urine with brick-dust sediment, or discharge of large quantities of blood with the urine.
5. Thick, purulent urine, with an intolerable smell of musk.

Sexual Organs.

Men. Heat, swelling, and excessive sensibility of the left testicle.
Women. Lancinations in the labia majora.
Swelling of the whole vulva.
Prolapsus vaginæ.
10. Engorgements of the mammary glands.
The tips of the breasts (nipples) are very painful; the least contact extorts a cry.
Engorgement of the mammary glands.
The breasts feel full and tense.
Swelling of the inguinal glands.
15. Numbness of the right thigh.

OLEANDER.

Mind and Disposition.

Absence of mind, want of attention.
Slowness of perception.
Indolence, aversion to do any thing.

Head.

Vertigo when rising from bed, or if looking fixedly at any object, or when looking down while standing.
5. Heaviness of the head; better when lying down.
Biting-itching on the scalp, as from vermin, principally on the back part of the head and behind the ears; relieved when first scratching it, which is followed by burning and soreness, which gives place to biting-itching; worse in the evening when undressing.
Humid, scaly, biting-itching eruption on the head, especially on the back part of the head.

Eyes.

When reading; burning and tension in the eyelids; lachrymation.
Double vision.

Ears.

10. Herpes and ulcers on and around the ears.

Face.

Pale, sunken face in the morning with blue rings around the eyes.
Alternate paleness and dark redness of the face.
Numbness of the upper lip.

Mouth and Throat.

Toothache only when masticating.
15. Drawing in the molar teeth at night when lying down, with anxiety, nausea and frequent micturition.
Bluish-white gums.
The papillæ are elevated, dirty-white.
Loss of speech.
Dryness of the mouth and white tongue.

Stomach and Abdomen.

20. Ravenous hunger with trembling of the hands and hasty eating without appetite.
Much thirst, especially for cold water.
Violent empty eructations, while eating.
Vomiting of food and bitter greenish water.
After vomiting ravenous hunger and thirst.
25. Sensation of emptiness in the stomach, even after eating.
Beating and pulsation in the pit of the stomach as if the beats of the heart were felt through the whole thorax.
Stitches and gnawing about the navel.
Rolling and rumbling in the intestines, with emission of a great quantity of fetid flatulence.

Stool and Anus.

Ineffectual urging to stool.
30. Almost involuntary discharge of undigested stool.
The food which he had taken on the previous day passes off undigested and almost without effort; imagines he is only emitting flatulence.
Chronic diarrhœa; undigested food, worse in the morning.
Burning at the anus before and after the stool.

Urinary Organs.

Urinary secretions increased with frequent micturition, especially after drinking coffee.
35. Brown, burning urine, depositing a white sediment.

Respiratory Organs.

Viscid mucus in the trachea.
Oppressed breathing when lying, as if the chest were too narrow, with long, deep breathing.
Violent shaking cough from tickling in the larynx.
Sensation of emptiness and coldness in the chest.
40. Dull stitches in the left side of the chest and in the sternum, worse when taking a long breath.
Violent, anxious palpitation of the heart; the chest feels expanded.

Extremities.

Upper. Swelling and stiffness of the fingers, with burning pains.
The veins on the hands are swollen.
Lower. Paralysis of the legs and feet; painless.
45. Great weakness of the legs, especially of the knees.
Constant cold feet.

Buzzing sensation in the legs, especially the soles of the feet.

Generalities.

Painful stiffness and paralysis of the limbs
Insensibility of the whole body.
50. Want of animal heat in the limbs.
Painless paralysis.
Faintish weakness of the whole body; when standing trembling of the knees, when writing trembling of the hands.
Fainting as from weakness, relieved by perspiration.

Sleep.

Frequent yawning, with chilliness and trembling of the muscles.
55. Restless, voluptuous dreams and frequent waking.

Fever.

Pulse very changeable and irregular; weak and slow in the morning, full and rapid in the evening.
Chilliness and chills over the whole body, periodically, with heat of the face and coldness of the hands.
Chilliness and want of animal heat.
External chilliness with internal heat without thirst.
60. Flushes of heat periodically, especially from bodily or mental exertion.

OLEUM ANIMALE.

Mind and Disposition.

Sadness.
Taciturn and thoughtful, absorbed in revery.
Frequent vanishing of thought.

Head.

Painful dizziness, early in the morning in bed.
5. Painful sensation of reeling and giddiness, in the open air, when stooping.
Numb and paralytic sensation in the left side of the head.
Pressure on the vertex, shifting to the occiput.
Boring in the left frontal protuberance.

Conditions.

70. The symptoms are caused or aggravated by mental excitement, wounded pride, and non-approval by others.
Aggravation on standing and from motion.
Amelioration when lying down, when lying on the left side.
The uterine and ovarian symptoms are similar to those of Platina and Argentum; but the mental symptoms of Platina are the reverse to those of Palladium, and Argentum has similar symptoms on the left side to those of Palladium on the right side of the abdomen, on the ovaries, and in connection with the prolapsus uteri.

PAREIRA BRAVA.

Urinary Organs.

Micturition difficult, with much pressing and straining only in drops, with the sensation as if the urine should be emitted in large quantities.
Violent pains in the bladder, and at times in the back; the left testicle is painfully drawn up; pain in the thighs, shooting down into the toes and soles of the feet.
Paroxysms of violent pain with the strangury; he cries out loud, and can only emit urine when he goes on his knees, pressing his head firmly against the floor; remaining in this position for ten to twenty minutes, perspiration breaks out, and finally the urine begins to drop off with interruptions, accompanied by tearing, burning pains at the point of the penis.
Urine smells strongly of Ammonium, and contains a large quantity of viscid, thick, white mucus.
5. The paroxysms appear generally from three to six A. M.; amelioration through the day.
Almost cartilaginous induration of the mucous membrane of the bladder.
Similar conditions of the bladder are to be found under Berberis vulgaris, but not the ammoniacal smell; and the pain under Berberis is in the hip, not, as under Pareira, in the thigh. Berberis has also paralysis of the bladder with discharge of great quantities of mucus, which deposits itself at the bottom of the vessel and is viscid.

33

PARIS QUADRIFOLIA.

Mind and Disposition.
Loquacious mania.
Silly conduct.

Head.
Vertigo when reading aloud, with impeded speech and difficult vision.
Pressing headache aggravated from mental exertion.
5. Headache from smoking tobacco.
Sensitiveness of the vertex to contact.
Stinging and stitches in the head.
Tension in the brain and on the forehead.

Eyes.
The eyeballs feel too large and too thick; swollen.
10. Wandering, unsteady looks.

Ears.
Sensation as if the ear were pressed out or torn out.
Sensation as if a burning heat were rushing out of the ears.

Nose.
Milk and bread smell like putrid meat.
Discharge of red and greenish mucus on blowing the nose.

Face.
15. Hot stitches in the left malar bone, painful when touched.
Violent itching, biting and burning on the edges of the lower jaw, frequently with red, small, easily-bleeding (miliary) eruption.
Tetters around the mouth.
Vesicles on the surface of the lower lip.

Mouth and Throat.
Dryness of the mouth in the morning.
20. Swelling, painfulness and peeling off of the roof of the mouth.
Tight, almost painless swelling of the size of a pigeon's egg on one side of the roof of the mouth.
White frothy mucus in the corners of the mouth in the morning.
Tongue rough, dry; feels too large.
Burning, stinging and scraping in the throat.
25. Sore throat, as if a ball were lodged in it.

Hawking of mucus.
Tart saliva.

Stomach and Abdomen.

Hunger very soon after a meal.
After eating, hiccough.
30. Heaviness in the stomach as from a stone; relieved by eructation.
Burning in the stomach, extending down in lower abdomen.
Weak, slow digestion.
Rumbling and rolling in the abdomen.

Stool and Anus.

Frequent soft stools.
35. Diarrhœic stools smell like putrid meat.

Urinary Organs.

Frequent micturition with burning when passing the urine.
Dark red urine, with a cloud in the middle, red sediment, and a greasy pellicle swimming on it.
Acrid, excoriating urine.
Burning and stinging in the urethra.

Respiratory Organs.

40. Trachea very dry in the morning on waking.
Hoarseness, with feeble voice, continuous hawking of mucus and burning in the larynx.
Periodical painless hoarseness.
Hawking up of viscid green mucus from the larynx.
Burning in the larynx. (Bronchitis.)
45. Cough as from vapor of sulphur in the larynx.
Cough, with expectoration of viscid mucus difficult to raise in the morning and evening on lying down.
Oppression of the chest, with desire to draw a long breath.
Stitches in the chest.
Palpitation of the heart on motion and when at rest.

Back and Neck.

50. Stitches in the back between the shoulder-blades, and pulsating stitch in the os coccygis when sitting.
Sensation as if the neck were stiff and swollen on turning it.
Sensation as if the nape of the neck were oppressed by a great, heavy load.

Generalities.

Stinging pains in all parts of the body, especially the limbs.
Sensation of spasmodic tension in the joints.
55. Sensation of heaviness in the body.

Fever.

Pulse full and slow.
Chilliness, mostly towards evening, with internal trembling.
Coldness on one side (right) with heat on the other side of the body (left).
During the chill, sensation as if the skin and other parts of the body were contracted.
60. Chilliness, with gooseflesh.
Cold feet all night in bed.
Heat extending from the neck down the back.
Heat, with perspiration on the upper part of the body.
Perspiration in the morning on waking, with biting-itching.

Conditions.

65. At every motion, sensation as if all the joints were broken.

PETROLEUM.

Mind and Disposition.

Excited, irritable, with inclination to anger and to scold; anxious and irresolute.
Sadness and despondency, inclination to weep.
Weakness of memory.
Delirium; imagination; thinks another person is lying with him in bed; or always and continuously delirious talk of the same distressing and unpleasant subject.

Head.

5. Headache when stooping or rising from bed.
Pulsation in the cerebellum.
Pressing stinging in the cerebellum.
Sensation as if every thing in the head were alive.
Headache in the forehead; every mental exertion causes him to become quite stupid.
10. Headache from anger.

Sensitiveness of the scalp on both sides, very sore to the touch, followed by numbness, and very sore on scratching, worse in the morning and on becoming heated.

Eyes.

Inflammation, with itching of the eye.
Fistula lachrymalis.
Like a veil before the eye.

Ears.

15. Dryness and disagreeable sensation of dryness in the ear.
Hardness of hearing.
Discharge of pus and blood from the ear.
Humid soreness behind the ear.

Nose.

Dryness and sensation of dryness in the nose.
20. Fluent coryza, with hoarseness.
Swelling of the nose, with discharge of pus, and pain at the root of it.

Face.

Yellow complexion.
Heat in the face after eating (sometimes with thirst).
Scurfs around the mouth.
25. Easily dislocated jaw, in the morning in bed, with much pain.
Swelling of the submaxillary glands.

Mouth and Throat.

Toothache from contact with the fresh open air, at night, and with swelling of the cheek.
Numbness of the teeth, they pain when biting on them.
Swelling of the gums, with stinging-burning pain when touching it.
30. Fistula dentalis.
Smell from the mouth like garlic.
Great dryness of the mouth and throat in the morning, with much thirst (for beer).
Stinging pain in the throat when swallowing.
Ulcers on the inner cheek, painful when closing the teeth.
35. Hawking of mucus in the morning.
When swallowing, the food enters into the posterior nares.
The tongue is coated white.

Stomach and Abdomen.

Taste, putrid, flat, mucous.
Violent thirst (for beer).

40. Ravenous hunger.
Aversion to meat and fat as well as all warm, cooked food.
Sour or bitter eructations and gulping up of.
Waterbrash.
After eating vertigo and giddiness.
45. Nausea, from riding in a carriage.
Nausea and vomiting of pregnant women.
Vomiting of bitter, green substances.
Pressure on the stomach; colic (at night).
Sensation of emptiness and weakness in the stomach.
50. Sensation of fulness or swelling of the pit of the stomach, with soreness when touched.
Pain in the pit of the stomach as if something were tearing off.
Cutting in the abdomen soon after eating.
Weakness of digestion.
Sensation of coldness in the abdomen.

Stool and Anus.

55. Stool insufficient, difficult, hard, in lumps.
Diarrhœa preceded by colic only during the day.
Stools of bloody mucus.
Itching herpes on the perinæum.

Urinary Organs.

Constant dripping of urine.
60. Frequent micturition, with scanty emission of brown, fetid urine.
Contraction of the urethra. Burning in the urethra.
Involuntary micturition, at night in bed.

Sexual Organs.

Men. Red, sore, moist scrotum and adjacent parts.
Itching and humid herpes on the scrotum and between the scrotum and thigh.
65. *Women.* Soreness and moisture on the sexual organs.
Aversion to an embrace.
Menses too early, the discharge causes itching.
During pregnancy diarrhœa and vomiting.
Itching and mealy covering of the nipples.

Respiratory Organs.

70. Cold air causes an oppressed feeling on the chest.
Oppression of the chest, at night.
At night, dry cough, coming deep from the chest, caused by a scratching in the throat.

Cough with stitches under the sternum.
Herpes on the chest.

Back and Neck.

75. Pain in the small of the back, preventing one from standing.
Weakness and stiffness in the back and small of the back.
Pain in the back, which does not allow him to move.
Herpes in the neck.

Extremities.

Upper. Brown or yellow spots on the arms.
80. Burning in the palms of the hands.
During the winter, chapped hands and fingers, full of deep, bloody rhagades.
Arthritic stiffness of the finger-joints.
Pain in the wrist-joint as if sprained.
Lower. Stitches in the knee.
85. Hot swelling of the soles of the feet with burning.
Painful swelling and redness of the heel (chilblains).
Ulcers on the toes, originating in blisters on the toes.
Herpes on the knees and ankles.
Feet swollen; cold.

Generalities.

90. Twitching in the limbs; epileptic attacks.
The limbs go to sleep and become stiff.
Cracking and arthritic stiffness in the joints.
Great debility with trembling.
Aversion to the open air; and from it chilliness.
95. Fainting, with ebullitions, heat, pressing on the heart and palpitation of the heart.

Sleep.

Sleep with distressing dreams, as if somebody were lying alongside of him in bed.

Fever.

Pulse full and accelerated from every exertion; as soon as reposing, the pulse becomes again slow.
Chill, especially toward evening, often with heat at the same time.
Chilliness through the whole body followed by itching.
100. Chilliness in the open air.
Chill with headache and excessive coldness of the face and hands.
Heat in the evening after the chill, with cold feet.
Heat after midnight and in the morning, in bed.

Sensation of heat over the whole body, with violent burning of the skin.
105. Flushes of heat.
Night-sweats.
The fore-arms and lower legs perspire easily.
Perspiration after the chill, no heat intervening.

Intermittent Fever.

Violent chilliness and coldness of the hands and face at ten A. M.; half an hour later, heat in the face, especially in the eyes, with thirst.
110. Shaking fits, seven P. M., followed by perspiration, first in the face, later all over, except in the legs, which are quite cold.

Skin.

Swelling and indurations of the glands; also after contusions.
Itching herpes.
Itching, sore, moist surfaces.
Brown or yellow spots on the skin.
115. The skin is hard to heal.
Ulcers with stinging pain or with proud flesh.

Conditions.

Many ailments originate or are aggravated during a thunderstorm.
After a walk in the open air, or after a slight fit of anger, flushes of heat, ebullitions and perspiration.
Complaints from riding in a carriage, or in a ship.
120. Bad effects from sprains and bruises (glands).
Amelioration from warmth, warm air.

PETROSELINUM.

Stool and Anus.

Stool whitish, like clay; chronic diarrhœa.

Urinary Organs.

Agglutination of the orifice of the urethra by mucus.
Albuminous yellow discharge from the urethra; gonorrhœa.
During micturition, burning and tingling from the perinæum through the whole urethra.
5. Drawing, afterwards itching in the fossa navicularis.

PHELLANDRIUM AQUATICUM.

Intolerable pains in the lactiferous tubes; much worse during the act of nursing.

PHOSPHORUS.

Mind and Disposition.

Great excitability; becomes easily vexed and angry, which makes him exceedingly vehement, from which he suffers afterwards.
Great anxiety and restlessness, especially when alone, or during a thunder-storm.
Zoomagnetic condition; clairvoyance.
Ecstacy.
5. Melancholy depression, sometimes with shedding of tears or with attacks of involuntary laughter.

Head.

Vertigo when rising from the bed in the morning; when rising from a seat, with fainting and falling to the floor; worse in the morning and after meals.
Stupefying headache in the morning when moving, and worse on stooping; ceasing for a short time after eating; better when lying down and in the cold air.
Congestion to the head, with burning, singing and pulsations in the head, red face, puffiness under the eyes; worse in the morning when sitting, and in the evening in bed.
Burning in the forehead, with pulsations in the morning and in the afternoon; after eating worse in the warm room, better when walking in the open air.
10. Sensation of emptiness in the head, with vertigo.
Sensation of coldness in the cerebellum, with sensation of stiffness of the brain.
Pulsation in the head, with singing and burning in it, mostly in the forehead, with nausea and vomiting from morning till noon; worse from music, while masticating and in the warm room.

Inflammation of the brain, with pulsations and singing in the head; the heat enters the head from the spine, and from it extends to the feet; worse in the warm room, better when moving about in the cold air.

Headache over the left eye.

15. Tension in the skin of the forehead and in the face, as if the skin was not large enough, frequently only on one side; worse from change of temperature and while eating; better after eating, with anxiety.

Itching on the scalp, worse from scratching, with dandruff.

Dry, painful heat of the scalp, compelling one to uncover the head, the temperature of the body not increased; better when lying down.

Clammy perspiration on the head only, and in the palms of the hands, with discharge of much turbid urine.

Falling off of the hair in large bundles on the forepart of the head, and on the sides above the ears.

20. The headache is aggravated from music, laughing, and in the warm room.

Eyes.

Burning in the eyes, with profuse lachrymation in the wind.

Agglutination in the eyes in the morning, with lachrymation in the open air; worse in the wind.

Inflammation of the eyes, with pressing and burning pains.

Pain in the bones of the orbit of the eye.

25. Aversion to light.

Pupils contracted.

Mistiness of sight; dim-sightedness (gauze before the eyes).

Halo around the candle.

Black motes floating before the eyes (muscæ volitantes).

30. Momentary loss of sight, as from fainting.

Cataracta viridis.

Ears.

Roaring before the ears.

Hardness of hearing, especially of the human voice.

Nose.

Bleeding from the nose, during stool; blowing of blood from the nose.

35. Swelling and redness of the nose.

Painful dryness of the nose.

Bad smell from the nose; foul smell.

Over-sensitiveness of smell.

Polypus of the nose (bleeding easily).
40. Profuse discharge of green (or yellow) mucus from the nose, without coryza.
Freckles on the nose.

Face.

Pale, hippocratic countenance.
The color of the face is very changeable.
Bloated face; puffiness under the eyes; eyes sunken, with a blue ring under them.
45. Circumscribed red spot on the cheeks.
Tearing and stinging in the facial bones.
Ulcerated corners of the mouth.
Bluish lips.

Mouth and Throat.

Pricking-stinging in the teeth; worse in the open air, and from warm food.
50. Necrosis of the (left) lower jaw; swelling of the jaw bones.
Swelled and easily bleeding gums; inflamed gums, with ulcers on them.
Toothache after washing clothes.
Tongue dry, white, coated with white mucus.
Stinging in the tip of the tongue.
55. Burning in the œsophagus.
Dryness of the throat day and night.
Spasmodic constriction of the œsophagus.
Tonsils and uvula are much swollen.
Saliva increased, saltish, sweetish; soreness of the mouth.
60. Spitting of blood.
Hawking of mucus in the morning.

Stomach and Abdomen.

Want of appetite, caused by a fulness in the throat.
Hunger soon after eating.
Immoderate hunger, especially at night (during an attack of gout), with great weakness, so great that he faints if the hunger is not soon allayed.
65. Thirst, with longing for something refreshing.
Taste saltish, sour, sweetish; bitter after eating.
After eating sleepiness.
Frequent empty and sour eructations.
Rising up of sour ingesta.
70. Throwing up of the ingesta by mouthfuls.
Vomiting of bile; of what has been drunk as soon as it becomes warm in the stomach; of blood; sour.

Painfulness of the stomach to the touch and when walking.
Loud rumbling and rolling in the intestines.
Great pressure in the stomach after eating.
75. Burning in the stomach; inflammation of the stomach.
Spasms of the stomach.
The cardiac opening of the stomach seems contracted (too narrow), the food scarcely swallowed comes up again.
The pains in the stomach are relieved by cold food (ice-cream, ice).
Soreness of the abdomen to the touch when walking.
80. Sensation of coldness in the abdomen.
Flaccidity of the abdomen.
Large yellow spots on the abdomen.

Stool and Anus.

Constipation; the small-shaped, hard stool is expelled with great difficulty.
Stools very soft, pap-like.
85. Painless, debilitating diarrhœa (worse in the morning).
Stools black or green; watery, with flakes of mucus; bloody; involuntary; indigested.
Discharge of blood from the rectum, also during stool.
Spasms in the rectum.
Paralysis of the lower intestines; of the sphincter ani.
90. Discharge of mucus out of the wide open anus.
Stinging or itching at the anus.
Hæmorrhoidal tumors easily bleeding.

Urinary Organs.

Increased secretion of watery, pale urine.
Frequent micturition, but a small quantity each time.
95. Hæmaturia.
Urine whitish, like curdled milk, soon becoming turbid with brick-dust sediment, with a variegated cuticle on the surface.
Twitching and burning in the urethra, with frequent desire to urinate.
Involuntary discharge of urine.

Sexual Organs.

Men. Sexual desire increased, with irresistible desire for coition.
100. Impotence.
Frequent involuntary seminal emissions.
Women. Menstruation too early and too profuse, and of too long duration, or too early and too scanty (and watery).

Stitches upward in the vagina into the pelvis.
During menstruation pains in the small of the back; palpitation of the heart.
105. Sterility on account of excessive voluptuousness, or if the menstruation comes on too late and is too profuse.
Leucorrhœa acrid, drawing blisters and excoriating.
Inflammation (erysipelatous), even after the formation of pus.
Ulceration of the mammæ, with hardness; bluish color; fistulous openings, with burning and stinging.

Respiratory Organs.

Hoarseness; loss of voice.
110. Great painfulness of the larynx, preventing talking.
Stitches, soreness, roughness and dryness in the larynx.
Croup; bronchitis.
Cough, with stitches over one eye; splitting headache; dryness and burning in the throat, hoarseness, aphonia, soreness, roughness and dryness in the larynx.
Cough, dry, from tickling in the throat and chest; from cold air; from reading aloud or from talking; from laughing; from eating and drinking; from a change in the weather, and from strong odors; from lying on the left side or on the back.
115. Cough, with expectoration in the morning, without expectoration in the evening; expectoration bloody, frothy, pale-red, rust-colored, streaked with blood, purulent, white and tough; cold mucus, tasting sour, salt or sweet.
Hollow, hacking, spasmodic tickling cough, especially if caused by tickling in the chest.
Cough worse in the evening and at night.
Respiration oppressed, quick, anxious.
Difficult inspiration; heaviness, fulness and tension on the chest.
120. Congestions to the chest; anxiety in the chest.
Constrictive spasms in the chest.
Inflammation of the lungs (left side), with stitches in the sides of the chest.
Pneumonia nervosa (lungs hepatized).
Tuberculosis (phthisis mucosa).
125. Palpitation of the heart from every mental emotion.
Yellow spots on the chest.

Back and Neck.

Pain in the back as if it were broken, impeding all motion.
Stiffness of the neck.
Stitches in the shoulder-blades.
130. Pain in the small of the back when rising from a stooping position.
Burning in the back or small of the back. Tabes dorsalis.

Extremities.

Trembling of the limbs from every exertion.
Upper. Rheumatic pains in the arms, especially in the joints.
Trembling of the hands, if holding any thing.
135. Burning in the palms of the hands; clammy perspiration in the palms of the hands (and on the head).
Numbness and insensibility of the fingers.
Lower. Rheumatic stiffness of the knee.
Rheumatic pain extending from the knee to the feet.
Swelling of the feet, with stinging.
140. Pains in the soles of the feet, as if bruised.
Nightly tearing pain in the feet of pregnant women.
Swelling of the tibia.
Numbness of the toes.
Corns and chilblains on the toes.

Generalities.

145. Great emaciation.
Great nervous debility; trembling in all the limbs from the least exertion.
Over-sensitiveness of all the senses.
Burning in the body and limbs internally and externally.
Sensation of dryness or of festering in internal parts.
150. Increased secretion of mucus.
Hemorrhages from internal organs.
Inflammation and stinging pain of inner parts.
Ebullitions and congestions.
Itching of inner parts.
155. Sprains, easy dislocations.

Sleep.

Sleepiness in day-time.
Sleeplessness before midnight; goes to sleep late.
Wakes frequently in the night.
Sleepiness with drowsiness (coma vigil).
160. Anxious, vivid dreams.

Frequent waking from feeling too hot, without perspiration.
Somnambulism.

Fever.

Pulse generally accelerated, full and hard; occasionally small and weak.

Chill, generally only in the evening, without thirst, with aversion to being uncovered and with swollen veins on the hands.

165. Internal chilliness and chill not relieved by the heat of the stove.

Chilliness and heat alternately during the night.

Chilliness in the evening till midnight, with great weakness, and sleep.

Chill at night with diarrhœa.

Chill running down the back.

170. Flushes of heat over the whole body, beginning in the hands.

Heat with anxiety and burning in the hands and face, in the afternoon and evening.

Heat at night disturbing the sleep.

Heat running up the back.

Heat with desire to sleep.

175. Perspiration most profuse on the head, hands and feet, with increased secretion of urine.

Perspiration only on the forepart of the body.

Profuse perspiration after midnight and in the morning-hours, followed by great debility.

Clammy perspiration.

The perspiration frequently smells of sulphur.

180. *Intermittent fever.* Heat and perspiration at night, with faintness and ravenous hunger, which could not be satisfied by eating; afterwards chilliness, with chattering of teeth and external coldness; the chilliness was succeeded by internal heat, especially in the hands, while the external coldness continued.

Chilliness in the afternoon, followed by heat and thirst with internal chilliness; heat and perspiration followed, lasting all night.

Fevers with soporous condition, dry black lips and tongue and open mouth. Typhus fever. Hectic fever.

Skin.

Blood-boils.

Fungus hæmatodes; small wounds bleed much.

185. Polypus.

Petechiæ. Red spots.
Dry herpes.
Burning in the skin.
Pustulous and scaly exanthema.
190. Yellow spots (chest and abdomen). Freckles (nose).
Swelling of the bones (left lower jaw, tibia).
Glandular diseases especially after contusions.
Chilblains (fingers, toes).
Corns.

Conditions.

195. Liability to take cold, and from it stinging and tearing in the limbs.
Sensitiveness to cool weather and to the open air.
The head and face symptoms are relieved by the cold air, but the chest symptoms are aggravated by it.
Aggravation; in the evening, at night, especially before midnight; after breakfast; when alone; after eating (something warm); when lying on the back or on the left side; when rising from a seat; from light; during a thunder storm; from a change of weather; from singing, laughing, strong smells (cough).
Amelioration; in the dark; while lying on the right side; from rubbing; after sleeping; from eating something cold.
200. Especially suitable for lean, slender persons.
In a condition of great debility the person is much easier beneficially affected by Phosphor., being mesmerized before taking the remedy.
Phosphor, is an antidote to over-doses of Camphor.

PHOSPHORICUM ACIDUM.

Mind and Disposition.

Perfect indifference.
Silent sadness.
Indifference, thoughtlessness, stupidity.
Disinclination to talk, even to answer a question.
5. Home-sickness with inclination to weep.
Low-spirited and anxiety about the future or about one's health.

OLEUM ANIMALE. 497

Sensation as if the blood were rushing to the occiput on entering a room.

Eyes.

10. Burning in the eyes in the open air or on waking or at candle light.
Spasmodic quivering of the lids.
Mistiness of sight, especially in the afternoon when writing.

Ears.

Sticking in the ears.
Boring in the ears with dryness of the throat.

Nose.

15. Itching burning of the tip of the nose.
Itching in the nostrils.
Pimples on the septum, with burning and oozing.

Face.

Pale, earthy complexion.
Redness of the cheeks, even when the skin is cold.
20. Cramp-pain in the (left) cheek.
Itching pimples and vesicles on the cheeks.
Itching of the lips.   Chapped lips.

Mouth and Throat.

Dryness in the mouth and throat also, on waking in the morning.
Greasy feeling in the mouth and on the palate.
25. Accumulation of a quantity of snow-white saliva in the mouth.
Choking and constriction of the throat, particularly in the morning and evening.
Dryness of the throat, especially perceptible during empty deglutition.
Dryness with sour taste in the mouth.
Hawking of tenacious mucus after a meal.

Stomach and Abdomen.

30. Desire for soft-boiled eggs.
Frequent empty eructations, relieving the nausea and the urging to vomit.
Bruised pain about the stomach.
Sensation as if the stomach were full of water.
Pressure in the pit of the stomach, also after drinking cold water.
35. Stinging in the stomach.
Sensation of coldness in the stomach.

32

Burning and heat from the stomach to the chest.
Pressure with sticking in the region of the liver and spleen.
Shifting of flatulence in the abdomen with rumbling.
40. Drawing from the groins into the testicles.

Stool and Anus.

Difficult stool even when natural.
Burning and stinging in the anus and rectum.

Urinary Organs.

Copious, clear, pale urine, also depositing a cloud.
Greenish urine.
45. Burning during micturition.
Itching in the urethra.

Sexual Organs.

Men. Burning-stinging about the root of the penis (afternoon).
Both testicles are drawn up and painful.
Pressing in the prostate gland.
50. Nocturnal erections and emissions.
Women. Menses too early, preceded and accompanied by colic.
Scanty menses, blood black.

Respiratory Organs.

Hoarseness with inability to talk loud.
Roughness in the throat, inducing dry, hacking cough.
55. Rushes of blood to the chest with dry heat of the face.
Pressure and crushing sensation about the heart.

Back and Neck.

Pain in the small of the back worse when sitting.
Cracking of the vertebræ on raising the head.

Extremities.

Upper. Numbness of single fingers.
60. Drawing and digging in the right thumb, as if it would ulcerate.
Lower. Sticking in the sole of the foot.
Tingling at one spot in the middle of the sole, in the evening.
Cramp in the toes.
Tearing in the big toe, which is painful as if ulcerated, particularly near the nail.
65. Lameness of the left lower limb and left arm.

Generalities.

Cramp-like drawing in different parts.
Languor with indolence; inclination to sit.
Fainting.

Fever.

Coldness after a walk in the open air.
70. Coldness of the whole left lower limb.
Shuddering from the vertex to the chest.
Dry, pricking heat, particularly in the face.
Perspiration during a meal.

OPIUM.

Mind and Disposition.

Vivid imagination, exaltation of the mind, increased courage, with stupefaction and dulness.
Stupid indifference; imbecility.
Stupefaction of the senses.
Illusions and frightful fancies; visions.
5. Loquacious delirium, with open eyes and red face; furious delirium.
Mania, with frightful or pleasing, delightful visions, alternating with stupor.
Delirium tremens; with diminished sensitiveness of the senses and stupor with snoring.
Stupor, must lie down; snoring sleep and half-open eyes.
Complete loss of consciousness and sensation, with relaxation of the muscles.
10. Apoplexy, with vertigo, buzzing in the ears, loss of consciousness, red, bloated, hot face, red, half-closed eyes, dilated, insensible pupils, foam at the mouth, convulsive movements of the limbs, and slow, snoring breathing.
Fright with fear; is followed by heat in the head and convulsions.
Grief over insults is followed by convulsions.

Head.

Stupefying vertigo when rising, compelling one to lie down.
Dulness and stupefaction of the head, as from drunkenness.
15. Congestion of blood to the head, with pulsation in it.

The headache is aggravated on moving the eyes.
Great heaviness of the head.

Eyes.

The lids hang down as if paralyzed.
The eyes are half open and are turned upwards.
20. The pupils are dilated and insensible to light.
Staring look.
Glassy, protruded, immovable eyes.
Swelling of the lower lids.
Obscuration of sight.
25. Sensation as if the eyes were too large for the orbits.

Face.

Face bloated, dark (brown) red, hot.
Face pale, clay-colored, sunken countenance and eyes, with red spots on the cheeks.
Bluish (purple) face.
All the muscles of the face are relaxed and the lower lip hangs down.
30. Trembling, twitching and spasmodic movements of the muscles of the face.
Corners of the mouth twitch; distortion of the mouth.
The veins of the face are distended.
Hanging down of the lower jaw.
Lockjaw.

Mouth and Throat.

35. Dryness of the mouth.
Ptyalism; spitting of blood.
Ulcers in the mouth and on the tongue.
Paralysis of the tongue and difficult articulation.
Black tongue.
40. Feeble voice, and requires a strong effort to talk loud.
Dryness of the throat.
Inability to swallow; daily attacks of distention and strangulation.

Stomach and Abdomen.

Violent thirst; aversion to food, or canine hunger without appetite.
Vomiting, with violent colic and convulsions; of green substance; of blood.
45. Vomiting of feces and urine.
Heaviness and pressure in the stomach.
Inactivity of the digestive organs.
Hard, bloated abdomen. Tympanitis.
Heaviness in the abdomen, as from a weight.

50. Lead-colic.
Incarcerated inguinal hernia.

Stool and Anus.

Constipation from inactivity of the intestines.
Spasmodic retention of the feces, especially in the small intestines.
Black, fetid stool.
55. Involuntary discharge of offensive stool; involuntary stools after fright.
Fluid, frothy, diarrhœic stools, with burning in the anus and violent tenesmus.
Suppression of urine, as from contraction or paralysis of the bladder.
Scanty, dark-brown urine, with brick-dust sediment.
Hæmatorrhœa.

Sexual Organs.

60. *Men.* Excitement of the sexual organs and violent erections; or impotence.
Women. Spasmodic, labor-like pain in the uterus.
Suppressed, false or spasmodic labor-pain.
Puerperal spasm, during and after parturition, with loss of consciousness and drowsiness or coma between the paroxysms.
Violent movements of the fœtus.

Respiratory Organs.

65. Hoarseness, with dry mouth and throat and white tongue.
Difficult, intermitting breathing, as from paralysis of the lungs: Pneumonia notha.
Rattling breathing.
Deep snoring breathing, with open mouth.
Tension and constriction of the chest.
70. Suffocative attacks during sleep, like nightmare.
Cough, with dyspnœa and blue face.
Cough, with frothy expectoration of blood and mucus.
Heat in the chest.
Burning about the heart.

Back and Neck.

75. Pulsating arteries and swollen veins on the neck.
The back is (spasmodically) bent backwards.

Extremities.

Upper. Twitching and spasmodic movements of the arms.
Paralysis of the arms.

Trembling of the arms and hands.
80. Distended veins on the hands.
Lower. Twitching and spasmodic movements of the legs.
Weakness, numbness and paralysis of the legs.
Heaviness and swelling of the feet.

Generalities.

Numbness and insensibility of the body and limbs.
85. Trembling of the whole body, with external coldness and jerking and twitching in the limbs.
Trembling of the limbs after fright.
Convulsions, with sudden loud cries.
Buzzing through the whole body.
Want of sensitiveness against the effects of medicines, with want of vital reaction.
90. Increased excitability and action in the voluntary muscles, with diminution of it in the involuntary muscles.
Paralysis without pain.
Convulsions and spasmodic motions, with foam at the mouth.
Convulsions, with sleep after the paroxysms.
Rigidity of the whole body.
95. Tetanic spasms, with bending the head or back backwards.
Epileptic convulsions, particularly at night or towards morning, with suffocative paroxysms.

Sleep.

Drowsiness, great inclination to sleep; dreams, and cannot be roused.
Coma vigil.
Stupefying, unrefreshing sleep.
100. Stupefying sleep, with the eyes half open and snoring.
During sleep, picking of bed-clothes (floccilegium); groanign; voluptuous dreams.

Fever.

Pulse varies very much; full and slow, with difficult, snoring breathing; quick and hard with heat, with quick and anxious breathing.
Chill and diminished animal heat, with stupor, and weak, scarcely perceptible pulse.
Rigidity and coldness of the whole body.
105. Coldness only of the limbs.
Heat with damp skin predominates, extending itself from the head or stomach over the whole body.

Burning heat of the whole body, which is in a perspiration, with great redness of the face, followed by sleep with snoring.
Heat, with inclination to be uncovered.
Profuse perspiration over the whole body, which is burning hot, with sleep and snoring.
110. In the morning, profuse hot perspiration, with desire to be uncovered.
Perspiration of the upper part of the body, with dry heat of the lower part.
Cold perspiration on the forehead.
Intermittent fever; first shaking chill, afterwards heat with sleep, during which he perspires much.
Falling asleep during the cold stage and no thirst; during the hot stage thirst and general copious perspiration.
115. Fever with stupor; snoring with the mouth open; twitches through the limbs and perspiration on the hot body.
Fever with sopor.

Skin.

Dropsical swelling of the whole body.
Redness and itching of the skin.
Blue spots on the skin.

Conditions.

120. Painlessness with all ailments; complains of nothing and asks for nothing.
Especially suitable for children and old persons.
All ailments are accompanied by sopor.
Reappearance and aggravation from becoming heated.
Suitable very often to persons addicted to drinking and aged persons.
125. Bad effects from fright.
Aggravation from brandy, wine; while perspiring; on rising; during and after sleep.

OXALICUM ACIDUM.

Mind and Disposition.

Great cheerfulness and clearness of mind.
Thinking of his ailments aggravates them.
Aversion to talk; with headache, fulness in the face.

Head.

Vertigo, with weakness and thirst; anxiety; headache and perspiration.
5. Vertigo while looking out of the window; when rising from a seat.
Vertigo, like swimming, on lying down.
Sensation of emptiness in the head.
Dulness in the forehead (morning).
Pain in the forehead and vertex; on the left side of the forehead, on waking.
10. Pressing pain on small spots.
Pressing, like screwing, behind both ears.
Headache after lying down, after sleeping, and on rising.
Headache relieved after stool.
Head affected by drinking wine.

Eyes.

15. Pain in the balls of the eyes; worse in the left.
Inclination to close the eyes.
Small, especially linear, objects appear larger; they are thought to be more distant than they really are.
Vanishing of sight, with giddiness and perspiration; with bleeding of the nose.

Nose.

Stitches in the right nostril on taking a long inspiration.
20. Pimples in the right side of the nose; the wing of the nose is swollen.
Sneezing, with chilliness.
Red, shining swelling of the right side of the nose, beginning at the tip of the nose and from there extending.

Face.

Face red, swollen, feeling full; hot or cold; covered by cold perspiration.
Face pale and livid, with open mouth and unconsciousness.
25. Pale color, with sunken eyes.

Mouth and Throat.

Pain in decayed molar teeth.
The gums bleed, and are painful in spots.
Small ulcers on the gums.
Tongue swollen, sensitive, red, dry, burning.
30. Tongue swollen, with a thick white coating.
Tongue coated white, with nausea, thirst and loss of taste.
Sour taste in the mouth.

Heartburn.
In the mouth, pain, accumulation of saliva, water, or mucus.
35. In the throat, scraping, increased accumulation of mucus.
Dryness in the throat (in the morning) after diarrhœa.
Painful deglutition, especially in the morning.
Difficult deglutition, with sour eructations.

Stomach and Abdomen.

Appetite increased.
40. Appetite wanting, with loss of taste, thirst and nausea.
Thirst, with vertigo, loss of appetite, nausea, colic.
The pain in the stomach is relieved by eating; soup is pleasant when there is gnawing at the stomach.
After eating, eructations, nausea, pains at the navel, colic, rumbling in the abdomen, urging to stool, weakness.
Eructations empty, sour.
45. Sudden hiccough, with eructations.
Nausea and thirst with colic,—after diarrhœa.
Sensation of emptiness in the stomach, compelling one to eat.
Burning in the stomach and throat.
Stomach sensitive to the touch.
50. Violent colic, waking one at night.
Continuous pain in the left hypochondrium, as if bruised; stitches.
Stitches in the liver relieved by taking a deep breath.
Colic, rumbling (evening and night).
Incarcerated flatulence (in the left hypochondrium).
55. Colic pain around the navel, as if bruised; stitches, with pressing and discharge of flatulence; worse on moving, better when at rest.
Burning in small spots in the abdomen.
Cutting pain in the abdomen.

Stool and Anus.

Morning diarrhœa; stools soft or watery, with colic around the navel and pressing in the rectum; returning as soon as one lies down again.
Stool of mucus and blood.
60. Before the stool and from the pain with the stool, headache.
During the stool micturition (fainting, vomiting).
After the stool nausea and tension in the calves; dryness in the throat; relief of the pain in the small of the back.
Diarrhœa as soon as one drinks coffee.
Constipation; no stool.
65. Pressing and straining in the rectum; tenesmus.

Urinary Organs.

Pain in the region of the kidneys.
Frequent micturition and profuse discharge of urine.
Burning in the urethra, as from acrid drops.
When urinating pain in the glans penis.

Sexual Organs.

70. Sexual desire increased. Erections (forenoon).
Sensation of contusion in the testicles; worse in the left testicle.
Heaviness of the testicles, with drawing pain, extending into the spermatic cords.

Respiratory Organs.

Hoarseness; the larynx feels swollen, contracted, raw, with tickling in it.
Dry cough on taking violent exercise.
75. Mucous secretion in the throat increased.
Mucus in small lumps, or hard or thick, yellowish-white phlegm, with black lumps in the centre of it.
Difficulty of breathing, with oppression of the chest (right side), when moving about in the evening.
Difficulty of breathing, with constrictive pain in the larynx and wheezing.
When breathing, stitches in the chest and pain above the hip.
80. Sudden lancinating pain in the left lung, depriving him of breath.
Dull, heavy, sore pain in the chest.
Pain in the middle of the chest, extending through to the back.
Pain in the heart; soreness, stitches from behind forward or from upwards downwards.
Palpitation of the heart, after lying down at night.
85. The beats of the heart intermit when thinking of it.

Back and Neck.

Pain in the back, under the point of the shoulder-blade, between the shoulders, extending from the shoulders to the loins.
Pain in the back, extending to the thighs.
Numbness, pricking, causing a sensation of coldness and weakness in the back; the back is too weak to support the body.
Pain in the small of the back, sensation of numbness, or as if broken.
90. Stitches extending from the chest into the shoulders.

Extremities.

Upper. Pain first in the left, later in the right deltoid muscle, with inclination to move.

The right wrist feels sprained, with inclination to stretch it and stitches in the ulnar region; cannot hold any thing.

Pain in the (right) metacarpus and fleshy part of the right thumb, with sensation of fulness, heat and numbness.

Heaviness of the hand; can move the fingers but slowly.

95. Hands are cold, as if dead.

Arthritic pains in the fingers; the fingers are drawn in.

Twitching of the fingers.

Dark nails.

Lower. Restlessness in the legs

100. The knees feel tired.

Weakness of the lower extremities; they are gone to sleep; paralysis, stiffness.

Pain in the limbs, with weakness and numbness.

Generalities.

The pains appear on small longitudinal spots.

The pains come on periodically.

105. Trembling, convulsions.

Paralysis of the left side.

Sleep.

Frequent yawning; sleepiness during the day.

Dreams, with fright and fear; sits up and looks around.

Fever.

Pulse more rapid in the morning; slower, irregular, weak.

110. Chilliness, ascending from below upwards.

Chilliness, with sneezing (evening).

Chill after diarrhœa (afternoon).

Shaking chill, with red face (evening).

Heat from every exertion.

115. Heat, especially in the face or on the hands.

Heat with perspiration.

Perspiration with weakness, or with giddiness.

Night-sweat clammy and cold.

Skin.

Skin very sensitive while shaving.

120. Marbled skin.

Itching on the neck or fingers.

Itching eruption with redness.

Warts.

Conditions.

Aggravation of the pains or ailments when thinking of them.
125. Motion and exercise increase the pains.
Sugar aggravates the pains in the stomach, and wine the headache.

OSMIUM.

Head.

Violent headache above and under the eyes, one-sided, extending to the ears; worst below the eyebrows; the eye waters.
Falling off of the hair.

Eyes.

Weakness of sight.
The flame of the candle looks larger and less distinct.
5. Burning of the eyes and lachrymation.

Ears.

Tingling and pain in the (right) ear.

Nose.

Sneezing and fluent coryza, with tickling in the larynx, with difficult respiration.
Discharge from the posterior nares of loose mucus.

Stomach and Abdomen.

Chronic vomiting, with pressure in the stomach.

Urinary Organs.

10. Diminution or suppression of the urinary secretions.

Sexual Organs.

Men. Violent pain on the point of the penis and prepuce.
Erections every night, after midnight or towards morning.
Discharge of semen larger and continues longer than usual.

Respiratory Organs.

Tickling in the larynx.
15. Mucous secretion increased; mucus hangs in the larynx like a string, causing hawking and coughing with straining to vomit; when sneezing the mucus becomes loose easily.

Dryness of the throat when coughing.
Spasmodic coughs in attacks (with twitching of the fingers, dryness of the throat and crying).
Cough with sneezing.
Cannot expectorate what has been coughed up; has to swallow it again.
20. Chronic dyspnœa. (Heaves in horses.)
Sensation of soreness of the sternum; it is painful to the touch.

Extremities.

Upper. Perspiration in the axillæ smelling like garlic.
Lower. Rash on the thighs and on the ankle.
The lower legs and feet feel too full, with restlessness in the legs till he lies down.

PÆONIA.

Head.

Vertigo on every motion, with constant reeling in the head.
Dulness, heaviness, vertigo and feeling of heat in the head.

Eyes.

Burning, itching and feeling of dryness in the eyes.

Face.

Burning heat in the face.
5. Tingling in the upper lip.

Throat.

Burning and heat in the throat.
Tenacious mucus in the throat, inducing hawking.

Stomach and Abdomen.

Pressure in the pit of the stomach, as from great anxiety.

Stool and Anus.

Papescent diarrhœa, with qualmishness in the abdomen, burning in the anus after stool, followed by internal chilliness.
10. Painful ulcer at the anus, with exudation of a fetid moisture, extending towards the perineum.

PALLADIUM.

Mind and Disposition.

Greatly inclined to use strong language and violent expressions.
Fond of the good opinion of others; also too much weight is laid on their judgment: therefore very excited in society, and her complaints worse on the next day.
Mental agitation, especially society, or musical entertainments, or excited conversation, or motion, aggravate the pain in the right ovary.
Excited and impatient (from headache).
5. Time passes too slow.

Head.

Headache is worse in the afternoon; pulsations over the whole body; he feels as if the head were shaken to and fro from behind forwards; better after sleep.
Morning headache, with weakness in the back.
Sensation of roughness on the forehead.

Eyes.

Dull, heavy pain in and behind the left eye, in the evening, after walking.
10. Sensation of dryness on the edges of the lids.
Dryness and itching of the eyes in the evening, which is not relieved by rubbing.

Face.

Itching pimples in the face, on the nose, behind the ears.
Soreness and painfulness of the right corner of the mouth.

Throat.

Accumulation of tough mucus in the throat, with slimy taste, which returns after rinsing out the mouth.
15. Dryness in the throat and on the tongue, without thirst.
Tongue red in the middle (morning).
Tickling, as if a crumb of bread had lodged in the throat.

Stomach and Abdomen.

Pain and soreness in the liver.
Pain in the left hypochondrium; relieved by eructations.
20. Pain in the region of the spleen.

Sensation as if the intestines were entangled and were turned into different directions.

Violent colic in the abdomen, more on the right side; growing worse under continuous eructations; can only endure the pain when lying on the left side; worse from sneezing, coughing and urinating, and in the afternoon; returning next day in the afternoon, with cold hands and feet, continuous chilliness, and passing of urine like blood mixed with water; after going to bed cramps in the legs, which prevents motion in bed; relieved by external heat (hot cloths).

Shooting pains from the navel to the pelvis.

Soreness in the abdomen with bearing down (on the right side).

25. Swelling and hardness in the right side of the abdomen (ovary).

Sharp pains, as darts with a knife, low down in the abdomen; better after stool.

Stool and Anus.

Distended abdomen from flatulency.

Constipation; stools hard, frequently whitish (like chalk).

Urinary Organs.

Single stitches through the bladder, with painful weakness in it.

30. Single stitches in the urethra, extending down to the corona glandis.

Frequent micturition; the bladder feels full, but little urine is passed.

Pressure in the bladder, as if it were very full.

Dark urine with brick-dust sediment, or coloring the vessel red.

Muddy (not dark) urine; urine like water mixed with blood.

Sexual Organs.

35. *Men.* Sensation as if the testicles were bruised, with pain in the abdomen.

Women. Pain and weakness, as if the uterus were sinking down; every motion was especially painful; she could not well stand.

Heaviness, like a weight in the pelvis. Bearing-down pain.

In the region of the right ovary, drawing down and forward; relieved by rubbing.

Swelling and induration of the right ovary, with soreness and a shooting pain from the navel to the pelvis; with

a heaviness and weight in the pelvis; worse from exertion and while standing up, better when lying on the left side.
40. Menstrual discharge while nursing.
Leucorrhœa, transparent, like jelly; worse before and after menstruation.

Respiratory Organs.

Stitches in the right side of the chest, through to the back; worse from taking a long breath, better when walking in the open air.
Pain in the region of the heart. Pressing deep in the left side of the chest periodical, as if in the heart.
Pain in the heart, with paralysis of the left arm.

Back.

45. Pain in the back and hips, with coldness of the limbs.
Tired feeling in the back.

Extremities.

Upper. Sudden stitches in the right shoulder-joint; rheumatic pains in the right shoulder.
Sensation as if sprained in the right shoulder-joint.
Stitches from the shoulders into the middle of the chest.
50. Pain in the right arm and temple.
Sensation of numbness in the left arm, as if paralyzed.
Lower. Rheumatic pains in the right hip.

Generalities.

Aversion to make any effort to exercise; must lie down.
Stitches! rheumatic pains, suddenly changing and often lasting but a short time; soreness, as if bruised.

Sleep.

55. Great sleepiness; in the afternoon, sleep relieving the symptoms, and early in the evening.

Fever.

Chilliness with cold hands and feet, with colic.
Coldness of the limbs, with pain in the back.

Skin.

Redness of the knuckles; warts on the knuckles.
Itching and crawling as from fleas, on different spots,—on the back, arms, abdomen, thighs, ankles.

PHOSPHORICUM ACIDUM.

Bad effects from grief, sorrow, unfortunate love, with great emaciation, sleepiness and morning sweat.

Quiet delirium with great stupefaction and dulness of the head (in typhus fever).

Head.

Stupefaction in the forehead, with somnolency without snoring, the eyes being closed.

10. Sensation as if intoxicated, in the evening in the warm room, with humming in the head, which feels as if it would burst when coughing.

Pressing tensive headache, especially on the side on which one lies.

Great heaviness of the head.

Stitches over one (the right) eye.

Morning headache.

15. The headache compels one to lie down, and is insupportably aggravated from the least shaking or noise.

The hair becomes gray early or flaxen and very greasy, falls off; also the hair of the beard, especially after grief and sorrow.

Pain in the bones of the skull; it feels as if somebody scraped the swollen and tender periosteum with a knife; worse at rest, better from motion. Caries of the skull with burning pain.

Eyes.

The eyes look glassy, but without lustre.

Pressing in the eyes as if the eyeball were too large.

20. Coldness of the internal surface of the eyelids.

Burning of the eyelids and the corners of the eyes, especially in the evening by candle-light.

Inflammation of the eyelids.

The eyes are dazzled on looking at bright objects.

Yellow spot in the white of the eye.

Ears.

25. Stitches in the ears, with drawing pains in the cheeks and teeth; aggravated only from musical sounds.

Every sound re-echoes loudly in the ears.

Intolerance of all sounds, especially music.

Shrill sound in the ears on blowing the nose.

Hardness of hearing at a distance.

Nose.

30. Discharge of bloody pus from the nose.

Swelling of the dorsum of the nose with red spots; scurfs on the dorsum of the nose.
Inclination to bore with the fingers in the nose.
Fetid smell from the nose.

Face.

Heat of that side of the face on which he is not lying.
35. Pale, sickly complexion, with lustreless, sunken eyes surrounded by blue margins, and pointed nose.
Hot tension on the skin of the face, as if the white of an egg had dried on it.
Lips dry, scurfy, suppurating.
Yellow-brown, crust-like eruptions with pus on the lower lip towards the corner of the mouth.
Pimples and scurfs on the vermilion borders of the lips.

Mouth and Throat.

40. Burning in the front teeth, especially at night, aggravated by the heat of the bed as well as from hot and cold things.
Violent aching in a hollow tooth when particles of food get into it, going off after they have been removed.
The teeth become yellow.
The gums are swollen, stand off from the teeth, and bleed easily.
Painful tubercle on the gum.
45. Ulceration of the soft velum, with burning pain.
Tough, clammy mucus in the mouth and on the tongue.
Swelling of the tongue, with pain on talking.
Nasal voice.
Dryness of the throat (palate) without thirst.
50. Bites himself involuntarily in the tongue at night.
Sore throat, with soreness, scraping and stinging, worse on swallowing food.
Hawking up of tough mucus.

Stomach and Abdomen.

Violent thirst from a sensation of dryness of the whole body.
Longing for something refreshing and juicy; bread is too dry.
55. Bad effects from sour food and drink.
Bitter eructations after eating sour things.
Continuous nausea in the throat; vomiting of food.
Pressing in the stomach as from a heavy load, with sleepiness, after every meal and when touching the pit of the stomach.
Rumbling in the intestines and noise as from water.

PHOSPHORICUM ACIDUM.

60. The flatulency is much augmented by sour food.
   The uterus is bloated as if filled with wind.

Stool and Anus.
Diarrhœa not debilitating.
Diarrhœic stools of mucus; undigested, greenish-white.
Difficult discharge of even the soft stool.

Urinary Organs.
65. Sudden, irresistible urging to urinate.
   Frequent profuse emission of watery urine, which forms a white cloud at once.
   Urine like milk, with bloody, jelly-like lumps.
   Diabetes melitus.
   Urging to urinate, with pale face, heat and thirst.
70. Burning in the urethra while urinating.
   Painful constriction in the bladder (without urging).
   Involuntary secretion of urine.

Sexual Organs.
Men. Pricking pain in the glans penis.
   Tingling and humid secretions at the frenulum.
75. Sycotic excrescences with heat and burning.
   Swelling of the testicles, with swelling and tension in the spermatic cords.
   The testicles are very tender to the touch; gnawing pain in the testicles.
   Inflammatory swelling of the scrotum.
   Sexual desire suppressed.
80. Bad effects from onanism.
   Frequent involuntary, very debilitating emissions.
   Women. Meteoristic distention of the uterus.

Respiratory Organs.
Shortness of breath and inability to speak long on account of great weakness of the chest.
Constriction in the throat-pit.
85. Hoarseness and roughness in the throat.
   Cough from tickling in the pit of the stomach and throat, with expectoration only in the morning.
   Cough with headache, nausea and vomiting of food, or with involuntary emission of urine.
   Cough with purulent, very offensive expectoration.
   Spasmodic tickling cough, caused by a sensation as from dust in the larynx and chest down to the pit of the stomach in the morning; expectoration of dark blood or of tough white mucus, tasting acid, herbaceous.

90. The cough is worse morning and evening; during rest, if one sits or lies long in the same position; after sleeping; from cold air; from loss of fluids.
Burning and pressure in the chest.

Back and Neck.

Formication in the back and small of the back.

Extremities.

Upper. Shrivelled dry skin of the hands and fingers.
Wen on the hand (between the metacarpal bones).
95. Stitches in the finger joints.
Trembling of the hands (when writing).
Sharply marked deadness of one half of the fingers.
Lower. Blood-boil on the nates.
Painful spasm in the hip-joint.
100. Weakness of the legs; he falls easily from a misstep, or on tripping.
Burning in the tibia and soles of the feet at night.
Ulcers on the lower extremities, with itching.
Swelling and burning, beating pains in the joint of the big toe.
Blisters on the balls of the toes.
105. Feet swollen; sweaty.

Generalities.

Sensation as if the body and the limbs were bruised, as from growing, especially in the morning.
Formication in different parts of the body.
Burning through the lower half of the body from the small of the back and pit of the stomach downwards, while the extremities are cold to the touch.
Weakness from loss of fluids without any other pain than burning.

Sleep.

110. Great drowsiness.
Deep and heavy sleep; can scarcely be roused in the morning.
Anxious dreams.

Fever.

Pulse irregular, sometimes intermitting one or two beats, generally small, weak or frequent, at times full and strong.
Violent ebullitions with great restlessness.
115. Swollen veins.
Chills with shuddering and shaking, always in the evening.

PHOSPHORICUM ACIDUM.

Chill and heat frequently alternating.
Sensation of coldness on one side of the face.
During the chill, a peculiarly strong sensation of coldness in the tips of the fingers and in the abdomen.
120. Internal dry heat without heat and without any complaint, at any time of the day.
General heat with loss of consciousness and somnolence.
Heat in the head, with cold feet.
Perspiration mostly on the back part of the head and in the neck, with sleepiness during the day.
Profuse perspirations during the night and in the morning, with anxiety.
125. Great inclination to perspire during day and night. Clammy perspirations.
Intermittent fevers.—Shaking chills over the whole body; the fingers being as cold as ice, without any thirst, followed by heat without thirst, or by excessive heat, depriving one almost of consciousness.

Skin.

Swelling of the glands.
Pain as if the periosteum of all the long bones were scraped with a knife.
Inflammation of the bones with burning at night.
130. Swelling of the bones.
Caries with smarting pains.
Formication on the skin.
Scarlet-like exanthems. Erysipelatous inflammations.
Blood-boils.
135. Chilblains, wens, sycotic excrescences.
Corns with stinging and burning.
Ulcers, flat, itching.
Smarting in the wounds, even in those of the bones.

Conditions.

Bad effects from sexual excesses (loss of fluids).
140. Bad consequences from grief, sorrow or unfortunate love.
Most of the pains are only felt during rest and are much ameliorated by motion.
Aggravation from suppression of cutaneous eruptions; from loss of animal fluids; from warm food; from talking.
Amelioration from motion and the nightly pains from pressure.

PHYTOLACCA DECANDRA.

Mind and Disposition.

Great indifference.

Head.

Vertigo and dimness of vision.
One-sided headache above the eyes with sickness of the stomach.
Shooting pain from the left eye to the vertex.

Eyes.

5. Burning and smarting sensation in the eyes and lids, with profuse lachrymation, which is relieved in the open air.
Purple-colored swelling of the eyelids (left eye in the morning.)

Ears.

Shooting pains in the (right) ear.

Face.

Pale face.
Heat in the face (left side) after dinner; with redness of the face, coldness of the feet, eruption in the upper lip (left side).

Mouth and Throat.

10. The mouth fills with water, the saliva is yellowish and has a metallic taste.
The tongue feels rough, with blisters on both sides, with a very red tip; great pain at the root of the tongue on swallowing.
The teeth feel elongated and are very sore.
Sensation of dryness in the throat and the posterior fauces.
Sensation of a lump in the throat, causing a continuous desire to swallow.
15. Roughness and rawness in the throat.

Stomach and Abdomen.

Nausea followed by violent vomiting of mucus, bile, of the ingesta, worms, blood.
Soreness and pain in the right hypochondrium (during pregnancy).

Stool and Anus.

Constipation, hard stools.
Stool with mucus and straining.

Urinary Organs.

20. Violent urging to pass urine.
Copious nocturnal urination.
Sediment like chalk; the dark-red urine leaves a stain in the chamber of a mahogany color.
Albuminous urine.

Sexual Organs.

Women. Menstruation too profuse and too frequent.
25. Inflammation, swelling and suppuration of the mammæ.

Generalities.

Pains are pressing, shooting and sore.
Syphilitic and mercurial rheumatism; nightly pains in the tibia, with nodes and irritable ulcers on the lower leg.

PLATINA.

Mind and Disposition.

Pride and over-estimation of oneself; looking down with haughtiness on others.
Illusion; every thing around her is very small and everybody inferior to her in body and mind.
Low-spirited, inclined to shed tears, worse in the evening.
Anxiety, horrified by the thought that he would die soon.
5. Great indifference.
After anger alternate laughing and weeping, with great anguish and fear of death.
Delirium, with fear of men, often changing, with over-estimation of oneself.
Mania; with great pride; with fault-finding; with unchaste talk; trembling and clonic spasms, caused by fright or from anger.
Pressing headache from without to within the forehead and temples, gradually increasing and decreasing, aggravated in the evening, from stooping, while at rest, in the room; ameliorated from exercise and in the open air.

10. Constrictive headache, as if a tape were tightly drawn around it, with sensation of numbness in the brain, flushes of heat and ill-humor, worse from stooping and exercise.

Formication in one temple, extending to the lower jaw, with sensation of coldness on that spot; worse in the evening and when at rest, better from rubbing.

Sensation of numbness in the head and externally on the vertex, preceded by a sensation of contraction of the brain and the scalp; worse in the evening and while sitting, better from motion and in the open air.

Eyes.

Sensation of coldness in the eyes.
Spasmodic trembling and twitching of the eyelids.
15. The objects appear smaller than they really are.

Ears.

Otalgia, with cramp pain.
Sensation of coldness in the ears, with sensation of numbness extending to the cheeks and lips.

Nose.

Numbness and cramp pain in the nose.

Face.

Redness and burning heat of the face, with violent thirst, especially towards evening.
20. Sensation of coldness, tingling and numbness in (one side of) the face.

Cramp pain and sensation of numbness in the (left) malar bone.

Benumbing, dull pressure in the malar bone.
Lockjaw.
Pale, sunken countenance.
25. Sensation of coldness, especially in the mouth.
Purple, net-like appearance on the chin.

Mouth and Throat.

Rhagades in the gums.
Cramp-like drawing in the throat, as if it were constricted.
Hawking of mucus, with scraping in the throat.
30. Sensation as if the tongue were scalded.
Sensation as if the palate were elongated.

Stomach and Abdomen.

Aversion to food on account of feeling low-spirited.
Thirstlessness.

Sweet taste on the tip of the tongue.
35. Ravenous appetite and hasty eating, with the inclination to detest every thing around himself.
Unsuccessful efforts to eructate.
Continuous nausea, with trembling weakness and anguish.
Pressure on the stomach, especially after eating.
Sensation of constriction in the pit of the stomach and in the abdomen.
40. Burning in the pit of the stomach, extending into the abdomen.
Pinching in the region of the navel.
Pressing and bearing down in the abdomen, extending into the pelvis.
Lead-colic.

Stool and Anus.

Constipation; after lead poisoning or while travelling; frequent urging, with expulsion of only small portions of feces, with great straining.
45. After an evacuation sensation of great weakness in the abdomen or chilliness.
Itching-tingling and tenesmus at the anus, especially in the evening.

Urinary Organs.

Frequent micturition, with slow flow of urine.
Urine red, with white clouds or turbid with red sediment.

Sexual Organs.

Men. Unnaturally increased sexual desire, with violent erections, especially at night.
50. *Women.* Painful sensitiveness of the genitals internally and externally.
Bearing down to the genitals and pressing down in the abdomen.
Nymphomania; unnatural excitement of the sexual desire, especially in lying-in-women, with voluptuous tingling in the external and internal sexual organs.
Induration of the uterus.
Menstruation too early and too profuse (lasting but a short time), with clotted, dark blood.
55. Metrorrhagia, with great excitability of the sexual system.
Spasms on the appearance of the menstruation.
Pressing down in the genitals during menstruation.

Respiratory Organs.

Difficult, anxious respiration.
Shortness of breath, as if the chest were constricted, with anxious warm rising.
60. Inclination to draw a long breath, prevented by a sensation of weakness in the chest.
Loss of voice (aphony).
Sensation of cramp-pain externally on the thorax, gradually increasing and decreasing.
Palpitation of the heart with anxiety.

Back and Neck.

Pains in the back, and small of the back, as if bruised, especially when pressing on it, or when bending backward.
65. Sensation of numbness in the os sacrum.
Stiffness of the neck.
Weakness, tension and numbness in the neck.

Extremities.

Upper. Cramp-like pains in the arms and hands.
Paralytic drawing and weakness in the arms.
70. Ulcers on the fingers.
Lower. Cramp-like pains in the legs.
Sensation of stiffness in the lower legs.
Ulcers on the toes.

Generalities.

Cramp-like pains, especially in the extremities and joints.
75. Dull, pushing or inward, pressing pains, as from the pressure of a plug.
Tension in the limbs, as if they were wrapped up tightly.
Paralytic sensation, numbness and stiffness in the limbs, generally accompanied by coldness.
Paralytic weakness in the limbs, especially when at rest.
Hysterical spasms, with full consciousness (at the dawn of day, morning).

Sleep.

80. Spasmodic yawning, especially in the afternoon.
Wakens (after midnight) with frightful dreams, want of consciousness.
At night and during sleep he lies with his arms thrown over his head, the thighs drawn up, and inclined to have his legs uncovered.

Fever.

Pulse small, feeble, frequently tremulous.
Chill in the evening, with trembling and tremulous sensation over the whole body.
85. Shaking chill when going from the room into the open, even warm, air.
Chilliness predominates, with low spirits, which ceases during the heat.
Heat, with sensation of burning in the face, without any visible change in the color of the face.
Flushes of heat, interrupted by chilliness.
Gradually increasing, and in the same manner gradually decreasing heat.
90. Perspiration only during the sleep, ceasing as soon one wakens.

Skin.

Sensation of soreness, tingling smarting and itching, or pricking, stinging burning, with inclination to scratch on different parts of the body.
Ulcers on the fingers and toes.

Conditions.

Is especially suitable for women.
Alternate appearance of the symptoms of the body and mind; as soon as the one group predominates the other ceases.
95. Aggravation of such symptoms in the evening and in the room as are ameliorated in the open air.
Most ailments are worse when at rest, and better during motion.
The pains begin slightly, increase gradually, and decrease in the same slow, gradual manner.

PLUMBUM.

Mind and Disposition.

Quiet and melancholy mood.
Anxiety, with restlessness and yawning.
Wild delirium, with distorted countenance.

Head.

Vertigo, especially on stooping and on turning the eyes upwards.
5. Stupefaction of the head, he falls down unconscious.
Heaviness of the head, especially in the cerebellum.
Congestions of blood to the head, with heat and beating in it.
Headache as if a ball were rising from the throat into the brain.
Great dryness of the hair, it falls off even in the beard.

Eyes.

10. Inflammation of the eyes, with congestion of blood to them.
Pressing in the eyes, as if the balls were too large.
Pupils contracted.
Paralysis of the upper eyelids.
Spasmodic contraction of the eyelids.
15. Yellow color of the white of the eye.
Cloudiness before the eyes, inducing one to rub them.

Ears.

Stitches and tearing in the ears.
Hardness of hearing; often sudden deafness.

Nose.

Erysipelatous inflammation of the nose.
20. Fetid odor before the nose. Much tough mucus in the nose, which can only be discharged through the posterior nares.
The nose is cold.

Face.

Face pale, yellowish, like a corpse.
Bloated face.
Swelling of one side of the face.
25. The skin of the face is greasy, shining.
Painless pealing off of the lips.
Lock-jaw.
Tearing in the jaws, relieved by rubbing them.

Mouth and Throat.

The teeth become black.
30. Yellow mucus on the teeth.
Teeth hollow, decayed, crumbling off, and smelling offensively.

Pale, swollen gums; purple-colored thin border on the gums nearest the teeth.
Hard, painful tubercles in the gums.
Grinding of the teeth.
35. Dryness in the mouth.
Aphthæ and dirty-looking ulcers and purple blotches in the mouth and on the tip of the tongue.
Sensation in the throat as from a plug or foreign body.
It rises in the throat like a ball (globus hystericus).
Constriction in the throat, as soon as the least effort is made to swallow, with great urging to do so.
40. Inflammation of the tonsils,—formation of consecutive, small, exceedingly painful abscesses in the tonsils.
Paralysis of the throat, with inability to swallow.
Accumulation of sweetish saliva in the mouth.
Froth in the mouth.
Inflammation, swelling, and heaviness of the tongue.
45. Tongue dry, brown, cracked, or coated yellowish or green.
Paralysis of the tongue preventing speech.

Stomach and Abdomen.

Violent thirst, especially for cold water.
Sweetish taste.
Sweetish eructations; gulping up of sweetish water.
50. Violent vomiting; of food and of discolored substances, with violent colic; or of greenish and blackish substances.
Vomiting of feces, with constipation.
Painful pressure in the stomach.
Violent colic; the abdomen drawn in, especially the navel, which seems to be drawn back by a string to the spinal column.
Constriction of the intestines; navel and anus are violently drawn in.
55. Colic and paralysis of the lower extremities.
Hard lump in the abdomen, as from internal indurations.
Rumbling in the abdomen.
Inflammation, ulceration and gangrene of the bowels.

Stool and Anus.

Constipation; stools hard, lumpy, difficult to expel.
60. Painful, fetid diarrhœa of yellow feces.
Bloody diarrhœa; watery diarrhœa, with vomiting and violent colic, especially pain in the umbilicus.
Painful contraction and constriction of the anus.
Prolapsus ani.

Urinary Organs.

Difficult emission of urine; only by drops.
65. Strangury.
Hæmaturia.

Sexual Organs.

Men. Genitals swollen and inflamed.
Constriction of the testicles.
The testicles are drawn up.
70. Increased sexual desire with violent erections.
Women. Miscarriage.

Respiratory Organs.

Spasmodic dyspnœa.
Constriction of the larynx.
Cough with expectoration of blood, or of pus (after hemorrhages from the lungs).
75. Dry, spasmodic cough.
Breathing heavy, difficult.
Stitches in the chest and sides.
Anxiety about the heart and violent palpitation.

Back and Neck.

Stitches in the back and small of the back, and between the shoulder-blades.
80. Tension in the neck, extending to the ears when moving the head.

Extremities.

Upper. Convulsive motions of the arms and hands, with pain in the joints.
Weakness and painful lameness of the arms.
Wens on the hand.
Lower. Paralytic sensation in the hip, knee and foot joints.
85. Paralysis of the lower limbs and feet.
Swelling of the feet.
Fetid foot-sweat.

Generalities.

Twitching in the limbs.
Paralysis of the limbs.
90. Sensation of constriction, with pain and spasms, in internal organs.
Epileptic attacks; convulsions.
Dropsical swellings.
Emaciation, especially of the paralyzed parts, followed by swelling of those parts.

Sleep.

Somnolency.
95. Great sleepiness during the day.
Sleeplessness at night from colic.

Fever.

Pulse very variable, generally contracted, small and slow; at times hard and slow, occasionally small and quick.
Chill predominates, increasing towards evening, with violent thirst and redness of the face.
Coldness in the open air and when exercising.
100. Heat with thirst, anxiety, redness of the face, and sleepiness.
Internal heat in the evening and at night, with yellowness of the buccal cavity.
Perspiration, anxious, cold and clammy.

Skin.

Sensitiveness of the skin to the open air.
The color of the skin is yellow or pale-bluish.
105. Dark-brown spots on the body.
Decubitus.
Burning in the ulcers; small wounds become easily inflamed and suppurate.
Gangrene.

Conditions.

The ailments develop themselves slowly and intermit for a time,—intermission every third day.
110. The pains in the limbs are worse at night and are relieved by rubbing.

PODOPHYLLUM PELTATUM.

Mind and Disposition.

Depression of spirits; imagines he is going to die or be very ill.

Head.

Giddiness, with the sensation of fulness over the eyes.
Delirium and loquacity during the fever, with excessive thirst.
Morning headache, with flushed face.

5. Headache alternating with diarrhœa.
   Rolling of the head during difficult dentition in children.
   Perspiration of the head during sleep, with coldness of the flesh during teething.

Eyes.

Pain in the eyeballs and in the temples, with heat, and throbbing of the temporal arteries.

Mouth and Throat.

Offensive odor from the mouth (at night).
10. The tongue is furred white, with foul taste.
    Dryness of the mouth and tongue in the morning.
    Grinding of the teeth at night.
    Dryness of the throat.
    Rattling of mucus in the throat.

Stomach and Abdomen.

15. Regurgitation of the food.
    After eating and drinking, diarrhœa.
    Vomiting of food with putrid taste and odor.
    Colic with retraction of the umbilical muscles.
    Fulness and pain in the region of the liver.

Stool and Anus.

20. Constipation, with flatulence and headache; feces hard and dry, and voided with difficulty.
    Morning diarrhœa; stools green (chronic diarrhœa).
    Feces yellow or dark-green; white, slimy, chalk-like and very offensive, with gagging and excessive thirst in children; frothy mucus; hot, watery; undigested.
    After stool extreme weakness and cutting pain in the intestines.
    Prolapsus ani (with diarrhœa).
25. Descent of the rectum from a little exertion, followed by stool or by the discharge of thick, transparent mucus, sometimes mixed with blood.

Urinary Organs.

Suppression of urine.
Frequent nocturnal urination during pregnancy.
Involuntary discharge of urine during sleep.

Genital Organs.

Women. Pain in the region of the ovaries.
30. Suppression of the menses in young persons, with bearing down in the hypogastric and sacral regions, with pains from motion; better from lying down.

Prolapsus uteri, with pain in the sacrum.
In the earlier months of pregnancy she can only lie comfortably on the stomach.
After-pains with strong bearing down.

Respiratory Organs.

Hooping-cough, with costiveness and loss of appetite.
35. Loose, hacking cough.
Palpitation of the heart, from physical exertions.

Sleep.

Sleepiness in day-time, especially in the forenoon, with rumbling in the bowels.
Unrefreshing sleep; feeling of fatigue on waking in the morning.

Fever.

Chilliness when moving about during fever.
40. Before the chill pain in the small of the back.
Chill with pressing pain in both hypochondria; dull aching pain in the knees, ankles, elbows and wrists; consciousness, but cannot talk, because he forgets the words.
Chill with thirst, which increases during the heat.
Heat, with violent headache, excessive thirst, delirium and loquacity.
Perspiration, with sleep.

POTHOS FŒTIDUS.

Face.

Above the nasal bone, swollen and red, forming a saddle, painful to the touch, especially on the left side of the nose; the cartilaginous part is cold and bloodless, with red spots on the cheeks; on the left side of the face small pimples.

Mouth.

Sensation of numbness of the tongue, cannot touch the teeth with it.
Papillæ elevated.
Red and sore on the tip and the edges.

35

Respiratory Organs.

5. Catarrh of aged persons.
Sudden anxiety, with dyspnœa and perspiration, followed by stool and relief of that and other complaints.
Inclination to draw a long breath, with the sensation of emptiness in the chest; later, constriction in the larynx and chest.
Asthma, aggravated or caused by dust. (Heaves in horses from dusty hay.)
The difficulty of breathing is better in the open air.

PRUNUS SPINOSA.

Mind and Disposition.

Restlessness, which does not allow one to remain quiet in one place, walks about constantly, with dyspnœa and short breathing.

Head.

Heaviness of the head, also with vertigo.
Pressing in the head, as if the brain were pressed out through the skull with a plug.
Stitches in the scalp.

Eyes.

5. Pain in the right eye as if it were torn asunder.
Itching in the corners of the eyes and in the edges of the lids.

Ears.

Pain as if pressed out in the right ear.

Nose.

Pain as from pressing asunder above the nasal bones.

Mouth and Throat.

Burning of the tongue as if scalded.

Stomach and Abdomen.

10. Sensation of repletion in the stomach; a very small quantity of food satisfies the appetite.

Sensation of fulness in the pit of the stomach, as after a full meal, or as from overlifting, with shortness of breathing.

Ascites, with loss of appetite, scanty urine, hard, knotty stool, which is difficult to pass.

Incarcerated flatulency (on the bladder, with spasms, compelling one to walk stooped).

Pain in the right inguinal region as if hernia would protrude.

Stool and Anus.

15. Stool hard, difficult to expel, in small pieces, with stitches in the rectum.

Diarrhœa with nausea, feces consisting of mucus, with burning in the rectum as from a wound.

Urinary Organs.

Tenesmus vesicæ.

Strangury; continuous urging to urinate, with burning-biting in the bladder and urethra; when the effort is made to urinate, burning in the urethra, so that one must bend double without being able to urinate.

Urgent desire to urinate; the urine only reaches the glans penis and causes there violent pains and spasms, also with tenesmus in the rectum; the pain in the bladder is momentarily relieved as soon as the urine descends in the urethra.

20. Scanty secretion of urine, brown; must always press a long time before passing any urine, and then in a feeble stream.

Spasms in the bladder, disturbing the sleep at night; burning in the sphincter vesicæ.

In the urethra burning-biting; great soreness, so that he can not touch it.

Sexual Organs.

Men. The prepuce is drawn behind the corona glandis, the penis becoming smaller.

Women. Tickling, itching in the region of the ovaries, not relieved by scratching and rubbing.

25. Menstruation too early, with violent pain in the small of the back.

Metrorrhagia of thin pale blood, becoming more watery the longer it lasts.

Leucorrhœa, excoriating, coloring the linen yellow.

Respiratory Organs.

Breathing difficult, caused by a sensation of heaviness in the lower part of the thorax.

Back.

Back and small of the back feel stiff as from overlifting.
30. Stitches between the shoulder-blades on drawing a long breath.
Pain in the small of the back when sitting.

Extremities.

Upper. Pressure on the right shoulder, extending to the deltoid muscle, preventing one from raising the arm.
Sensation as if sprained in the right thumb, hindering one from writing; cannot hold the pen.
Lower. Pain in the hip, worse in the forenoon, and free from it after midnight.
35. Pain in the first joint of the big toe, as if it were pulled out.
Restlessness in the legs, has to change the position continually.

Fever.

Chilliness in the evening, must go to bed, is inclined to stretch himself.
Dry heat over the whole body, with pain in the corona glandis and redness of the prepuce; burning on the genitals, relieved by perspiration, and ceasing when going to bed.
Perspiration during sleep, only in the face.

PSORINUM.

Mind and Disposition.

Anxiety about the future.
Despair of recovery, thinks to be very ill, and in great danger not to survive the sickness; hopelessness.
Great anxiety, full of fears.
Religious melancholy.
5. Impatience; ill humor.

Head.

Vertigo with headache; it presses the eyes out.

Congestions of blood to the head, with red-hot cheeks and nose, redness of the eruption on the face, with great anxiety every afternoon after dinner (during pregnancy fifth month).

Fulness in the vertex as if the brain would burst out, with formication in the head; before the headache flickering before the eyes; the objects dance before the eyes, or black spots and rings appear before the eyes; afterwards very heavy sleep.

Congestion of blood to the head with heat, wakened him in the night, was stupefied, could not recollect what happened, and after sitting for a while had to rise to collect his senses.

10. Fulness and heaviness in the head.

Morning headache with pressing in the forehead, with stupefaction, vertigo and soreness of the eyes.

At night (1 A. M.) sensation as if one received a heavy blow on the forehead, awakens him.

Dry hair, with loss of lustre.

The hair glues together and becomes entangled, has to comb it continually.

15. Dry and humid fetid eruptions on the head.

Large humid blotches on the head, with scabby eruptions on the face.

Suppurating, fetid, humid eruption on the head with humid soreness behind the ears (in children).

Great aversion to have the head uncovered, even in the hottest weather does he persist in wearing a fur cap.

Eyes.

Aversion to light.

20. Every thing gets dark before the eyes.

Heat and redness of the eyes, with pressing pains.

Eyelids bloated; swollen; inflamed.

Ears.

Singing, humming and ringing in the ears, with hardness of hearing.

Discharge of pus from the ear, with headache.

25. Scurfs on the ears; and humid scurfs behind the ear.

Herpes extending from the (left) temple extends over the whole ear down to the cheek, at times throwing off innumerable scales, and again showing painful rhagades with humid yellow discharges, forming scurfs; fetid, humid, intolerable itching, especially in the evening till midnight.

Nose.

Loss of smell.

Soreness of the nose; sensitiveness of the mucous membrane when inhaling air.

Face.

Pimples on the forehead.

30. Red small pimples on the face, especially on the nose and chin, and in the middle of the cheeks.

Burning heat and redness of the face.

Ulcers in the face.

Humid eruptions on the face. The whole face is covered with humid scurfs or crusts, with swelling of the lips and eyelids, with humid soreness behind the ears.

Lips dry, brown, black.

35. Ulcers on the lips.

Mouth and Throat.

Sensation of soreness of the teeth.

Stinging in the teeth (while eating).

Looseness of the teeth.

Ulcers on the gums (right side).

40. Tough mucus in the mouth and throat with much hawking.

Burning in the throat; sensation as if it were scalded.

Sensation of a lump (plug) in the throat which impedes the hawking up of mucus.

Dryness in the throat with thirstlessness.

Loss of taste, with coryza.

45. Tongue dry; dry on the tip, feels as if scalded, coated white, yellow.

Taste bitter.

Stomach and Abdomen.

Eructations, smelling like rotten eggs.

Nausea in the morning, with pain in the small of the back.

Nausea all day, with vomiting of sweetish mucus.

50. Deep-seated, heavy pain in the region of the liver, worse when pressing on it and when lying on the right side, when walking, coughing, laughing, and taking a long breath.

Stitches in the region of the spleen.

Emission of fetid flatulence.

Inguinal hernia.

Stool and Anus.

The soft stool is discharged with great difficulty.

55. Constipation; with pain in the small of the back; with discharge of blood from the rectum.
Frequent liquid stools (with tinea capitis).
Stools of mucus mixed with blood.
Discharge of large quantities of blood from the rectum, with hard, difficult stool.
Burning, hæmorrhoidal tumors.

Urinary Organs.

60. Urinary secretion profuse.
Involuntary micturition, cannot hold the urine.
Urine thick, whitish, turbid, depositing a red sediment and forming a cuticle swimming on it.

Sexual Organs.

Men. Impotence.
Excessive, uncontrollable sexual instinct.
65. Hydrocele.
Discharge of painless mucus from the urethra. (Gonorrhœa secundaria.)
Drawing pains in the testicles and spermatic cords.
Sycotic excrescences on the edges of the prepuce, itching and burning.

Respiratory Organs.

Shortness of breath.
70. The thorax expands itself with great difficulty when breathing.
Anxious dyspnœa, with palpitation of the heart.
The dyspnœa is worse when sitting up to write, better when lying down.
Asthmatic attacks with hydrothorax.
Cough from tickling in the larynx.
75. Cough, with stitches in the chest, or with sensation of weakness in the chest.
Dry cough, with soreness of the sternum.
Burning pressing pain in the chest.
Suppuration of the lungs. (Phthisis pulmonalis.)
Pain in the chest, as if raw, as from subcutaneous ulceration.
80. Cutting as from knives in the chest.
Stitches in the chest (left side).
Palpitation of the heart, with anxiety.
Pain (stitches) in the heart, worse when lying down.

Back and Neck.
Painful stiffness of the neck.
85. Pain in the small of the back, worse on motion.

Extremities.
Upper. Attacks of lameness and soreness in the right shoulder, extending to the hand.
Lower. Pain in the hip-joints as if dislocated, worse when walking, with weakness of the arms.
The feet go to sleep often.
Pain in the legs, especially on the tibia and in the soles of the feet, as from over-exertion in walking, with great restlessness in the legs, better on rising.
90. Heat and itching in the soles of the feet.
Ulcers on the lower legs, with intolerable itching over the whole body.
Arthritis.

Generalities.
Very weak from the least exertion.
Great debility from loss of fluids or after severe acute diseases (Typhus).
95. Rheumatism and arthritis.
Dropsical diseases.

Sleep.
Sleepiness in day-time.
Sleeplessness at night, from dyspnœa, from intolerable itching.
Wakens from congestions to the head.

Fever.
100. Chilliness in the evening on the upper arms and thighs, with thirst; drinking causes cough.
Heat in the afternoon or evening, feels as if he should lose his senses, with thirst.
Heat, with perspiration on the face; heat when riding in a carriage.
Heat at night, and dryness in the mouth.
Want of perspiration, dry skin.
105. Profuse, colliquative perspiration.
Perspiration profuse when taking the slightest exercise; at night.
Perspiration after typhus fever.
Perspiration in the palms of the hands.

Skin.
Itching and stinging in the skin in many parts at the same time.

PULSATILLA PRATENSIS. 553

110. Intolerable itching from getting warm; in the evening in bed, scratches himself till he bleeds.
Urticaria, with eruptions on the head.
Itching pustules on the forehead, chin, chest.
Dry itch on the arms and chest, but most severe on the finger-joints.
Itch on the elbow and wrist.
115. Herpes, with biting-itching, with meal-dust, humid.
Old ulcers, with fetid pus.
Violently itching ulcers.
Suppressed itch, eruptions.
Rash on the neck and back.

Conditions.

120. Psor. is an indispensable remedy if debility remains after violent acute diseases; if profuse perspirations remain after typhus fever; in the evil consequences of suppressed itch, especially after large doses of sulphur; if the patient is hopeless, despairing of his recovery.
Many ailments are worse or come on when riding in a carriage, and when exercising in the open air, and relieved by rest and in the room.
Aggravations in the evening and before midnight.
Sitting aggravates the dyspnœa (asthma) and pain in the heart; these and other ailments are relieved while lying down.

PULSATILLA PRATENSIS.

Mind and Disposition.

Mild, bashful, yielding disposition, with inclination to weep.
Peevishness, which increases to tears, with chilliness and thirstlessness.
Gloomy, melancholy, full of cares.
Mistrust; anthropophobia.
5. Anguish about the heart, even to desire for suicide.
Tremulous anguish, as if death were near.
Covetousness.

Head.

Vertigo, as if intoxicated, when rising from a seat; when stooping; after eating; when lifting up the eyes.

Giddiness, with heat, with nausea and loss of sight, in the evening.
10. Intellectual labor fatigues him.
Frightful visions, delirium.
Stupefaction in the evening, in the warm room, with chilliness.
Fright, followed by diarrhœa, with internal heat and external coldness of the body.
Stupefying headache, with humming in the head, worse when lying or sitting quiet, or in the cold.
15. Soreness as from subcutaneous ulceration in one or both temples; worse in the evening, when at rest, and in the warm room; relieved by walking in the open air.
Pulsation in the head in the evening; worse from mental exertion and stooping.
Twitching-tearing in the temple on which one lies, and going to the other side when turning on it; worse in the evening and on raising the eyes upwards.
Tension in the forehead, as if it were in a vice.
Stitches in one side of the head, generally in one temple or in the back part of the head, with vertigo, ringing in the ears, and vanishing of sight.
20. Pain in the head, as if the brain were lacerated, on or soon after waking.
Congestion of blood to the head, with stinging pulsation in the brain, especially when stooping.
Pain, as if the head would burst.
Headache from the abuse of mercury or after eating fat food.
The headache is worse in the evening, after lying down; is aggravated by lifting up the eyes, by meditation, in the warm room, and is ameliorated from compression, and when walking slowly in the open air.
25. Tumors on the scalp, suppurating and affecting the skull; more painful when lying on the opposite well side.
Tingling, biting-itching on the scalp, mostly on the temples and behind the ears, followed by swelling and eruptions, paining sore, worse in the evening when undressing and on getting warm in bed.
Fetid, frequently cold perspiration, at times only on one side of the head and face, with great anxiety and stupor; worse at night and towards morning, better after waking and rising.
Disposition to take cold on the head, which is exclusively perspiring, especially on the head becoming wet.
Drawing pain in the scalp on brushing the hair backwards.

Eyes.

30. Pressing, tearing and stinging in the eyes.
    Painful inflammation of the eyes and of the meibomian glands. Styes, especially on the upper eyelid.
    Swelling and redness of the eyelids.
    Lachrymation in the open air and in the wind.
    Burning and itching in the eyes, inducing rubbing and scratching.
35. Dryness of the eyes and lids, with the sensation as if it were darkened by some mucus hanging over the eye which ought to be wiped away.
    Inflammation of the eye, with secretion of large, thick mucus and nightly agglutination.
    Stitches in the eyes, especially from light and in the sunshine.
    Fistula lachrymalis, discharging pus on pressing upon it.
    Dimness of sight, especially on getting warm from exercise.
40. Over-sensitiveness to light.
    Obscurations of the cornea.
    Like a veil before the eyes, better on rubbing and wiping them.
    Incipient cataract.
    Amaurosis; paralysis of the optic nerve.

Ears.

45. Otalgia, with darting, tearing pains.
    Inflammation of the external and internal ear, with redness, heat and swelling.
    Flow of mucus or thick pus from the (left) ear.
    Hardness of hearing, as if the ears were stopped up, especially from cold, from having the hair cut or after suppressed measles.
    Hardened, black cerumen.
50. Humming and tingling in the ears.

Nose.

The nose feels sore internally and externally.
Ulceration of the external wing of the nose, emitting a watery humor.
Bleeding of the nose,—blood coagulated; with dry coryza.
Green fetid discharge from the nose (like old catarrh).
55. Smell before the nose as from old catarrh.
    Coryza, with loss of smell and taste, or of long standing, with a heavy yellowish-green discharge.

Face.

Alternate redness and paleness of the face.
Color of the face pale or yellowish, with sunken eyes.
Face bloated, purple.
60. Puffiness of the cheeks and nose.
Sweat in (one side of) the face and on the hairy scalp.
Erysipelas in the face with pricking pain.
Painful sensitiveness of the skin in the face.
Gnawing and smarting around the mouth.
65. Lower lip swelled and cracked in the middle.

Mouth and Throat.

Toothache, tearing, jerking, as if the nerve were strung and suddenly released.
Jerking and stinging in the teeth, extending to the ears and eyes.
Looseness of the painful teeth.
Toothache from cold (in the first warm spring days), with otalgia, paleness of the face and chilliness.
70. Toothache aggravated in the evening and at night, from the heat of the bed, from warm air, in the warm room, from taking warm things in the mouth; relieved in the cool open air; from taking cold water in the mouth.
Pulsating and stinging in the gums, aggravated by the heat of the stove; gums pain as if they were sore.
Putrid smell from the mouth, especially in the morning.
Dryness in the mouth in the morning.
Ptyalism, the increased saliva tastes sweet.
75. Tongue coated yellow or white, and covered with tough mucus.
The tongue feels dry and clammy; feels in the middle as if burned.
Pain in the throat, as if sore and raw; stinging, with pressing and tension, or empty swallowing.
Inflammation of the throat, with veins distended.
Dryness of the throat in the morning, with tough mucus in the throat, especially in the night and morning.

Stomach and Abdomen.

80. Taste, putrid, bitter, especially after swallowing food or drink; sweetish (beer tastes sweet).
Thirstlessness, with moist tongue, or thirst for beer and strong alcoholic drink.
Aversion to fat food (butter), meat, bread and milk.
Hunger and desire to eat, without knowing what.

PULSATILLA PRATENSIS.

Eructations; tasting and smelling of what has been eaten; like bile in the evening.
85. Nausea felt in the upper part of the abdomen, especially in the evening, after eating and drinking, with rumbling in the abdomen.
Morning sickness (during pregnancy).
Vomiting of mucus; of bile; of bitter-sour fluids; of ingesta after each meal, especially in the evening and at night; of blood.
Disordered stomach (digestion) from eating fat food (pork).
Cold in the stomach from ice cream and fruit.
90. Colic, with nausea, ceasing after vomiting.
Pressure in the pit of the stomach after each meal, with vomiting of the ingesta.
Sensible pulsation in the pit of the stomach.
Inflammation of the abdomen, with great sensitiveness of the integuments to pressure.
Stitches and cutting in the abdomen in the evening; worse on sitting still.
95. Colic and labor-like pains in pregnant women.
Colic with chilliness, while the menstruation is suppressed.
Sensitiveness and inflammation of the abdominal walls.
Incarcerated flatulence, and from it colic in the evening.
Colic and rumbling of wind, especially in the upper abdomen.
100. Painless rumbling of flatulence in the upper abdomen.

Stool and Anus.

Constipation, especially if the feces are hard and large, after suppressed intermittent fever by Chininum Sulph.
Frequent soft, diarrhœic stools, consisting of yellow mucus or mixed with blood, preceded by cutting in the abdomen, or with pains in the small of the back.
Nightly diarrhœa, discharges watery or green like bile, after previous rumbling in the abdomen.
Difficult soft stool, with straining and backache.
105. Stools consisting only of mucus, or acrid, or bloody, or very offensive, or white.
Dysentery, with pain in the back.
During stool, congestions of blood to the anus.
Hæmorrhoidal tumors, with great soreness.

Urinary Organs.

Ischuria, with redness and heat in the region of the bladder.
110. Incontinence of urine; the urine is discharged by drops when sitting or when walking; involuntary discharge of urine when coughing, when passing wind, during sleep.

Tenesmus vesicæ.
Hæmaturia, with burning at the orifice of the urethra, and with constriction in the region of the navel.
During micturition burning in the urethra.
Scanty red-brown urine.
115. Sediment of the urine reddish, bloody or mucous.
Thick gonorrhœic discharge from the urethra.

Sexual Organs.

Men. Sexual desire too strong.
Itching-burning on the inner and upper side of the prepuce.
Inflammation and swelling of the testicles, with swelling of the scrotum (from a contusion or after suppressed gonorrhœa).
120. Burning in the testicles, without swelling.
Hydrocele.
Inflammation of prostate gland.
Women. Menstruation too late and too scanty, and of too short duration, with cramps in the abdomen; blood thick, black, clotted, or thin and watery.
Suppressed menstruation, especially from cold, getting the feet wet.
125. First menstruation delayed.
Metrorrhagia (discharge now stopping, and then stronger again) of coagulated, clotted blood, or with false labor-pains.
Labor-pains too weak, spasmodic or ceasing.
After-pains of long duration.
Suppression of the lochial discharges.
130. Suppression of or very scanty secretion of milk.
Leucorrhœa, acrid, burning, like milk, and painless.

Respiratory Organs.

Hoarseness, which does not permit one to speak a loud word.
Breathing, groaning or rattling.
Dyspnœa, especially when lying on the back, at night, with giddiness and weakness in the head.
135. Difficulty of breathing when walking.
Asthma at night, as from vapors of sulphur.
Dyspnœa, as from spasmodic tension in the lower part of the chest, below the false ribs.
Tickling on the sternum.
Short dry cough, as soon as he gets warm.
140. Dry cough, whenever he wakens from sleep, disappearing while sitting up in bed, and returning as soon as lying down again.

Dry, severe cough, mostly in the morning, with retching and desire to vomit, and sensation as if the stomach were turned inside out.
Cough, with expectoration of black, clotted blood (during the suppression of the menstruation).
Cough, with copious expectoration of yellow, bitter mucus.
Cough caused by dryness and scraping in the chest, with nausea and straining to vomit.
145. Expectoration salty, offensive, tasting like the discharge in chronic catarrh.
Acute suppuration of the lungs.
Cough, with expectoration in the morning or during the day only, without expectoration at night.
Anxious and spasmodic tightness of the chest, as if it were too full, and the larynx constricted, especially in the evening and at night.
Violent spasmodic hooping-cough, in two consecutive coughs, caused by itching, scraping, with dryness, as from the vapors of sulphur, in the larynx and chest.
150. Pain in the chest, as from subcutaneous ulceration.
Tension in the chest, especially on drawing a long breath.
Stitches in the chest, especially when coughing and drawing a long breath.
Attacks of burning in the chest.
Violent attacks of palpitation of the heart, often accompanied by anguish and vanishing of sight.
155. Burning pain in the heart.

Back and Neck.

Curvature of the spine (upper part).
Stitches in the small of the back.
Pains in the back and chilliness from suppressed menstruation.

Extremities.

Upper. Pressing heaviness or tearing and drawing in the shoulder-joint, extending to the fingers.
160. Swelling of the elbow after a contusion.
Swelling of the veins on the fore-arms and on the hands.
Itching chilblains on the hands.
Lower. Coxalgia.
Hot, inflammatory swelling of the knee.
165. Drawing pain in the tibia.
Varices on the lower extremities.
Red-hot swelling of the feet, extending up to the calf, with stinging pain.

Swelling of the top of the foot.
Sensation of soreness in the soles of the feet.
170. Chilblains.
The complaints are worse when one allows the feet to hang down.

Generalities.

Pain as from subcutaneous ulceration or as from inward festering.
Tension in inner parts or in the joints.
Burning-stinging pains.
175. Rheumatic red-hot swelling, with stinging pains.
Pains (rheumatic) shifting from one place to another.
Congestions to single parts.
Inflammation of internal organs, with disposition to suppurate.
Diseases (inflammation) of the mucous membranes.
180. Pulsations through the whole body.
Frequent anxious trembling of the limbs.
Hysterical complaints.
Chlorosis.
Attacks of fainting, with great paleness of the face.
185. Epileptic attacks (after suppressed menstruation), with violent beating of the limbs; later they become relaxed, with nausea and eructations.

Fever.

Pulse weak and small, but accelerated.
During the evening, heat; the veins are enlarged.
Coldness predominates.
Continuous internal chilliness, even in the warm room.
190. Increased chilliness towards evening.
Chilliness with the pains.
Sensation of coldness and numbness on one side of the body.
Thirst before the chill or heat, seldom during the hot stage.
The chill is followed by heat, with anxiety and heat of the face.
195. Internal general dry heat without external heat, in the evening or at night.
Heat of the face or heat of one hand, with coldness of the other.
Heat of the body with coldness of the extremities.
Profuse perspiration at night or in the morning.
Perspiration during sleep, soon ceasing when waking.
200. Perspires easy during the day.

One-sided perspiration, sometimes only in the face and the head.
Night-sweat with stupor.
Smell of the perspiration sour, musty, like musk.
Perspiration at times cold.
205. Perspiration only on (one side of the) face and scalp.
Intermittent fever, chilliness without thirst, then slight thirst, then heat without thirst, accompanied by vertigo and stupor.
First heat; afterwards violent chilliness.
Chilliness (4 P. M.) without thirst, accompanied by anxiety and dyspnœa; this is followed by a drawing pain extending from the back into the head, three hours later heat of the whole body without any thirst, with sweat on the face, drowsiness without any sleep and unconsciousness; in the morning perspiration over the whole body.
Intermittent fevers, with the prevalence of gastric and bilious symptoms or consequent upon the abuse of Chinin., with bitter taste of the food and constipation.
210. Vomiting of mucus when the cold stage comes on, absence of thirst during the hot stage and during the perspiration.
Mucous diarrhœa during the apyrexia, with nausea and loss of appetite.

Skin.

Pale skin.
Eruptions from eating much pork, itching violently in bed.
Eruptions like measles.
215. Exanthemata; itching-stinging, chapped.
Chilblains, inflamed, itching.
Rhagades.
Suppurating wounds,—pus thick and too profuse.
Ulcers; bleeding easily, burning or stinging in the circumference, itching, or very hard or red around the ulcers.
220. Fistulous ulcers.
Pus copious and yellow.
Inflamed varices.

Conditions.

Especially suitable for slow, phlegmatic, good-natured, timid temperaments; for women, and especially during pregnancy.
The symptoms are often accompanied by chilliness, thirstlessness and oppression of the chest.

225. The more severe the pain the stronger is the chill.
Serves as an antidote for the abuse of China, Chinin., Mercury, Sulphur, or Chamomilla tea.
Aggravation in the evening; in twilight; when rising after sitting long; on beginning to move; from changing the position; while lying on the left or on the painless side; when lying with the head low or in a warm room; while exhaling; from having eaten fruit, ice-cream, pork, pastry or warm food.
Amelioration from slow motion; in the open air; in a cold place; while lying on the painful side; from eating cold things.
After Pulsatilla follow well Sepia, Kali bichr., Sulphur.

RANUNCULUS BULBOSUS.

Mind and Disposition.

Angry mood and quarrelsome.
Obtuseness of the senses.
Vanishing of thought on reflection.

Head.

Pressing headache in the forehead and on the vertex, as if pressed asunder, with pressure on the eyeballs and sleepiness; worse in the evening or while entering a room from the cold air or vice versa.
5. Congestion of blood to the head, sensation of fulness and enlargement of the head.
Headache with nausea and sleepiness.
The headache is caused or aggravated by a change of temperature.

Eyes.

Sensation of soreness and smarting in the eyes and corners of the eyes.
Pressure in the eyes.

Ears.

10. Stitches in the ears (in the evening).
Spasmodic sensation in and around the ears.

Nose.

Redness and inflammatory swelling of the nose, with tension.
Scabs in the nostrils.

Face.

Dry heat in the face, with redness of the cheeks.
15. Tingling in the face, especially on the nose and chin.
Spasms of the lips.

Mouth and Throat.

White saliva in the mouth, tasting like copper.
Accumulation of tough mucus in the throat.
Scraping burning in the throat, and on the roof of the mouth.

Stomach and Abdomen.

20. Spasmodic hiccough.
Nausea in the afternoon and evening, sometimes with headache.
Sensation of soreness and burning in the pit of the stomach, especially to the touch.
Sensation of soreness in the hypochondria, especially to the touch.
Stitches in the region of the liver, extending up into the chest.
25. Pulsations in the left hypochondrium.
Colic and cutting pains in the abdomen, and when pressing on it the sensation as if every thing were sore and bruised.
Burning soreness in the abdomen (chronic inflammation).
Great tenderness of the abdomen to the touch.

Urinary Organs.

Ulcers in the bladder.

Sexual Organs.

30. *Women.* Acrid, corroding leucorrhœa.

Respiratory Organs.

Breathing short and oppressed, with pains in the chest, and inclination to draw a long breath.
Pains in the chest as if sore, as from subcutaneous ulceration, or rheumatic soreness of the intercostal muscles.
Stitches in the chest (right side of the chest, extending to the liver).

The external soreness of the chest is aggravated by touch, motion, and from stretching the body.
35. Adhesion of the lungs (after inflammation).

Back.
Stitches in and between the shoulder-blades.

Extremities.
Upper. Spasmodic, rheumatic pains in the arms.
Stitches in the arms and hands.
Herpes in the palms of the hands.
40. Herpes or blue blisters on the fingers.
Tingling in the fingers.
Cold hands.
Lower. Cracking in the joints (knee).
Drawing pains in the thighs, extending downwards.
45. Stinging and soreness in the feet and toes.

Generalities.
Rheumatic and arthritic soreness, with stitches over the whole body.
Trembling of the limbs, with dyspnœa (after anger).
Twitching of the muscles.
Epileptic attacks.
50. Sudden weakness, with fainting.

Sleep.
Sleeplessness often from dyspnœa, heat and ebullitions.
Cannot lie on the side.

Fever.
Pulse full, hard and rapid in the evening; slower in the morning; chill predominates, with heat in the face; worse in the afternoon and evening.
Chilliness and heat in the face after dinner.
55. He feels the chilliness, especially in the open air, and on the well-covered chest.
The fever consists only of a chill.
Heat in the evening, especially on the face; frequently only on the right side, with cold hands (and feet).
Heat, with internal chill at the same time.
Perspiration very scanty, and only in the morning on waking.

Skin.
60. Vesicular eruptions, as from burns.
Burning, itching, dark-blue vesicles in clusters, and a herpetic scurf, like horn.

Flat, burning, stinging ulcers, with ichorous discharge.
Horny excrescences.
Herpes over the whole body.

Conditions.

65. Aggravation in the evening, and after eating; from change of temperature, from touch, motion, from stretching the body.

RANUNCULUS SCELERATUS.

Mind and Disposition.

Indolence and aversion to mental occupation in the morning, and low spirited, depressed in the evening.

Head.

Vertigo, with loss of consciousness.
Gnawing headache in (a small spot of) the temples or on the vertex.
Sensation as if the head were enlarged and too full.
5. Tension of the scalp.
Biting-itching on the scalp.

Eyes.

Biting-gnawing in the eyes and corners of the eyes.
Painful pressing in the eyeballs.
Pain in the eyeballs on moving them quickly.

Ears.

10. Otalgia (right ear), with pressing or gnawing pain in the head, and drawing pain in the teeth.

Face.

Sensation as if the face were covered with carbuncles.
Twitches in the face; sardonic laughter.
Drawing in the face, with sensation of coldness.

Mouth and Throat.

Drawing, stinging in the teeth.
15. Burning in the throat.
Swelling of the tonsils, with shooting stitches in them.
Scraping in the throat.
Tongue coated white, inflamed, red and burning.

The tongue cracks and peels off.
20. Shooting in the tip of the tongue.

Stomach and Abdomen.

Fulness in the pit of the stomach, aggravated by external pressure, and in the morning.
Sensation of soreness and burning in the pit of the stomach.
Inflammation of the stomach.
Dull pressure in the region of the liver, aggravated by drawing a long breath.
25. Stitches in the region of the liver.
Pressure and stitches in the region of the liver, spleen, or kidneys.
Sensation of a plug behind the navel in the morning.
Twitching in the abdominal integuments.
Pain in the stomach, with fainting fits.

Stool and Anus.

30. Frequent soft or watery, fetid stools.

Sexual Organs.

Stitches at the glans penis.

Respiratory Organs.

Dyspnœa from gnawing behind the sternum.
Pain in the chest as if bruised, with sensation of weakness, periodically returning in the evening.
Stitches in the chest and the intercostal muscles.
35. Gnawing in the chest; behind the sternum (with dyspnœa).
Painful sensitiveness of the external chest, especially of the sternum.

Extremities.

Upper. Stinging, boring and gnawing in the arms, especially violent in the fingers.
Swelling of the fingers.
Lower. Stinging, boring and gnawing in the legs, especially violent in the big toe.

Generalities.

40. Boring, gnawing, stinging, tingling pains in various parts, aggravated in the evening and before midnight.
Convulsive twitches of the limbs.
Fainting with the pains.

Sleep.

Sleeplessness after midnight; with anxiety, heat and thirst, or with restlessness and tossing about.

Fever.

Pulse quick, full, but soft, with the heat at night.
45. Chill and chilliness during meals.
Heat in the evening in the room after walking in the open air.
Dry heat at night, with violent thirst and ebullition, mostly after midnight.
Heat predominates.
Perspiration after the heat, towards morning, mostly on the forehead.
50. Intermittent fever after midnight; heat and violent thirst, with full, soft, quick pulse, followed by general perspiration, mostly on the forehead.

Skin.

Vesicular eruptions, with acrid, thin, yellowish discharges.

Conditions.

The pains become worse towards evening, and decrease after midnight, and then sleeplessness, with tossing about.

RAPHANUS SATIVUS.

Head.

Vertigo, with dimness of sight.
Pressure above the eyes, with difficulty of sight, going off after vomiting.
Pressure above the root of the nose.
Stitches on the vertex.

Eyes.

5. Œdema of the lower lids.

Mouth and Throat.

Tongue coated thick white.
Tongue pale and purplish, with a deep furrow and pale red points in the middle.
White, tenacious mucus in the throat after heavy sleep.

Stomach and Abdomen.

Vomiting of food and white mucus, with oppression of the chest, heaving of the stomach and coldness.

10. Vomiting of bile and mucus, of a green, bitter liquid.
Pain in the stomach, obliging one to eat all the time.
Distention of the abdomen.
Gurgling in the abdomen (at night).
No emission of flatulence either by the mouth or rectum.

Stool and Anus.

15. Frequent, liquid, copious stools, passing out with great force.
Diarrhœa, stools green, liquid, with mucus and blood.

Urinary Organs.

Copious micturition, turbid urine, sediment like yeast.
During micturition, burning in the urethra.

RATANHIA.

Head.

Painful sticking in the head here and there.
Headache, as if the head were in a vice.
Dull, deep stitches on the vertex.
Pain in the middle of the forehead, as if the brain would fall out while straining to stool.

Eyes.

5. Twitching in the right eye and right upper eyelid.
Sensation of a white speck before the eyes, impeding sight in the evening by candle-light, with constant urging to wipe the eyes, and amelioration after wiping.

Ears.

Violent stitch in the right ear.
Chirping in the right ear.

Nose.

Dryness of the nose.
10. Dry coryza, with complete stoppage of the nostrils.
Bleeding of the nose.

Mouth and Throat.

The gums exude sour blood on sucking them.
Shooting, pulsating pain, with sensation of elongation in one left upper incisor (which is painful to the touch), in the evening; worse after lying down, compelling one to rise and to walk about.

RHEUM.

The molars feel elongated, with the sensation as if coldness rushed out of them.
15. Burning at the tip of the tongue.
Painful, spasmodic contraction in the throat, during which he is unable to speak a loud word.

Stomach and Abdomen.
Constant desire to eat.
Contractive pain in the stomach.
Ulcerative pain in the region of the stomach.

Stool and Anus.
20. Hard stool, with straining; ineffectual urging to stool.
Burning in the anus before and after soft diarrhœic stools.
Protrusion of varices after hard stool, with straining.
Bloody diarrhœa. Discharge of blood from the rectum, with or without stool.

Urinary Organs.
Frequent urging to urinate, with scanty discharge.
25. The scanty urine soon becomes turbid and cloudy.

Sexual Organs.
Women. Menstruation too early, too profuse, and of too long duration, with pains in the abdomen and small of the back.
Metrorrhagia.

Respiratory Organs.
Dry cough, with tickling in the larynx and great soreness in the chest.
Congestion of blood to the chest, with heat and dyspnœa.
30. Stitches in the chest, especially when ascending the steps.

RHEUM.

Mind and Disposition.
Restlessness, with inclination to weep.
The child demands various things with vehemence and weeping.
Indolent and taciturn.

Head.
Heaviness in the head, with heat rising to it.

5. Dull, stupefying headache, with bloated eyes.
Pulsation in the head, ascending from the abdomen.

Eyes.

Pulsation in the eyes.
Swimming eyes, full of water, especially in the open air.
Contracted pupils.
10. Convulsive twitching of the eyelids.
Eyes weak and dull, especially when looking intensely on an object.

Ears.

Pulsation in the ears.
Dulness of hearing, as from relaxation of the tympanum.

Nose.

Stupefying drawing in the root of the nose, extending to the tip of the nose, where it tingles.

Face.

15. Tension of the skin of the face.
The muscles of the forehead are drawn together and wrinkled.
Cool perspiration in the face, especially around the nose and mouth.

Mouth and Throat.

Painful sensation of coldness in the teeth, with accumulation of much saliva.
Difficult dentition of children.
20. The tongue becomes numb and insensible.

Stomach and Abdomen.

Aversion to coffee if not exceedingly sweetened.
Hunger without appetite.
Longing for various things, but the first morsel satisfies; he rejects it at once.
Nausea as from the abdomen, with colic pain.
25. The food tastes bitter while in the mouth.
Tension in the region of the stomach.
Fulness in the stomach as if it were overloaded.
Tension and bloatedness of the abdomen.
Violent pain in the abdomen, with cutting, compelling one to lie doubled up; much worse when standing.
30. Twitching in the abdominal muscles.
Cutting and rumbling in the abdomen as from flatulence.

Stool and Anus.

Frequent ineffectual urging to stool, worse on motion and when walking.

Thin, papescent, sour-smelling diarrhœic stools, with straining before, and colicky, constrictive cutting in the abdomen after, and chilliness during the stool.

Mucous diarrhœa.

35. Stools brown, mixed with mucus.

Diarrhœa of lying-in women; of children.

Urinary Organs.

Increased secretion of urine.
Urine, red or greenish-yellow.
The bladder is weak, one has to press hard to pass the urine.

40. Burning in the bladder.

Respiratory Organs.

Dyspnœa, as from a load on the upper part of the chest.
Stitches in the nipples.
The milk of nursing women is yellow and bitter; the infant refuses the breast.

Back.

Stiffness in the sacrum and hips, which does not allow one to walk straight.

Extremities.

45. *Upper.* Twitching in the arms, hands and fingers.
Swelled veins on the hands.
Cold perspiration on the palms of the hands.
Bubbling sensation in the elbow-joint.
Lower. Twitching of the muscles on the thighs.
50. Sensation of fatigue in the thighs.
Bubbling sensation from the bend of the knee to the heel.
Stiffness in the bend of the knee with pain on motion.

Generalities.

Bubbling sensation as from small bubbles in the muscles and joints.
The limbs on which one lies go to sleep.
55. Weakness and heaviness in the whole body, as if one were waking from a heavy sleep.
The joints pain on moving them.

Sleep.

Restless sleep at night, with tossing about, crying, moaning and groaning, or with convulsive twitching of the eyelids, muscles of the face and fingers, especially in children.

After sleep on waking, headache, bad odor from the mouth, and unconsciousness.

The hands are stretched over the head when going to sleep and during sleep.

Fever.

60. Chilliness alternating with heat.
One cheek is red and the other pale.
Internal chilliness with external heat.
Heat over the whole body, mostly on the hands and feet, with cold face.
Heat predominates, without thirst.
65. Perspiration from slight exertions.
Cold perspiration around the nose and mouth.
Perspiration on the forehead and scalp.
The perspiration colors yellow.

Conditions.

Especially suitable for children, especially nursing infants or during dentition.

RHODODENDRON.

Mind and Disposition.

Great indifference, with aversion to all occupation or labor.

Head.

Sensation of stupefaction and drowsiness in the head on rising in the morning.
Pain in the forehead and temples when lying in bed in the morning; worse from drinking wine and in wet, cold weather; better after rising and moving about.
The scalp feels sore and as if bruised.
5. Violent drawing and tearing in the bones and the periosteum of the cranial bones; worse when at rest, in the morning, during a thunder-storm and during wet, cold, stormy weather; better from wrapping the head up warmly, from dry heat and from exercise.

Biting-itching on the scalp, especially in the evening.

Eyes.

Periodically returning dry burning in the eyes, especially in the bright daylight, and from looking intensely on an object.
Spasmodic contraction of the eyelids.
Dimness of vision when reading and writing.

Ears.

10. Otalgia (right ear); violent twitching pain.
Sensation in the ear, as from a worm.
Buzzing in the ear, aggravated when swallowing.

Nose.

Diminished sense of smell.
Bleeding of the nose.

Face.

15. Chilliness over the face.
Dry, burning lips.
Vesicles on the inner side of the under lip, with soreness when eating.

Mouth and Throat.

Smarting vesicles under the tongue.
Increased accumulation of saliva in the mouth, with dryness of the throat.
20. Constriction and burning in the throat.
The food has no taste.
Easily satisfied with a small quantity of food; he feels very uncomfortable afterwards.
Nausea, pressure at the stomach and waterbrash, relieved by belching.
Pressure in the stomach at night.
25. Heaviness in the stomach after drinking water.
Constriction and pressure at the pit of the stomach, with dyspnœa.
Pain as from tension under the short ribs.
Stitches in the spleen from walking fast.
Tension in the region of the spleen when stooping.
3   Distention in the upper part of the abdomen, with dyspnœa, evening and morning.
Painful incarceration of flatulence in the hypochondria and in the small of the back.
Much rumbling in the abdomen, with eructations and discharge of fetid flatus.

Stool and Anus.

Soft, papescent stools, difficult to evacuate, with previous violent pressing.
Diarrhœa after eating fruit, or from wet, cold weather.
35. Pulsation in the anus.
Drawing extending from the rectum to the genitals.

Urinary Organs.

Frequent urging to urinate, with drawing in the region of the bladder.
Increased secretion of very offensive urine.

Sexual Organs.

Men. Sensation of soreness between the genitals and thighs.
40. The testicles are drawn up and are swollen.
Sensation of soreness in the testicles extending to the abdomen and the thighs.
Scrotum wrinkled, or itching, or sweating.
Induration and swelling of the left testicle.
Hydrocele.
45. Swelling of the testicles after gonorrhœa.
Aversion to an embrace.
Women. Menstruation too profuse and too early.
Suppressed menstruation.

Respiratory Organs.

Dyspnœa from constriction of the chest.
50. Dry, exhausting cough in the morning and evening, with oppression of the chest and roughness in the throat.

Back and Neck.

Rheumatic pains in the back and shoulders.
Stiffness of the neck and rheumatic pains in the muscles of the neck.

Extremities.

Upper. Tearing in the fore-arms, as if it were in the periosteum, during wet, cold weather.
Sensation as if the blood ceased to circulate in the arms.
55. Increased warmth in the hands.
Sensation as if the wrists were sprained.
Lower. Sensation of soreness in the thighs near the genitals.
Sensation of coldness, the skin wrinkles on the lower legs.
Dropsical swelling of the lower legs and feet.

60. Rheumatic pains in the lower extremities and feet, as if it were in the periosteum, worse when at rest and during wet cold weather.
Unusual coldness of the feet.

Generalities.

Rheumatic and arthritic pains (drawing and tearing) in the limbs, mostly on the periosteum, caused by stormy weather, and worse when at rest; mostly in the forearms and lower legs.
Sensation of formication in the limbs.
Sensation in the joints as if sprained, with swelling and redness, with arthritic nodosities.
65. Dropsical swellings.

Sleep.

Great sleepiness during the day, with burning in the eyes.
Deep, heavy sleep before midnight, with sleepiness early in the evening, but sleeplessness after midnight; the morning sleep is disturbed by restlessness in the body and by pain.

Fever.

Pulse slow and weak.
Chilliness in the morning, in bed, and during the day, if cold air blows on him.
70. Chilliness and heat alternating.
Ice-cold feet in the evening after lying down, continuing long.
Heat in the evening, with cold feet.
Sensation of heat, especially in the hands, although they feel cold to the touch.
Feverish heat in the evening, with burning in the face.
75. Profuse debilitating perspiration, especially when exercising in the open air.
Offensive smelling perspiration in the axilla.
The perspiration smells of spice.
While perspiring the skin itches and tingles, like formication.

Skin and Bones.

Drawing in the periosteum.
80. Dropsical swellings.

Conditions.

Most complaints appear in the morning.
Aggravation of the pains during rest, during a thunderstorm.
The pains are caused and aggravated by wet, cold air.

RHUS TOXICODENDRON.

Mind and Disposition.

Restlessness which does not permit one to sit quiet, and compels him to throw himself about in bed.
Anxiety and apprehensiveness (at twilight).
Fear; that he will die; of being poisoned.
Desire to commit suicide (to throw himself into the water).
5. Disgust for life.
Absence of mind.
Inclination to weep, especially in the evening, with desire for solitude.
Illusions of the fancy; visions.
Mild delirium, with insensibility.

Head.

10. Stupefaction, with tingling in the head and pain in the limbs, ameliorated on motion.
Giddiness, as if intoxicated; when rising from the bed, with chilliness and pressure behind the eyes.
Fulness and heaviness in the head, especially in the forehead; as if a weight were falling forward, on stooping, with heat in the face.
Rush of blood to the head with burning-tingling and beating in the brain, bright redness of the face, great restlessness of the body, in the morning, when at rest, worse after eating.
Stinging headache, extending to the ears.
15. Stinging pain at the root of the nose, extending to the malar bones, with painfulness of the teeth.
Painful tingling in the head, especially of the occiput.
Burning in the forehead when walking.
When stepping, sensation as if the brain were loose, also when shaking the head.
Liability to take cold from having the head wetted.
20. Humid, suppurating eruption on the head, forming heavy crusts, eating off the hair, offensive smell and itching, worse at night.
Great sensitiveness of the scalp, worse on the side on which he does not lie, worse from combing the hair back, from becoming warm in bed and from the touch.

Erysipelatous swelling of the head and face, with vesicles drying up and forming burning itching scabs.
The hair falls off from suppurating eruptions.
The headache is worse in the morning, while lying; from cold, from drinking beer, relieved by heat, and when moving about.

Eyes.

25. Inflammation of the eyes and lids, with redness, and agglutination of the lids at night.
Erysipelatous swelling of the eyes and around them.
Swelling of the eyelids.
Eyes full of water (bleareyedness).
Styes on the lower eyelids.
30. Heaviness of the eyelids.
Aversion to light.

Ears.

Discharge of bloody pus from the ears.
Otalgia with pulsation in the ear at night.
Inflammatory swelling of the parotid gland (left side).
35. Suppuration of the parotid glands (with scarlet fever).

Nose.

Redness of the tip of the nose, with soreness when touched.
Inflammation of the nose.
The nose feels sore internally.
Bleeding of the nose at night, or when stooping (coagulated blood).
40. Discharge of green offensive pus from the nose.
Puffiness of the nose.
Spasmodic sneezing.
Discharge of mucus from the nose without coryza.
Dryness of the nose.

Face.

45. Face pale, sunken, with blue rings under the eyes, and pointed nose.
Erysipelatous swelling of the face, with burning, tingling, and stinging.
Erysipelas, with vesicles containing yellow water.
Milk crust; acnea rosacea; Impetigo on the face or on the forehead.
Exanthema on the cheeks, on the chin, around the mouth.
50. Stiffness in the articulation of the jaws.
Cracking in the articulation of the jaw.

Mouth and Throat.

Looseness of the teeth.

Toothache, tearing, stinging, often at night, worse in the open air, better from external heat and in the warm room.

Dryness of the mouth, with much thirst.

55. Accumulation of much saliva in the mouth (saliva bloody).

Putrid taste in the mouth.

Offensive smell from the mouth.

Tongue dry, red, and cracked.

Much tough mucus accumulates in the mouth and throat.

60. Sore throat, as from an internal swelling, with bruised pain; also when talking, with pressure and stinging when swallowing.

Difficult deglutition of solid food, as from contraction.

Stomach and Abdomen.

Want of appetite, with unquenchable thirst.

Food tastes bitter; especially the bread.

Putrid taste, especially in the morning and after eating.

65. Metallic taste.

Thirst, especially in the night, from dryness in the mouth, and mostly for cold water or cold milk.

Hunger without appetite.

When eating sudden vomiting.

Longing for oysters.

70. After eating great sleepiness, fulness in the stomach or giddiness.

Heaviness in the stomach as from a stone, after eating.

Stinging or pulsation in the pit of the stomach.

Nausea, with inordinate appetite and inclination to vomit, worse after eating and drinking and at night.

Eructations, with tingling in the stomach, worse when rising up while lying.

75. Colic, compelling one to walk bent.

Visible contraction in the abdomen above the navel.

Sensation as if something were torn off in the abdomen.

Pains in the abdomen at night.

Sensation of soreness in the walls of the abdomen, especially in the morning, when stretching.

80. Bloated abdomen, especially after eating.

From drinking ice-water pain in the stomach and nausea.

Stool and Anus.

Diarrhœa, stools watery or consisting of mucus or bloody, or frothy, or white.

Tenesmus, with nausea, tearing and pinching in the abdomen. Dysentery.
Nightly diarrhœa, with violent pain in the abdomen, which is relieved after an evacuation, or when lying on the abdomen.
85. Involuntary stools, especially at night while asleep.
During stool shortness of breath.

Urinary Organs.

Frequent urging to urinate day and night, with increased secretion.
Involuntary discharge of urine at night, or while sitting, or when at rest.
Diminished secretion of urine, although he drinks much.
90. Urine hot, white and muddy, or pale, with white sediment.
Urine dark, which soon becomes turbid.
Tenesmus vesicæ, with discharges of only a few drops of blood-red urine.
The urine is emitted in a divided stream.

Genital Organs.

Men. Eruption on the genitals, closing the urethra by swelling.
95. Swelling of the glans and of the prepuce; prepuce dark-red.
Paraphymosis.
Humid vesicles on the glans.
Red blotches on the inner surface of the prepuce.
Stinging-itching on the inner surface of the prepuce.
100. Humid eruptions on the scrotum.
The scrotum becomes thicker and harder, with intolerable itching.
Erysipelas of the scrotum.
Violent erections at night, with urging to urinate.
Women. Bearing down pain (when standing).
105. Prolapsus uteri from overstraining, overlifting.
Catamenia too early, too profuse, and too protracted.
Discharge of blood during pregnancy.
Hemorrhage, blood clotted, with labor-like pains.
Soreness and stitches in the vagina.
110. The menstrual blood is acrid.
The lochia become bloody again and smell offensively.
After-pains of too long duration, after severe labor, with much and excessive straining.
Galactorrhœa, or suppression of the milk, with burning over the body.

Respiratory Organs.

Sensation of coldness in the larynx when breathing.
115. Hoarseness, with roughness in the larynx, and roughness and soreness in the chest.
Hot air rises from the trachea.
Cough, from tickling in the bronchia; short, dry, especially in the evening and before midnight.
Cough in the evening, with vomiting of the ingesta.
Cough in the morning soon after awaking.
120. Cough, with expectoration of (pale or clotted) blood, or with pains in the abdomen.
Cough, with stitches in the chest, profuse general perspiration, and pain in the stomach.
Hooping-cough; spasmodic violent cough, caused by tickling in the larynx and chest, with expectoration (except in the evening) of acrid pus or grayish-green cold mucus, of putrid smell, or of pale, clotted, at times brown blood.
Dyspnœa from pressure and painfulness in the pit of the stomach.
Hot breath.
125. Stitches in the chest and sides of the chest, worse when at rest, and while sneezing and breathing.
Inflammation of the lungs, also pneumonia nervosa.
Tingling in the chest, with tension in the intercostal muscles, worse when at rest.
Sensation of weakness and trembling of the heart.
Violent palpitation of the heart on sitting still.
130. Stitches in the heart, with painful lameness and numbness of the left arm.

Back and Neck.

Painful tension between the shoulder-blades.
Pain in the shoulders and back, as from a sprain.
Rheumatic stiffness of the neck, with painful tension when moving.
Curvature of the dorsal vertebræ.
135. Pain in the small of the back, when sitting still or when lying; relieved when lying on something hard, or from exercise.

Extremities.

Upper. Tearing and burning in the shoulder, with lameness of the arm.
Paralysis of the arm, with coldness and insensibility.

Erysipelatous swelling of the arm.
Tension in the elbow-joint.
140. Painful swelling of the axillary glands.
Rhagades on the back of the hands.
Swelling of the fingers; hot swelling of the hands in the evening.
Warts on the hands,—hangnails.
Swollen veins on the hands.
145. *Lower.* Pain in the hip when rising from a seat, or after over-exercise; involuntary limping.
Pain as if sprained in the hip, knee and foot-joint.
Spasmodic twitching in the limbs when stepping out.
Painful swelling above the knee.
Swelling of the feet (in the evening).
150. Corns, with soreness and burning.

Generalities.

Great debility, weakness and soreness, especially when sitting, and when at rest.
Rheumatic tension, drawing and tearing in the limbs, mostly with sensation of numbness, especially when at rest.
Tension, stiffness and stitches in the joints; worse when rising from a seat.
Tearing and weakness of the joints.
155. In inner parts sensation of fulness; or as if they were grown together (adhesion), or as if something in them were torn loose.
Numbness in the extremities, with previous twitching and tingling in them.
Painless paralysis of the limbs.
Burning and stinging pains in external parts.
Inflammatory swellings.
160. The parts on which one lies go to sleep.
Restlessness of the body; inclination to move the affected parts.
Pain as if sprained in outer parts; disposition to sprain a part by lifting heavy weights.

Sleep.

Spasmodic yawning, without inclination to sleep, and with stretching of the limbs, and pain as from dislocation of the articulation of the jaw.
He falls asleep late; sleeplessness before midnight.
165. At night he can only lie on his back.
Vivid dreams.

Fever.

Pulse irregular; generally accelerated but weak, soft; sometimes it cannot be felt, or is intermittent.

Constant chilliness, as if cold water were poured over him, or as if the blood were running cold through the veins.

Sensation of coldness when he moves.

170. Chills running over the back.

Chills with increased pains, especially in the limbs.

Chilliness, worse in the evening.

Coldness, with paleness of the face, alternating with heat and redness of the face.

Heat after the chill, often with perspiration and amelioration of the concomitant symptoms.

175. General heat, as if hot water were thrown over him, or as if the blood were flowing hot through the veins.

Heat with nettle-rash.

Evening fever, with diarrhœa.

Perspiration; with the pains; when sitting; often accompanied with violent trembling.

General perspiration, frequently already during the heat, and then often not in the face.

180. Perspiration, with violent itching of the eruption.

Night-sweat, with miliary itching eruption.

Intermittent fever. First drowsy, weariness and yawning; afterwards (at 10 A. M.) excessive heat in the body, without thirst.

Chilliness 7 P. M., as if he had cold water poured over him; after going to bed, heat with inclination to stretch the limbs; sweat towards morning.

Quotidian fever about midnight, with pressure and swelling at the pit of the stomach, and anxious palpitation of the heart during the day.

185. First headache (throbbing in the temples); afterwards chilliness, with thirst and tearing pains in the limbs as from fatigue; afterwards general warmth, with slight chills during motion, and livid face; finally profuse, sour-smelling perspiration.

Tertian fever with nettle-rash, which disappears after the attack; during the apyrexia, burning and redness in the sclerotica.

Skin.

Itching over the whole body, especially on the hairy parts.
Stinging and tingling on the skin, burning after scratching.
Erysipelas; vesicular; Zona.

190. Humidity of the skin.
Rhagades.
Hardness of the skin, with thickening.
Swelling (hard) of the affected parts.
Sensation of coldness in the skin.
195. Exanthema, burning, erysipelatous, itching, with swelling, pox-shaped, black, purulent; nettle-rash with burning-itching.
Milk crust.
Pustulous eruptions.
Warts.
Herpes, alternating with pains in the chest and dysenteric stools.
200. Inflammation, swelling, induration and suppuration of the glands.
Inflammation and swelling of the long bones.
Pain as if the flesh were torn loose from the bones, or as if the bones were being scraped.
Burning in the ulcers.

Conditions.

Bad consequences from getting wet, especially after being heated; from excessive bodily exercise; from bruises and sprains; from heavy falls; concussion of the body.
205. Great sensitiveness to the open air.
From cold bathing, convulsive twitches.
Aggravation in the morning; after midnight; during the winter; while at rest, reposing, lying down; on rising from a seat or after rising from the bed; from stepping heavily on the ground; on change of the weather; in wet weather; from getting wet; in cold air, and from cold in general; from cold water; from uncovering the head; from drawing up the limbs; from drinking beer.
Amelioration, when continuing to walk; from moving the affected parts; from stretching out the limbs; from warmth, warm air, wrapping oneself up warmly (the head) in dry (warm) weather.
Rhus follows well after Bryonia, or vice versa; but causes bad results when given after Apis, and vice versa.

RUMEX CRISPUS.

Mind and Disposition.
Low-spirited, with serious expression of the face.
Irritable,—disinclined to mental exertions.

Head.
Dull feeling in the head (with the cough).
Dull pain in the forehead (worse on motion).

Eyes.
5. Pain in the eyes, as from dryness and inflammation of the lids, especially in the evening.

Ears.
Itching, deep in the ears.

Nose.
Violent sneezing; with fluent coryza, worse in the evening and at night.

Face.
Heat of the face, with pulsation over the whole body.

Mouth and Throat.
Bitter taste in the mouth (in the morning).
10. Dryness on the tip of the tongue, and hot on the forepart.
Tongue white, or coated yellow-brown or reddish-brown.
Accumulation of mucus near the posterior nares.
Discharge of yellow mucus through the posterior nares.

Stomach and Abdomen.
Fulness in the stomach after breakfast.
15. Colic pain around the navel.

Stool and Anus.
Constipation, feces brown, hard, tough.
Itching at the anus.

Respiratory Organs.
Voice, higher, or as with catarrh; or nasal voice; or hoarse, especially in the evening.
Soreness and rawness in the larynx when coughing.
20. Hawking of mucus from the upper part of the larynx and throat; with burning soreness; extending later to the bronchus of the left chest; and can be renewed by a stronger exhalation and scraping.

Tickling in the throat-pit, causing cough.
Pressure on the throat causes cough.
Cough from tickling in the throat-pit, extending to behind the sternum and the stomach.
Cough dry, worse when walking, from tickling in the throat-pit, with soreness in the larynx and behind the upper part of the sternum, and pain in the chest.
Cough, with violent coryza, and rawness in the upper part of the sternum.
25. Tickling cough from irritation behind the sternum.
Cough, as soon as he turns on the left side.
Cough, with pain in the stomach, soreness behind the sternum; stitches in the left lung.
Cough from pressure on the throat; with soreness in the larynx and chest, and with hoarseness.
Hoarse, barking cough; every night several attacks, the first generally at 11 P. M., and two more at 2 and 5 A. M., lasting a long time (in children).
30. Breathing causes soreness behind the sternum.
Pain in the centre of the left lung.
The sternum feels sprained.
Burning in the region of the heart.

Extremities.

Upper. Coldness of the hands when coughing.
35. *Lower.* Sensitiveness of the feet, and stinging pain in the corns.

Generalities.

Great debility, with aversion to occupation and general indifference about his surroundings.

Fever.

Pulse accelerated, especially when ascending steps.
Chilliness, especially in the back, with colic, nausea and stitches near the middle of the chest.
Flushes of heat, especially in the cheeks.
40. Perspiration on awaking from sound sleep.

RUTA GRAVEOLA.

Mind and Disposition.

Melancholy disposition towards evening.
Anxious and low-spirited, with mental dejection.
Inclination to quarrel and contradict.

Head.

Giddiness; in the morning when rising; when sitting, and when walking in the open air.
5. Great heat in the head, with much restlessness.
Headache as if a nail were driven into the head.
Headache after excessive use of intoxicating drinks.
Ulcers and scabs on the scalp.
The head is externally painful, as if bruised or beaten.
10. Pain in the periosteum of the cranium as from a fall.
Large painful swellings on the scalp, as if originating in the periosteum, the place pained previously (tearing), and felt sore to the touch.
Biting, itching (ulcers) on the scalp.
Humid scabs on the head, with scald-head.

Eyes.

Spasms of the (lower) eyelids.
15. Watering eyes, they are full of tears in the open air, not in the room.
Heat in the eyes in the evening when reading with candle-light.
Spots on the cornea.
Pains in the eyes as if they had been strained too much.
Obscurations of sight from reading too much, with clouds, or like a veil before the eyes.
20. A green halo appears around the light in the evening.
Bad effects of overstraining the eyes, from reading too much, from sewing, especially fine work at night.

Ears.

Pain as if bruised in the cartilages of the ear.

Nose.

Bleeding of the nose, with pressure at the root of the nose.
Perspiration on the dorsum of the nose.

Face.

25. Erysipelas and swelling on the forehead.
Pains in the face as from contusion in the periosteum of the facial bones.

Mouth and Throat.

Pain in the lower teeth.
Gums painful, and bleed readily.
The lips are dry and sticky.
30. Sensation as from a lump in the throat on empty deglutition.
Spasm of the tongue, with difficulty of speech.

Stomach and Abdomen.

Violent thirst in the afternoon.
Sudden nausea while eating, and vomiting of food.
Colic, with burning or gnawing pain.
35. Gnawing, pressing pain in the region of the liver.
Gnawing sensation in the stomach, as from emptiness or hunger.
Painful swelling of the spleen.
Colic in children from worms.
Gnawing and eating pain about the navel.

Stool and Anus.

40. Soft stool, which is discharged with difficulty from inactivity of the rectum.
Constipation, alternating with mucous, frothy stools.
Frequent urging to stool, with small, soft discharges.
Frequent unsuccessful urging, with prolapsus ani.
Prolapsus ani with every (soft or hard) stool.

Urinary Organs.

45. Frequent pressure to urinate, with scanty discharges of green urine.
Pressure on the bladder, as if continually full; the pressure to urinate continues after micturition.
Frequent micturition at night.
Involuntary micturition at night in bed, and during the day when walking.

Sexual Organs.

Women. Menstruation irregular, followed by leucorrhœa.
50. Corrosive leucorrhœa after the menstruation has ceased.

Respiratory Organs.

Dyspnœa, with anxiety from stitches in the chest.
Sensation of coldness or heat in the chest.

Corrosive eating or gnawing in the chest.
Sensation in the larynx as from a bruise.
55. On the sternum a painful spot, which is painful to pressure.
Violent cough, with expectoration of tough mucus and nausea.
Cough, with copious expectoration of thick yellow mucus.
Expectoration of thick yellow mucus, almost without cough, with sensation of weakness in the chest.
Phthisic after mechanical injuries of the chest.

Back and Neck.

60. Pain in the back and on the os sacrum, as if bruised.
Stitches in the small of the back when sitting, walking or stooping, relieved by pressure and when lying-down.

Extremities.

Upper. Lameness and stiffness of the wrist after a sprain, worse in cold wet weather.
Sensation as from a sprain, and stiffness in the wrist.
Numbness and tingling in the hands after exercise.
65. *Lower.* Lameness and pains in the ankles after a sprain.
Sensation as if the tendons under the knee were shortened, and weakness in them, especially on descending.
Fistulous ulcers on the lower legs.

Generalities.

Sensation of soreness. or as from a contusion, bruise or fall or from a blow, especially in the limbs and joints.
Sensation of soreness of the parts on which one lies.
70. Lameness after sprains, especially the wrists and ankles.
Worm complaints of children.

Fever.

Pulse only accelerated during the heat.
Internal chilliness and shaking even near the warm stove.
Coldness running over one side of the head.
75. Chilliness principally in the back, and running up and down.
Chilliness with heat in the face, and violent thirst.
Heat over the whole body, mostly in the afternoon, without thirst, but with anxiety, restlessness and dyspnœa.
Heat in the face, with red cheeks, and cold hands and feet.
Frequent attacks of flushes of heat.
80. Cold perspiration on the face in the morning in bed.
Perspiration all over when walking in the open air.

Skin.

The skin becomes easily chafed from walking and riding, also in children.
Inflammation of the ulcers.
Pain in the long bones as if they were broken.
85. Bruises and other mechanical injuries of the bones and the periosteum.
Dropsy; warts, with sore pains.

Conditions.

The pains in the limbs are aggravated during rest and cold wet weather, and principally while sitting, and are ameliorated by motion.

SABADILLA.

Mind and Disposition.

Anxious restlessness.
Startled from the noise.
Imagines himself sick or having imaginary diseases.

Head.

Vertigo with fainting, every thing becomes black before the eyes (when rising from a seat).
5. Stupefying headache with coryza, itching and burning of the scalp and general heat of the whole body; worse in the forenoon.
The headache begins in the right side, and from there it extends.
Burning and tingling-itching on the scalp, as from lice.

Eyes.

The eyes are filled with water from pain and other causes; when looking in the light, from cough, yawning, &c.

Ears.

Tickling in the ears.

Nose.

10. Itching-tingling in the nose.
Bright-red blood comes from the posterior nares, and is expectorated.
The smell is very sensitive to garlic.

Face.

Burning heat and redness of the face (after drinking wine).
Cracking of the articulation of the jaw on opening the mouth wide.

Mouth and Throat.

15. Bluish gums.
Burning dryness in the mouth, without thirst.
Tongue thick, yellow-coated; soreness of the tip of the tongue.
Sensation of a lump in the throat with inclination to swallow.

Stomach and Abdomen.

Violent desire for sweet things, honey or pastry.
20 Aversion to coffee, wine, meat and acids.
Thirstlessness or thirst only in the evening for cold water.
Nausea before eating; better afterwards.
Vomiting of lumbrici.
Burning or coldness in the stomach or abdomen.
25. Cutting in the abdomen as from knives.
Colicky pains from worms.

Stool and Anus.

Fluid, thin stool mixed with mucus and blood floating on the water.
Discharges of worms (lumbrici, tape-worm).
Violent itching and tingling in the rectum.

Urine.

30. Thick, turbid, hot urine.

Respiratory Organs.

Hot breath; wheezing breathing.
Cough as soon as one lies down.
Cough, dry, with perspiration and water in the eyes; with stitches in the vertex, vomiting and pain in the stomach.
Burning and stitches in the chest.
35. Pain in the right shoulder, extending to the chest, with the sensation as if a tape prevented the circulation of the blood.
Red spots on the chest.

Extremities.

Upper. Convulsive motion of the arms.
Red spots, points and stripes on the arms and hands.
Lower. Swelling of the feet, with tenderness or profuse perspiration of the soles of the feet.

Generalities.

40. Great debility with relaxation or heaviness of the body.
Inflammation of internal organs.
Ailments dependent on worms.

Sleep.

Unrefreshing, restless sleep.
In the morning he starts up from his sleep as from a fright.

Fever.

45. Pulse small, but spasmodic.
Sensation as if the circulation were suspended.
Chilliness in the evening always at the same hour, frequently not followed by heat; the chills run up the body.
Chilliness, especially in the extremities, with heat of the face.
Heat, principally in the head and in the face, often interrupted by chilliness, always returning at the same hour.
50. Perspiration, frequently already during the heat; in the morning hours with perspiration.
Hot perspiration in the face with coldness of the rest of the body.
Intermittent fever which returns at the same hour; chill, then thirst, then heat with headache.
Thirst only between the cold and hot stage.
Fevers where the gastric symptoms prevail, with dry, convulsive cough in the cold stage (Quartan ague).

Skin.

55. Pain in the bones and joints especially, as if somebody were scraping and cutting inside with a knife.
Parchment-like dryness of the skin.
Red blotches and stripes more permanent in the cold.

Conditions.

Many complaints go from the right to the left (sore throat).
Sensitiveness to the cold, which aggravates the pains.
60. Reappearance or aggravation of the pains in the forenoon and in the hours before midnight and during rest.
The complaints (fever) always at the same hour.
Many complaints appear, especially during the new and full moon.
Sensitiveness to the cold which also aggravates the complaints.

SABINA.

Mind and Disposition.
Hypochondriacal mood.
Low-spirited and joyless.

Head.
Giddiness, with congestions to and heat in the head.
Headache, especially in temporal eminences (right side), suddenly appearing and slowly disappearing.

Face.
5. Pale face; eyes lustreless, with blue rings around them.
Black pores in the face and on the nose.

Mouth and Throat.
Drawing toothache, almost only caused by masticating.
Toothache at night as if the tooth were burst; worse from the heat of the bed.
Swelling of the gums around the broken teeth.
10. White saliva, becoming frothy when talking.
Desire for acids, especially lemonade.
Bitter taste of the food, of the milk and coffee.
Vomiting of bile, of undigested food eaten on the previous day.
Stitches in the pit of the stomach, extending to the back.
15. Tympanitis; bloatedness of the abdomen.
Labor-like pains in the abdomen.
Soreness of the abdominal muscles.
Pressing down towards the genitals.

Stool and Anus.
Diarrhœa, with much flatulence.
20. Discharge of blood and mucus; bleeding hæmorrhoids.

Urinary Organs.
Frequent violent urging to urinate, with profuse discharge.
Retention of urine, with discharge by drops, with burning.

Genital Organs.
Men. Inflammatory gonorrhœa, with discharge of pus.
Cartilaginous swelling on the penis.
25. Sycotic excrescences, with burning soreness.

Painfulness of the prepuce, with difficulty in drawing it back.
Sexual desire increases, with violent continuous erections.
Women. Menstruation too early and too profuse.
Hemorrhages, with partly pale-red, partly clotted or of very thin, discolored, offensive-smelling blood; worse on the least motion; has to lie perfectly quiet to avoid a profuse discharge after miscarriage.
30. Miscarriage, especially in the third month.
Very offensive-smelling leucorrhœa after suppressed menstruation.
Stitches deep in the vagina.
Inflammation of the uterus after parturition.
Increased sexual desire, almost amounting to nymphomania.

Back.

35. Labor-like pains drawing down into the groins.

Extremities.

Upper. Arthritic stiffness and swelling of the wrist-joint, with tearing and stinging, made almost insupportable when the hand hangs down.
Lower. Stinging pains in the hip-joints in the morning and when breathing.
Ulcers with a bottom like lard on the tibia.
Swelling, redness and stitches in the big toe (gout).

Generalities.

40. Red, shining swelling of the affected parts.
Arthritic complaints; tearing, stinging in the joints after they become swollen; arthritic nodosities.
Chronic ailments of women.
Twitching pulsation in the blood-vessels.

Sleep.

Sleeplessness and restlessness after midnight, with heat and profuse perspiration.
45. Lies on the left side during sleep.

Fever.

Pulse unequal; generally quick, strong and hard.
Violent beating of the veins in the whole body.
Chill in the evening, with attacks of chilliness.
Great chilliness through the day.
50. Chilliness, with obscuration of sight, followed by sleepiness.
Sensation of coldness in the whole (right) leg.

Insupportable burning heat, with restlessness, in the whole body.
Flushes of heat in the face, with chilliness over the whole body and coldness of the hands and feet.
Perspiration every night.

Skin.

55. Black pores in the skin.
Drawing pains through the long bones.

SAMBUCUS NIGRA.

Mind and Disposition.

Periodical delirium, with visions and hallucinations.
Very easily frightened; trembling, anxiety and restlessness.
Fright followed by suffocative attacks, with bluish, bloated face.

Head.

Tension in the head; when moving it sensation as if it were filled with water.
5. Sudden jerks through the head.
The head is bent backwards.

Face.

Face bloated, dark blue. Heat and perspiration in the face.
Red, burning spots on the cheeks; great heat of the face; circumscribed redness of the face.
Numb tension, as from swelling in the cheeks and on the nose.

Mouth.

10. Tearing and stinging in the teeth, with the sensation of swelling of the cheeks.
Dryness of the throat and mouth, with thirstlessness.

Stomach and Abdomen.

Vomiting, first of food, later of bile.
Colic pain, with discharge of much flatulence, from taking cold.
Painful pressure in the abdomen, with nausea, when leaning against a hard edge.

Urinary Organs.
15. Frequent urging to urinate, with profuse discharge of urine

Respiratory Organs.
Breathing through the nose impeded, with dry coryza, especially in infants.
Quick, wheezing, crowing breathing.
Suffocative attacks when waking after midnight out of a slumber, with half-open eyes and mouth, with bloated blue hands and face, and heat without thirst.
Oppression of the chest, with pressure in the stomach, and nausea.
20. Nightly suffocative attacks, with great restlessness; shedding of tears and throwing about of the arms.
Hoarseness, with much tough mucus in the larynx.
Inflammation of the larynx and trachea; croup; accumulation of mucus in the larynx.
Attacks of suffocative cough in children, with crying.
Hooping-cough; suffocative, hollow, deep (hooping) cough, caused by a spasm in the chest, with expectoration only during the day of small quantities of tough mucus.
25. The cough is worse at or soon after midnight, during rest, when lying in bed, or with the head low, from dry cold air.

Extremities.
Upper. Paralytic heaviness in the elbow-joint.
Trembling of the hands when writing.
Stitches in the wrists.
Dark-blue bloatedness of the fore-arms and hands.
30. *Lower.* Sharp, deep stitches in the tibia.
Œdematous swelling of the feet, extending to the legs.
Sensation of coldness, numbness and deadness in the middle of the (right) tibia.
Icy-cold feet, with warmth of the body.

Generalities.
Dropsical swellings of the body.
35. General trembling, with anxiety and ebullitions of blood.

Sleep.
Sleepiness without sleep.
Frequent awakening, as in a fright, with anxiety, trembling, dyspnœa, as if he would suffocate.
Slumber with the eyes and mouth half-open.
During the sleep dry heat, after awakening profuse perspiration.

Fever.

40. Pulse generally small and very quick, at times intermitting.
Chilliness over the whole body, with tingling here and there.
Chill, with very cold hands and feet.
Dry heat over the whole body as soon as one falls asleep after lying down, with aversion to be uncovered, and without thirst.
Burning heat in the face, with very cold feet.
45. Profuse perspiration day and night, but only when awake; first breaking out in the face.
Very debilitating perspiration.
Night-sweats, except on the head, increasing towards morning.
Continued perspiration while awake, changing into dry heat as soon as one goes to sleep.
Intermittent fever; chills over the whole body, with cold hands and feet; followed by intolerable dry heat, without any thirst, accompanied by dread of being uncovered, afterwards copious sweat, without any thirst; the sweat even continues during the apyrexia.

Skin.

50. Bloatedness and dark-red swelling, with tension after contusions.

Conditions.

Most ailments appear while the body is at rest, and are relieved by motion.
Sitting up in bed gives relief.

SANGUINARIA CANADENSIS.

Mind and Disposition.

Angry irritability; moroseness.
Anxiety preceding the vomiting.

Head.

Vertigo, when moving the head rapidly and looking upward, with nausea; ringing in the ears.
Congestion of blood to the head, with ringing in the ears; flushes of heat; accumulation of water in the mouth.

5. Headache, with rheumatic pains and stiffness of the limbs and neck.
Sick headache, with vomiting (of bile), beginning in the morning, increasing during the day; worse from motion, stooping, noise, and light; only endurable when lying still, and relieved by sleep or after vomiting; especially severe over the right eye,—the headache returns periodically.
Pains in the head, in spots.
Pulsations in the head, with bitter vomiting, worse from motion.
The headache rises up from the neck.
10. Feeling as if the head were drawn forward.
Distention of the veins on the head, especially on the temples, perceptible to the touch.

Eyes.

Burning and watering of the right eye, which is painful to the touch, followed by coryza.
Dim eyes, with the sensation as if hairs were in them.
Frequent obscuration of vision.

Ears.

15. Burning of the ears, with redness of the cheeks.

Nose.

Heat in the nose; coryza, rawness in the throat, pain in the breast, cough, and finally diarrhœa.
Loss of smell. Dislike to the odor of syrup.
Nasal polypus.

Face, Mouth and Throat.

Stiffness of the articulation of the jaws.
20. Pain in hollow teeth, especially when touched by food.
Toothache from picking the teeth.
Pain in the carious teeth after cold drinking.
Looseness of the teeth (with salivation).
Feeling of dryness of the lips.
25. Pricking on the point of the tongue.
Tongue feels as if burned, or as if sore; is coated white.
Ulcerated sore throat.
Feeling of swelling in the throat on swallowing.
Feeling of dryness in the throat, not relieved by drinking.
30. Heat in the throat alleviated by the inspiration of cold air.
Loss of smell and taste.

Stomach and Abdomen.

Craving for he knows not what, with loss of appetite; craving for piquant food.
Burning in the stomach, with headache.
Sensation of emptiness in the stomach soon after eating.
35. Inflammation of the stomach.
Nausea, which is not diminished by vomiting.
Extreme nausea, with great salivation and constant spitting.
Nausea, with headache, and with chill and heat.
Spasmodic eructation of flatus.
40. Hiccough (while smoking tobacco).
Vomiting preceded by anxiety.
Vomiting, of bitter water; of worms; with craving to eat, in order to quiet the nausea.
Vomiting and diarrhœa.
Pain in the left hypochondrium; worse by coughing, better by pressure and lying on the left side.
45. Hot streaming from the breast towards the liver.
Beating in the abdomen.
Sensation as if hot water poured itself from the breast into the abdomen, followed by diarrhœa.
Flatulent distention of the abdomen, in the evening, with the escape of flatus from the vagina (the os uteri being dilated).
Indurations in the abdomen.
50. Colic, with torpor of the liver.

Stool and Anus.

Ineffectual urging to stool, then vomiting.
Urging to stool (in the afternoon), but only discharges of flatus.
Frequent discharges of very offensive flatus. Diarrhœic stools, with much flatulence.
Colic, followed by diarrhœa.
55. Diarrhœa and termination of the coryza, catarrh, or pains in the chest.
Stools undigested.
Dysentery.
Hemorrhoids.

Urinary Organs.

Frequent and copious nocturnal urination, urine as clear as water.

Sexual Organs.

60. *Women.* Menstruation too early, with a discharge of black blood.
Amenorrhœa; uterine hemorrhage.
Stitches in the mammæ.
The nipples are sore and painful.

Respiratory Organs.

Dryness in the throat, and sensation of swelling in the larynx; with expectoration of thick mucus.
65. Tickling in the throat in the evening, with cough and headache.
Dry cough, awakens him from sleep, which did not cease until he sat upright in bed, and flatus was discharged both upwards and downwards.
Cough, with circumscribed redness of the cheeks, with pain in the chest; with coryza, then diarrhœa.
Pulmonary consumption; expectoration and breath exceedingly offensive.
Croup. Hooping-cough. Hydrothorax. Asthma. Pneumonia. Hæmoptysis.
70. Typhoid pneumonia, with very difficult respiration, cheeks and hands livid, pulse full, soft, vibrating, and easily compressed.
Burning and pressing in the chest, followed by heat through the abdomen and diarrhœa.
Palpitation of the heart.

Back and Neck.

Pain in the sacrum, from lifting; the pain in the sacrum is alleviated on bending forward.
Soreness of the nape of the neck on being touched.
75. Rheumatic pains in the nape of the neck, shoulders, and arms.

Extremities.

Upper. Rheumatic pain in the right arm and shoulder: worse at night in bed; cannot raise the arm; motion (turning in bed) makes it much worse.
Burning of the palms of the hands.
Stiffness of the finger-joints.
Ulceration at the roots of the nails on all the fingers of both hands.
80. *Lower.* Rheumatic pain in the left hip.
Rheumatic pain inside of the right thigh.

Bruise-like pain in the thigh, alternating with burning and pressure in the chest.
Stiffness of the knees.
Burning of the soles of the feet and palms of the hands (at night).
85. Rheumatic pains in the limbs; pain in those places where the bones are least covered with flesh, but not in the joints; on touching the painful part, the pain immediately vanished and appeared in some other part.

Generalities.

Great debility and weakness in the limbs, whilst walking in the open air.
Weakness and palpitation of the heart; fainting weakness.
Convulsive rigidity of the limbs.

Sleep.

Sleeplessness at night; awakens in a fright as if he would fall.

Fever.

90. Pulse too frequent and full.
Chill and shivering in the back, in the evening in bed.
Shaking chill.
Chill with nausea, headache.
Heat flying from the head to the stomach.
95. Fever heat and delirium.
Burning heat, rapidly alternating with chill and shivering.
Intermittent fevers; marsh fevers; nervous fever.

Skin.

Heat and dryness of the skin.
Itching and nettle-rash before the nausea.
100. Old indolent ulcers, with callous borders, and ichorous discharge.
Nasal polypi; fungus excrescences.
Jaundice.

Conditions.

Constant change of symptoms, when a new one arises the earlier cease.
Aggravation morning and evening; from light, noise, and motion.
105. Amelioration when lying still, in the dark room after vomiting.

SARSAPARILLA.

Mind and Disposition.

Changeable disposition.
Morose, with inclination to work.
The mental depression is caused by the pains.

Head.

Giddiness; when looking long at an object; or with nausea and sour vomiting.
5. Headache, with nausea and sour vomiting.
Stinging or pressing, stinging or pulsating headache.
Sound in the head as if a bell were striking, when talking.
Sensitiveness of the scalp; falling off of the hair.

Eyes.

Stitches in the eyes.
10. The eyes pain from the light of day.
The internal corners of the eye have a blue color and are bloated.
The white paper looks red in the evening.
Obscuration before the eyes as from a fog.

Ears.

Burning, itching scab on the lobe of the ear.

Nose.

15. Scabby eruption on and under the nose.

Face.

Eruption on the face like milk-crust.
Itching eruption on the forehead, with burning, and becoming humid on scratching.
Stiffness and tension in the muscles and articulation of the jaw.
Herpes on the upper lip.

Mouth and Throat.

20. Sensitiveness of the upper front teeth.
Tearing in the teeth from cold air and cold drink.
Spasmodic contraction of the throat with dyspnœa.
Aphthæ on the tongue and on the roof of the mouth.
Dryness and roughness in the throat in the morning.

Stomach and Abdomen.
25. Want of appetite, the thought of food causes him disgust.
Bitter eructations during and after eating.
Burning in the stomach, especially after eating bread.
After eating, the stomach has no sensation, feels as if he had eaten nothing.
Sensation of emptiness and rumbling in the abdomen.
30. Burning (or sensation of coldness) in the abdomen.

Stool and Anus.
Difficult and painful stool, with fainting attacks.
Stool retarded, hard and insufficient.

Urinary Organs.
Frequent, inefficient urging to urinate.
Diminished secretion of urine.
35. Tenesmus of the bladder, with discharge of white, acrid pus and mucus.
Painful constriction of the bladder.
Frequent, profuse discharge of pale urine, without any sensation in the urethra.
Burning in the urethra during every micturition.
Urine, red fiery; turbid, containing long flakes.
40. At the end of micturition some blood passes.
Stones in the bladder.
Sand (pale) in the urine (the infant cries before and during micturition, passes large quantities of sand).

Sexual Organs.
Men. Intolerable stench on the genital organs.
Herpes on the prepuce.
45. Painful seminal emissions at night.
Bad effects from gonorrhœa suppressed by mercury.
Women. Menstruation too late, too scanty and acrid.
During menstruation urging to urinate; soreness of the inside of the thighs.

Respiratory Organs.
Great shortness of breathing, compelling one to loosen the neck-cloth and vest to enable him to breathe.
50. Dyspnœa as from a spasm.

Back.
Stitches in the back from the least motion.

Extremities.
Upper. Stitches in the joints of the arms, hands and fingers, principally on motion.

Deep rhagades on the fingers, with burning pains.
The tips of the fingers feel bruised and sore.
55. *Lower.* Stitches in the legs, especially from motion.
Weakness in the thighs and knees.
Red spots on the calves.
Icy coldness of the feet.

Generalities.

Arthritic pains, after taking cold in the water, from suppressed gonorrhœa, with decreased secretion of urine.
60. The limbs are immovable, as if paralyzed.
Trembling of the hands and feet.
Great emaciation, the skin becomes shrivelled or it lies in folds.

Fever.

Pulse accelerated (in the evening).
Chilliness predominating (day and night).
65. Frequent shuddering, mostly in the forenoon, running from the feet upwards.
Heat in the evening, with ebullitions and palpitation of the heart.
Perspiration during the heat in the evening only on the forehead.

Sleep.

Sleeplessness at night; awakens frequently.

Skin.

Dry, red pimples, only itching when exposed to the heat.
70. Rash as soon as he goes from the warm room into the cold air.
Urticaria. Herpes. Warts.
Rhagades, deep, burning.
Ulcers, after the abuse of mercury.
Shrivelled skin.

Conditions.

75. During the chilliness the sensations are worse, and an amelioration occurs as soon as he becomes warm.
Bad effects from the abuse of mercury.

SCILLA MARITIMA.

Mind and Disposition.
Great anxiety of the mind, with fear of death.
Angry over trifles.

Head.
Vertigo (in the morning) with nausea.
Headache in the morning on waking, with pressing pains.
5. Painful sensitiveness of the vertex every morning.
Pulsation in the head when raising it.
Stinging headache.

Eyes.
Staring look, with the eyes wide open.
The left eye is much smaller than the right eye; the upper eyelid is swollen.
10. Contraction of the pupils.

Nose.
Nostrils painful as if sore, with violent coryza (in the morning).
Humid eruptions under the nose, with stinging-itching.

Face.
Changeable expression and color of the face.
During the heat redness of the face, followed by paleness, without coldness.
15. Distorted countenance, with red cheeks, and without thirst.
Humid, spreading eruption on the upper lip.
Black, cracked lips and black teeth.

Mouth and Throat.
Open, dry mouth.
Accumulation of much viscid mucus in the mouth.
20. Burning in the mouth and throat.
Dryness in the throat.

Stomach and Abdomen.
Insatiable appetite.
Longing for acids.
Thirst for cold water, but the dyspnœa compels her to take but a sip at a time.

SCILLA MARITIMA.

25. The food tastes bitter, especially the bread; or it tastes sweet, especially soup and meat.
Constant nausea in the pit of the stomach, alternating with pain, as for diarrhœa in the abdomen.
Pressure in the stomach, as from a stone.
Nausea during the morning cough.
Cutting pain in the abdomen, as from flatulence.
30. Painful sensitiveness of the abdomen and the region of the bladder.
Frequent discharge of very fetid flatulence.

Stool and Anus.

Painless constipation.
Diarrhœa, stool very offensive; watery (during the measles) or looking black.

Urinary Organs.

Frequent urging to urinate, with profuse discharge of pale (limpid) urine.
35. Continuous, painful pressure on the bladder.
Inability to retain the urine.

Respiratory Organs.

Moaning breathing, with the mouth open.
Wheezing breathing.
Shortness of breath from every exertion, especially when ascending.
40. Difficulty of breathing, with stitches in the chest when breathing and coughing.
Heaviness on the chest; congestion of blood to the chest.
Peumonia or pleurisy.
The pain in the chest is worse in the morning.
Cough in the morning, with copious expectoration of thin, frequently reddish-colored mucus.
45. Dry cough morning and night.
Cough caused by tingling in the chest; from drinking something cold; from every exertion.
Cough with stitches in the sides of the chest; pain in the abdomen; sensation of internal heat; dyspnœa; headache; pressure on the bladder and involuntary spirting out of the urine.
The morning cough, with even difficult expectoration, is much more severe and causes more suffering than the dry evening cough.
Especially suitable in pneumonia after blood-letting.

Back and Neck.
50. Stiffness of the neck.
Perspiration in the arm-pit.

Extremities.
Upper. Convulsive twitching of the arms; cold hands.
Lower. Convulsive twitching of the legs.
Cold foot-sweat.
55. Perspiration only on the toes.

Generalities.
Dull rheumatic pains; worse when exercising, relieved while at rest.
Convulsive twitchings and motions of the limbs; convulsions.

Sleep.
Frequent yawning without sleepiness.
Restless sleep, with much tossing about.

Fever.
60. Pulse small and slow, slightly hard.
Chill internally at night, with external heat.
Chilliness towards the evening when walking, not while sitting.
Heat, dry, burning, internally predominates.
Heat of the whole body, with cold hands and feet, with aversion to be uncovered.
65. Great sensation of heat in the body in the afternoon and evening, generally with cold feet.
Whenever he uncovers himself during the heat he suffers from chilliness and pain.
Perspiration wanting, even during the violent burning heat.

Skin.
Soreness in the bends of the joints.
Eruptions like itch, with burning-itching.
70. Gangrene.

Conditions.
Most complaints are worse in the morning and from motion.

SECALE CORNUTUM.

Mind and Disposition.
Great anxiety.
Madness, with inclination to drown oneself.
Mania, with inclination to bite.
Fear of death.

Head.
5. Stupefaction and unconsciousness.
Giddiness, as from intoxication.
Stupefaction, with tingling in the head and pain in the limbs, which are worse from motion.
Unconsciousness with heavy sleep, preceded by tingling in the head and limbs (in hemorrhages from the uterus).
Dull pain in the back part of the head.
10. Falling off of the hair.

Eyes.
Wild, staring look.
Distortion of the eyes.
The eyes are pushed back far into the sockets.
Double vision.
15. Obscuration of sight.

Ears.
Humming and roaring in the ears, with occasional deafness.

Nose.
Bleeding of the nose.

Face.
Pale, yellowish, sunken countenance, with deep-sunken eyes, surrounded by a blue circle.
Dark redness of the face.
20. Spasmodic distortion of the mouth and lips.
Formication in the face.
Locked jaw.

Mouth and Throat.
The teeth become loose and fall out.
Grinding of the teeth.
25. Bloody or discolored foam before the mouth.
Spitting of blood.
Painful tingling in the throat and on the tongue.
Swelling of the tongue.

Discolored, brown or blackish tongue.
30. Tongue coated with mucus.
Feeble, stuttering, indistinct speech, as if the tongue were paralyzed.

Stomach and Abdomen.

Violent, unquenchable thirst.
Insatiable hunger, especially for acids.
Continuous nausea; worse after eating.
35. Vomiting of bile, of mucus, of black bile, of lumbrici, or of the food, with great weakness, or painless, without any effort.
Violent pressure in the stomach, as from a heavy weight.
Great anxiety and pressure in the pit of the stomach, with great sensitiveness to the touch.
Inflammation and gangrene of the stomach.
Inflammation and gangrene of the liver.
40. Burning (or coldness) in the abdomen.
Burning in the spleen.
Colic, with convulsions.
Pain in the loins, as from false-labor pains.
Rumbling in the abdomen.

Stool and Anus.

45. Frequent diarrhœa; discharges watery and of mucus.
Very debilitating diarrhœa, with sudden sinking of strength.
Involuntary, very watery stools.
Offensive watery diarrhœa (in child-bed).
Cholera; diarrhœa after the Cholera.

Urinary Organs.

50. Urinary secretions suppressed.
Pale, watery urine.
Hemorrhage from the urethra.

Sexual Organs.

Women. Menstruation too profuse and of too long duration.
Discharge of blood during pregnancy.
55. Hemorrhage from the uterus of black, liquid blood; the discharge is increased by motion.
Labor ceases, and instead twitchings and convulsions.
Abortion, especially in the third month (after abortion the os uteri does not contract).
Lochia of too long duration.
Too long and too painful after-pains.
60. Swelling of and warts on the half-open uterus.

SECALE CORNUTUM.

Inflammation of the uterus from suppressed lochia or menstruation.
Cancer and gangrene of the uterus.

Respiratory Organs.

Heavy, anxious breathing, with moaning.
Spitting of blood, with or without cough.
65. Hollow, hoarse voice.
Violent palpitation of the heart, with contracted and frequently intermittent pulse.

Back.

Tingling in the back, which is numb (void of feeling), extending to the tips of the fingers.

Extremities.

Numbness and insensibility of the hands.
The fingers are bent backward, or spasmodically contracted.
70. Burning in the hands.
Gangrenous deadness of the fingers.
Swelling of the hands, with black pustules.
Lower. Violent cramps in the calves.
Burning in the swollen feet.
75. Tingling in the toes.
Gangrenous deadness of the toes.
Gangrena senilis.

Generalities.

Convulsive twitching in the limbs.
Spasmodic distortion of the limbs, relieved by stretching them out.
80. Tetanic spasms.
Drawing and tearing in the limbs, with tingling.
Numbness of all the limbs.
Burning in all parts of the body, as if sparks were falling on them.

Sleep.

Great sleepiness; deep, heavy sleep; stupor.

Fever.

85. Pulse unchanged, even with the most violent attacks.
Pulse generally slow and contracted, sometimes intermittent or suppressed; only slightly accelerated during the heat.
Violent chill of short duration, soon followed by violent internal burning heat, with violent thirst.
Disagreeable sensation of coldness in the back, in the abdomen and in the limbs.

Violent and long-continued dry heat, with great restlessness and violent thirst.
90. Perspiration, especially on the upper part of the body.
Cold, clammy perspiration over the whole body.

Skin.

Discolored, dry, shrivelled skin.
Numbness and sensation of deadness of the skin.
Formication under the skin.
95. Desquamation of the whole skin.
Gangrenous blood-vesicles.
Petechiæ.

Conditions.

Aggravation from motion; from touching the affected parts; during walking; from warmth; from getting warm in bed; from being covered; from warm applications to all the variously affected parts; during pregnancy, parturition and confinement.

Amelioration in the cold air, from getting cold; from rubbing; from stretching out the limbs; while standing.

SELENIUM.

Mind and Disposition.

Talkativeness and fond of conversing.
Mental labor fatigues him much.
Great forgetfulness when awake, with distinct recollection during half sleep.

Head.

Vertigo, when rising from a seat, on raising himself in bed, on moving about.
5. Paroxysms of vertigo, most violent an hour after breakfast and dinner.
Headache from lemonade, tea and wine.
Violent stinging pain over the left eye, caused by walking in the sun and from strong smells; with increased secretion of urine, and melancholy.
Headache every afternoon.

The hair falls off when combing the head, even of the eyebrows, whiskers and on the genitals, with tingling-itching on the scalp in the evening, oozing after scratching, and with tension and sensation of contraction of the scalp (with emaciation of the face and hands).

Eyes.

10. Itching vesicles on the edges of the eyelids and on the eyebrows.

Spasmodic twitching of the left eyeball.

Ears.

Increased secretion of wax, which is hardened in the ear in which he is deaf.

Nose.

Itching in the nose and on the borders of the wings.
Inclination to bore with fingers in the nose.
15. Yellow, thick, jelly-like mucus in the nose.

Face.

Greasy, shining skin of the face.
Twitching of the muscles of the face.
Great emaciation of the face.

Mouth and Throat.

Toothache, with inclination to pick till they bleed.
20. Teeth covered with mucus.

Stomach and Abdomen.

Want of appetite in the morning, with white-coated tongue.
Aversion to food much salted.
Great longing for spirituous liquors (brandy).
After eating, pulsations through the body, especially in the abdomen.
25. Pain in the liver, especially in taking a long breath, with sensitiveness to external pressure.
Red, itching rash in the region of the liver.
Stitches in the spleen when walking.

Stool and Anus.

Constipation; hard feces, with discharge of mucus or blood when passing the last portion of it; stool so hard and impact that it has to be removed by mechanical aid.
Papescent stools, with tenesmus.

Urinary Organs.

30. Dark, scanty urine.
Red urine in the evening.

Red, sandy, coarse-grained sediment.
Involuntary dripping of urine when walking.
Dripping of urine after micturition and after stool.

Sexual Organs.

35. Slow and insufficient erections, with too rapid emission of semen and long continued voluptuous thrill.
Discharge of prostatic fluid during sleep and stool.
Impotence, with lasciviousness.
Gonorrhœa (secondary).

Respiratory Organs.

Hoarseness, when beginning to sing, or from singing; talking long or reading; voice hoarse and husky.
40. Frequent deep breathing, with moaning.
Hawking up of mucus in globules, with blood.
Cough in the morning, straining the chest, with expectoration of mucus and blood.

Back and Neck.

Pain as from lameness in the small of the back, in the morning.
Stiffness of the neck on turning the head.

Extremities.

45. *Upper.* Tearing in the hands at night, with cracking in the wrists.
Itching vesicles on and between the fingers.
Emaciation of the hands.
Lower. Cracking of the knee-joint on bending it (at night).
Flat ulcers on the lower legs.
50. Emaciation of the legs.
Itching of the feet around the ankle, and especially in the evening.
Cramps in the calves, and soles of the feet.

Generalities.

Great emaciation, especially in the face and on the thighs and hands.
Great aversion to a draught of air.

Sleep.

55. Light sleep at night, the least noise wakens him.
Goes to sleep late in the evening.
Awakens early and always at the same hour.
Dreams of quarrels and unnatural cruelties.

Fever.

Pulse very little accelerated.
60. Chilliness, alternating with heat.
External heat, with burning in the skin, and only in single spots.
Very profuse perspiration, especially on the chest, arm-pits and genitals.
Perspiration from the least exertion.
Perspiration as soon as he sleeps, day or night.
65. The sweat makes yellow or white, stiff blotches in the linen.

Skin.

Red rash (region of the liver).
Frequent tingling on small spots of the skin, with great irritation to scratch.
The spots which one scratches remain humid very long.

Conditions.

China causes violent complaints, and much aggravates those already present.
70. Cannot endure any draft of air.
Aggravation after sleep, especially on hot days, from lemonade, wine and tea; from very salt food; in the sun, from draft of air.

SENEGA.

Mind and Disposition.

Great anxiety, with rapid breathing.
Melancholy mood, with great irritability of temper.
Hilarity, with great irritability, changing to anger and wrath.

Head.

Dulness and stupefaction of the head, with pressure in the eyes, and obscuration of sight.
5. The headache always extends to the eyes, is aggravated in the warm room, and relieved in the cold air.
Shuddering on the hairy scalp.

Eyes.

The eyes pain as if they were pressed out, as if the eyeballs were being expanded, especially in the evening at candle-light.
Congestion of blood to the eyes, with pulsation in them on stooping.
Swelling of the eyelids, with tingling in them.
10. Hardened mucus in the morning in the eyelashes.
Lachrymation in the open air, and when looking intensely on an object.
Obscuration of the cornea.
Sensitiveness of the eyes to the light.
Obscuration of sight, with glistening before the eyes, worse from rubbing them.

Ears.

15. Painful sensitiveness of hearing.

Nose.

Smell of pus before the nose.

Face.

Heat in the face.
Burning blisters on the upper lip, and in the corners of the mouth.

Mouth and Throat.

Burning in the throat, mouth and on the tongue.
20. White-coated tongue.
Inflammation and swelling of the throat and pallet.
Dryness in the throat and accumulation of tough mucus in the throat, which it is difficult to hawk up.
Metallic taste in the mouth, or taste like urine.

Stomach and Abdomen.

Violent thirst.
25. Gnawing hunger, with sensation of emptiness in the stomach.
Eructations (relieving the mucus and hawking of mucus from the thorax).
Nausea, as from the stomach, with vomiturition and straining to vomit.
Burning in the stomach.
Colic, with pressing pain.
30. Warmth and oppression in the upper part of the abdomen when inhaling.
Gnawing in the upper part of the abdomen.

Stool and Anus.
Hard, retarded, and insufficient stool.
Diarrhœa, with vomiting and great anxiety.
Urinary Organs.
Urinary secretions diminished.
35. At night, in bed, involuntary micturition.
Urine contains strings of mucus, foaming when getting cold, turbid and cloudy.
Burning and stinging in the urethra during and after micturition.
Respiratory Organs.
Dyspnœa as from stagnation in the lungs.
Oppressed breathing, as if the chest were not wide enough, especially in the open air and when stooping.
40. Congestion of blood to the chest.
Shortness of breath from accumulation of mucus in the chest and trachea.
Dry, shaking cough from tickling in the larnyx, especially in the open air.
Cough with copious expectoration of tough mucus.
Shaking cough, like hooping-cough, from burning and tickling in the larnyx, in the morning, with copious expectoration of tough, white mucus (like the white of an egg).
45. The cough is worse in the evening and at night, during rest, in the warm room, when sitting, when lying on the (left) side.
Pressing pain in the chest, worse during rest.
Great sensitiveness to the inner chest, also to the touch.
Stitches in the chest when coughing and breathing.
Soreness in the chest, aggravated by pressure, coughing and sneezing.
50. Accumulation of mucus in the chest, in the larynx, and trachea.
Phthisis mucosa : Hydrothorax.
Hoarseness; bronchitis.
The most chest symptoms are aggravated during rest and do not affect the breathing.
Violent palpitation of the heart.
Extremities.
55. *Upper.* Sensation as if the wrist were sprained.
Lower. Sensation of great weakness or debility in the legs; the joints feel as if lame.

Back.

Pain under the right shoulder-blade as if the chest should burst, when coughing or drawing a long breath.

Generalities.

Great bodily and mental lassitude.
Great weakness, which seems to originate in the chest.
60. Diseases of mucous membranes.
Dropsy of internal organs (especially after inflammation).
Inflammation of internal organs.

Sleep.

In the evening, as soon as one lies down, heavy sleep; in the morning one wakens frequently from dyspnœa.

Fever.

Pulse hard and frequent.
65. Chilliness and chill almost only in the open air, with weakness in the legs and dyspnœa.
Shudders over the back, with heat in the face and chest symptoms.
Sudden flushes of heat.
Perspiration wanting.

Skin.

Bites of poisonous animals or animals when in a state of rage.

Conditions.

70. Especially suitable for plethoric, phlegmatic persons.
Most symptoms, especially those of the chest, are aggravated when at rest and are relieved when walking in the open air.

SENNA.

Abdomen and Stool.

Painful colic from incarcerated flatulence (particularly in young children).
Diarrhœic stools, followed by tenesmus and burning at the anus.

SEPIA.

Mind and Disposition.

Sadness with weeping.
Great indifference, even to one's family.
Restlessness, fidgety.
Great excitability in company.
5. Dread of being alone.
Is easily offended and inclined to be vehement.
Sadness about one's health and her domestic affairs.
Anxiety, with flushes of heat.
Aversion to one's occupation.
10. Heavy flow of ideas.
Weak memory.

Head.

Stupefaction in the head (which disables him from performing any mental labor).
Vertigo; when walking in the open air, as if all the objects were moving around one, or as if suspended in the air, with unconsciousness; when rising from the bed; in the afternoon.
Paroxysms of hemicrania, stinging pain as from within to without, in one side of the forehead or side of the head (mostly in the left side), with nausea (and vomiting) and contraction of the eye; worse in the room and when walking fast, better in the open air and when lying on the painful side.
15. Boring headache from within to without, from the forenoon till evening, worse from motion and stooping, relieved by rest, when closing the eyes, from external pressure, and sleep.
Pressing headache, as if the head should burst and the eyes fall out, with nausea.
Sensation of coldness on the vertex; worse from moving the head and stooping, better when at rest and in the open air.
Pulsating headache in the cerebellum, beginning in the morning, worse in the evening, from the least motion, when turning the eyes, when lying on the back, better when closing the eyes and when at rest.

Headache, as from commotion of the brain when stepping or when shaking the head, better when sitting up or from slow exercise.

20. Shooting pains, especially over the left eye, extorting cries.

External coldness of the head.

Eruptions on the vertex and back part of the head, dry, offensive stinging-itching and tingling, with cracks, extending behind the ears, feeling sore when scratching them.

Swelling on one side of the head above the temple, with itching; sensation of coldness and tearing in it; worse when touching it; better when lying on it, or after rising from the bed.

Involuntary jerking of the head backwards (or forward), principally in the forenoon and when sitting.

25. Sensitiveness of the roots of the hair; worse in the evening, to contact, cold north wind, when lying on the painless side, and burning after scratching.

Fontanelles remain open, with jerking of the head, pale bloated face, stomacace, green diarrhœic stools.

Perspiration on the head, smelling sour, with faintish weakness; worse in the evening before going to sleep.

Disposition to take cold on the head from dry, cold wind, and if the head gets wet.

Itching on the head (nose and eyes).

30. Falling off of the hair.

Small red pimples on the forehead; rough forehead.

Eyes.

Pressure on the eyeballs.

Inflammation of the eyes, with redness and stinging pain.

Burning of the eyes in the morning.

35. Lachrymation in the morning and evening.

The eyelids pain in the morning when awaking, as if they were too heavy, and as if he could not keep them open.

Inability to open the eyelids at night.

Heaviness and falling down of the upper eyelids as if they were paralyzed.

Inflammation of the eyelids; nightly agglutination of the eyes.

40. Eyelids red, swollen; styes on them.

Great sensitiveness of the eyes to the light of day.

Yellow color of the white of the eyes.

Black spots hovering and swimming before the eyes.

Sparks before the eyes.
45. Green halo around the light of the candle.
Pustules or fungus hæmatodes on the cornea.

Ears.

Stinging in the (left) ear.
Discharge of thin matter from the ear.
Much itching in the affected ear.
50. Over-sensitiveness to music.
Swelling of and eruptions on the external ear.
Tetters on the lobe of the ear, behind the ear (and on the neck).

Nose.

Nose swollen and inflamed, especially on the tip.
Tip of the nose scurfy.
55. Ulcerated nostrils.
Stoppage of the nose; dry coryza.
Violent bleeding of the nose, and blowing of blood from the nose.
Loss of smell, or fetid smell before the nose.
Ozœna; blowing of large lumps of yellow green mucus or yellow green membranes, with blood, from the nose.

Face.

60. Pale yellow puffiness of the face, with blue margins around the eyes.
Yellow color of the face (and of the white of the eyes).
Yellow saddle across the nose and face.
Yellowness around the mouth.
Tetters around the mouth.
65. Moist, scaly eruptions in the red parts of the lips and on the chin.
Swelling of the under lip.
Erysipelas and swelling of one side of the face from the root of a decayed tooth.
Herpes, scurfs and black pores in the face.
Neuralgic pains in the face (left side, from abuse of tobacco).

Mouth and Throat.

70. Toothache; stinging, pulsating, extending to the ear during pregnancy, with shortness of breath, with swelled face and swelling of the submaxillary glands, aggravated from every cold draft of air, when touching the teeth, and when talking.
The teeth are dull, loose, bleed easily and decay rapidly.

Gums painfully swollen, bleeding without any cause.
Bad smell from the mouth.
Tongue and cavity of the mouth feel as if scalded.
75. Tongue coated white.
Soreness of the tip of the tongue.
Dryness of the throat, with tension and scraping.
Soreness and stinging in the throat, with swelling of the submaxillary glands.
Sensation as of a plug in the throat.
80. Hawking up of mucus in the morning.

Stomach and Abdomen.

Taste putrid or sour.
Food tastes too salt.
Canine hunger and sensation of emptiness in the stomach.
Thirst in the morning or thirstlessness.
85. After eating, acidity in the mouth and bloatedness of the abdomen.
Aversion to meat and milk, which cause diarrhœa.
Eructations, sour or like rotten eggs, or bitter.
Eructations which cause blood to rise in the mouth.
Water-brash after drinking or eating.
90. Acidity of the stomach (with disgust for life).
Nausea, especially in the morning and while fasting, or when riding in a carriage.
Nausea and vomiting after eating.
Vomiting of pregnant women, sometimes of milky water.
Vomiting, of bile and food, in the morning, with headache.
95. Painful sensation of emptiness in the stomach and abdomen.
Pain in the stomach after eating.
Pressure in the stomach, as from a stone, especially after eating or at night.
Cutting, boring, from the region of the stomach towards the spine.
Burning in the stomach.
100. Pulsation in the pit of the stomach.
Rumbling in the abdomen, especially after eating.
Soreness of the abdomen in pregnant women.
In the abdomen, pressing, cutting, stinging, burning, coldness.
Stitches in the liver and left hypochondrium.
105. Pot-belliedness of mothers.
Brown spots on the abdomen.

Stool and Anus.

Constipation; urging to stool ineffectual, with discharge of mucus or flatulence only.

Stool insufficient, retarded, like sheep-dung.
Insufficient stool, with straining and tenesmus.
110. Constipation during pregnancy.
Difficult discharge even of the soft stool.
Diarrhœa; stools green, smelling sour, very debilitating; after eating boiled milk.
Small jelly-like stools, with tenesmus.
Discharge of blood with the stool.
115. Prolapsus ani (during stool).
Pain in the rectum, as from contraction.
In the rectum and anus, itching, burning and stinging.
Oozing from the rectum.
Discharge of mucus, with stinging and tearing.
120. Prolapsus of the hæmorrhoidal tumor.

Urinary Organs.

Frequent urging to urinate, from pressure on the bladder.
Frequent micturition; even at night he has to rise frequently.
Involuntary discharge of urine at night, especially in the first sleep.
Burning in the bladder and in the orifice of the urethra.
125. Smarting in the urethra when urinating.
Urine: turbid, with sediment of red sand; blood-red, with white sediment and a cuticle on the surface; very offensive, with much white sediment.

Sexual Organs.

Men. Continued erections at night.
The prepuce ulcerates and itches continually.
Weakness of the genitals; they perspire profusely, especially the scrotum.
130. Scrotum swollen.
Cutting in the testes.
After coition great weakness in the knees.
Women. Pressure, as if every thing would protrude (with oppression of breathing).
Prolapsus of the uterus, of the vagina.
135. Induration of the neck of the uterus.
Violent stitches in the vagina, upwards.
Redness, swelling and itching humid eruption on the labiæ.
Catamenia too early and too profuse, or too scanty, or suppressed.
During menstruation, depression, toothache, headache, bleeding of the nose, and soreness in the limbs.

140. Leucorrhœa, of yellow or greenish water, like pus, or of bad-smelling fluids.
Inclination to miscarriages.

Respiratory Organs.

Roughness and soreness of the larynx and throat.
Hoarseness, with coryza and dry cough from titillation in the throat.
Sensation of dryness in the larynx.
145. Dry cough, especially in the evening, in bed till midnight, frequently with nausea and bitter vomiting.
Cough, especially evening and morning, with salty expectoration; with rattling of mucus in the chest; with expectoration only in the morning, or only during the night; cough only during the day, or cough which wakens one at night.
Expectoration, profuse, purulent, offensive, whitish, green, tasting salt.
Cough, with soreness in the chest; stitches in the chest or back.
Expectoration difficult, or being obliged to swallow again what had been raised.
150. Attacks of spasmodic cough, like hooping-cough; coughs in frequent succession, caused by tickling in the chest or from tickling extending from the larynx to the abdomen, with expectoration only in the morning, evening and at night of yellow, greenish-gray pus, or of milk-white, tough mucus, tasting salt, bitter, putrid or disagreeably sweet, which has to be swallowed again.
Cough worse when at rest, when lying on the (left) side; from acids.
Itching and tickling in the chest.
Sensation of emptiness in the chest.
155. Stitch in the left side of the chest and scapula when breathing and coughing.
Dyspnœa; oppression of the chest and shortness of breath when walking.
Congestion of blood to the chest, with violent palpitation of the heart.
Brown spots on the chest.
Soreness of the nipples.
The chest symptoms cease and are relieved by pressure of the hand on the thorax.

Back and Neck.

160. Pressure and stitches in the right shoulder-blade.
Stiffness in the small of the back and neck.

Stitches posteriorly above the right hip; she could not lie on the right side, and when touched it felt sore.
Weakness in the small of the back when walking.
Pulsation in the small of the back.
165. Stitches in the back when coughing.
Perspiration in the back and arm-pit.
Humid tetter in the arm-pit.

Extremities.

Upper. Paralytic drawing and tearing in the arm and arm-pit to the fingers.
Pain as from dislocation in the shoulder-joint.
170. Stiffness of the elbow-joint.
Stitches in the joints of the arm, hands and fingers.
Swelling and suppuration of the axillary glands.
Burning in the palms of the hands.
Cold perspiration on the hands.
175. Cold hands (and feet).
Herpes (scaling off) on the elbows.
Painless ulcers on the joints and tips of the fingers.
Itch and scabs on the hands (soldiers' itch).
Lower. Cramp pain in the hip-joint.
180. Pain as if bruised in the right hip-joint.
Stiffness of the legs up to the hip-joint, after sitting for a short time.
Swelling of the limbs and feet; worse when sitting or standing, better when walking.
Stiffness of the knee-joint and ankle.
Spasms in the buttocks at night, in bed, when stretching out the limb.
185. Restlessness in the legs every evening, with formication in them.
Coldness in the legs and feet, especially in the evening in bed.
Burning in the feet.
Profuse perspiration of the feet.
Stinging in the heels and in the corns.
190. Tension in the tendo-Achilles.
Ulcer on the heel from a spreading blister.
Painless ulcers on the joints and tips of the toes.

Generalities.

Heaviness in the body.
Stiffness of the joints (hands, knees and feet).
195. Arthritic pains in the joints.
Tearing in the muscles.

Excessive sensitiveness of the body to pain.
Sensation of contraction in outer parts.
Sore pain in inner and outer parts.
200. Burning pain, especially in inner parts.
Bleeding from inner parts.
Congestions at night, with palpitation of the heart and pulsation all over.
Jerking and twitching of the head and limbs during the day.
Twitching in the muscles.
205. Inflammatory swellings.
Stinging pains in the limbs, inner parts, bones.
Tingling in outer parts.
The limbs go to sleep easily after manual labor.
Vibrations like dull tingling in the body.
210. Sensation as of a ball in inner parts.
Fainting, after getting wet; from riding in a carriage, and while kneeling in church.
A short walk fatigues much.
Aversion to the open air.
Want of natural heat.
215. Weakness of the joints.
Hysterical spasms.

Sleep.

Great sleepiness in day-time.
Frequent awaking from sleep without cause.
Talks aloud during sleep.
220. Twitching of the limbs during sleep.
Awakens in the morning at 3 o'clock and cannot go to sleep again.
Ebullitions at night, with restlessness.
Nightly delirium.

Fever.

Pulse full and quick during the night and then intermitting; during the day slow.
225. The pulse is accelerated by motion and being angry.
Pulsation in all the blood-vessels.
Chill frequently setting in after previous heat.
Chilliness in the open air, in the evening, and from every movement.
During the chill more thirst than during the heat.
230. Chilliness with the pains.
Flushes of heat at intervals during the day, especially in the afternoon and evening, while sitting or in the open air, generally with thirst and redness of the face.

SEPIA. 625

Profuse perspiration, more after than during exercise.
Continuous, debilitating sweats.
Continuous night and morning sweats.
235. Perspiration only on the upper part of the body.
Perspiration smelling sour or offensive.
Intermittent fever, with thirst during the chill; pain in the limbs; hands and feet icy cold; the fingers feel as if they were dead; followed by violent heat and inability to collect one's senses; this is followed by profuse perspiration.

Skin.

Itching in the face, on the arms, hands, hips, feet, abdomen and genitals, changing to burning when scratching.
Soreness of the skin and humid places in the bends of the joints.
240. Brown spots, or claret-colored, tetter-like spots on the skin.
Pemphigus; ring-worms; boils; blood-boils.
Ulcers, painless (knuckles, finger-joints, tips of the fingers, joints and tips of the toes), or itching, stinging and burning.
Humid tetters, with itching and burning.
Lymphatic swellings.
245. Crippled nails.

Conditions.

The pains extend from other parts to the back.
Especially suitable for persons with dark hair and for women, especially during pregnancy, in childbed, and while nursing.
Aggravation in the forenoon and evening; from mental exertion, from washing in water, from stretching the affected limb, when at rest, sitting, on bending down, after sexual excesses, after eating.
Amelioration from warm air, on and after rising from the bed or seat and drawing up the limbs; from violent exercise, except riding on horseback.
250. Bad effects from masturbation.
Sepia follows well after Pulsatilla.

40

SILICEA.

Mind and Disposition.

Desponding, melancholy, tired of life.
Yielding, anxious mood.
Compunction of conscience about trifles.
The child becomes obstinate and headstrong; cries when kindly spoken to.

Head.

5. Vertigo, as if one would fall forward; when stooping, riding, raising the eyes upwards; ascending from the neck to the head, with nausea.

Burning in the head, with pulsation and perspiration of the head; worse at night, from mental exertion and talking, relieved by wrapping the head up warm.

Pressing headache, as if the head would burst, ascending from the neck to the forehead.

Pulsating and beating, most violent in the forehead and vertex, with chilliness.

Tearing headache, frequently only on one side of the head, with stitches through the eyes and in the cheek-bones; heat in the forehead and great restlessness; worse from a draught of air and motion.

10. Heaviness in the head, pressing out in the forehead; worse from evening till night, from stepping up hard, from uncovering the head, or if the head becomes cold in the open air.

Stitches in the forehead and in the temples, principally in the right, from within to without; worse at night, from moving the eyes, from talking and writing.

Most all the headaches are aggravated from mental exertion, stooping, talking and cold air, and are relieved in the warm room, and from wrapping the head up warmly.

Eruption on the back part of the head and behind the ears dry, offensive smelling, scabby, burning-itching; when scratching it, burning feeling, more sore, and discharging pus.

Itching pustules and bulbous swellings on the hairy scalp and on the neck; very sensitive to pressure, touch, and when lying on it; better when wrapping it up warm.

SILICEA.

15. Sensitiveness of the scalp to pressure (of the hat) and to contact; worse in the evening and when lying on the painful side; burning after scratching.

Open fontanelles; the head is too large and the rest of the body emaciated, with pale wax color of the face; hot, swollen abdomen, and fetid stools.

Burning and itching, mostly on the back part of the head; worse from scratching, which causes burning and soreness; worse when undressing in the evening and on getting warm in bed.

Tearing pain in the scalp worse at night, and from pressure.

Profuse, sour-smelling perspiration, on the head only (in the evening), with great sensitiveness of the scalp, with pale face and emaciation.

20. Tendency to take cold in the head, which cannot possibly be uncovered.

Eyes.

Lachrymation in the open air.
Agglutination of the eyes.
Swelling of the tear-gland.
Ulcers (and fungus hæmatodes) on the cornea.

25. Redness of the eyes with biting pains in the corner of the eye.
Spots and cicatrices on the cornea.
When reading the letters run together, look pale.
Obscuration of sight, as from a gray cover.
Black spots and fiery sparks before the eyes.

30. Aversion to light; day-light dazzles the eyes.

Ears.

Otalgia, with stitches out of the ears.
Itching in the ears.
Stoppage of the ears, which open at times with a loud report.
Difficult hearing, especially of the human voice and during the full moon.

35. Over-sensitiveness of the hearing to noise.
Swelling of the external ear, with discharge of pus from the ear.
Scabs behind the ear.
Increased secretion of very thin cerumen.
Hard swelling of the parotid gland.

Nose.

40. Painful dryness of the nose.
Gnawing pain and ulcers high up in the nose, with great sensitiveness of the place to contact.

Acrid, corroding discharge from the nose and stoppage of the nose.
Loss of smell.
Scabs and ulcers in the nose.
45. Bleeding of the nose.
Frequent violent sneezing.
Long-continued stoppage of the nose from hardened mucus.

Face.
Pale, earth-colored face.
White or burning red spots in the face, especially on the cheeks.
50. The skin of the face cracks.
Blood boils on the cheek.
Ulcerated corners of the mouth.
Scabby eruptions on the lips, which smart.
Ulcers in the vermilion border of the lower lip.
55. Herpes on the chin.
Swelling and caries of the lower jaw.
Painful swelling of the submaxillary glands.
Scirrhous indurations of the face and upper lip.
The articulation of the jaw is spasmodically closed (lockjaw).

Mouth and Throat.
60. Toothache from warm food and from drawing cold air in the mouth.
Tearing in the teeth; worse at night, or only when eating.
Stinging in the teeth, preventing sleep.
Painful inflammation, swelling, soreness, and easily bleeding gums.
Dryness of the mouth.
65. Accumulation of mucus in the mouth.
Sensation as if a hair were lying on the forepart of the tongue.
Soreness of the tongue.
One-sided swelling of the tongue.
Tongue coated with brown mucus.
70. Sore throat with much mucus in the throat.
When swallowing, soreness and stitches in the throat (Quinsy).
Swelling of the palate.
Difficult deglutition, as if the throat were paralyzed.
When swallowing, the food easily gets into the posterior nares.

Stomach and Abdomen.
75. Ravenous hunger, with want of appetite.

SILICEA.

Want of appetite and excessive thirst.
Aversion to warm, cooked food; he desires only cold things.
Loss of taste.
Bitter taste in the morning.
80. Aversion of the child to the mother's milk; refuses to nurse, and if it does it vomits.
After eating, sour eructations, fulness and pressure in the stomach; water-brash and vomiting.
Eructations tasting of the food eaten, or sour.
Water-brash, with chilliness.
Continuous nausea and vomiting; worse in the morning.
85. Vomiting whenever he drinks.
Sensitiveness of the pit of the stomach to pressure.
Abdomen bloated and hard (especially in children).
Pain in the abdomen; colic in children from worms.
Cutting pain in the abdomen (colic), with constipation.
90. Colic, with yellow hands and blue nails.
The region of the liver swollen and hard. (Inflammation and induration of the liver).
Beating soreness in the liver; worse on motion and when walking, or when lying on the right side, or when breathing.
Pressure in the abdomen, especially after eating.
Painful inguinal hernia.
95. Incarcerated flatulency; difficult discharge of flatulence very offensive flatulence.
Much rumbling of flatulence in the abdomen.

Stool and Anus.

Constipation; difficult, hard stool; the feces are large, and if partly expelled slip back again, as if there were not power enough to expel them; even the soft stool is expelled with much difficulty.
Frequent papescent, fetid smelling stools.
Itching in the anus and rectum; also during stool.

Urinary Organs.

100. Strangury.
Continuous urging to urinate, with scanty discharge; also at night.
Involuntary micturition at night.
Sediment of red sand or deposit of yellow sand.

Sexual Organs.

Men. Red spots and itching on the corona glandis.

105. Itching, humid spots on the genitals, especially on the scrotum.
    Prepuce red and itching; swollen and itching humid pimples on it.
    Hydrocele.
    Increased sexual desire; frequent violent erections.
    Discharge of prostatic fluid when urinating and passing stool.
110. After coition soreness in the limbs, and sensation in one side of the head as if paralyzed.
    Women. Menstruation too early and too scanty (or too profuse).
    Suppressed menstruation.
    Discharge of menstrual fluid while nursing.
    Itching on the genitals.
115. Abortion.
    Leucorrhœa, during micturition, acrid, corroding.
    Inflammation of the nipples.
    Suppuration of the mammæ.

Respiratory Organs.

Hoarseness, with roughness and soreness of the larynx.
120. Deep sighing-breathing.
    Shortness of breath and panting, from walking fast or from manual labor.
    Dyspnœa when at rest; when lying on the back.
    Stitches in the chest and sides of the chest, through to the back.
    Pulsation in the sternum.
125. Phthisis pulmonalis.
    Cough, with copious expectoration.
    Suffocative cough at night.
    Hollow, spasmodic, suffocative cough from tickling in the throat, especially the throat-pit, with expectoration only during the day of profuse, yellowish-green pus, or of tough, milky, acrid mucus, at times of pale, frothy blood, generally tasting greasy and offensive smelling.

Back and Neck.

Spasmodic pain in the small of the back, which does not allow one to rise.
130. Swelling and curvature of the vertebræ.
    Inflammatory abscess on the psoas muscle.
    Sensation of soreness between the shoulder-blades.
    Glandular swellings on the neck and arm-pits, with suppuration.

SILICEA.

Extremities.

Upper. The arms go to sleep when lying on them, or when laying them on the table.
135. Heaviness and paralytic weakness of the (fore) arms, with trembling from the least exertion.
Blood-boils and warts on the arms.
Stitches in the wrist at night, extending to the arm.
Paralysis of the hands.
Burning in the tips of the fingers.
140. Panaritium.
Yellow, crippled, brittle finger-nails.
Lower. Blood-boils on the thighs and calves.
Swelling of the knee.
Red, smarting spot on the tibia.
145. Ulcers on the lower leg, on the tibia.
Caries of the tibia.
Cramps in the calves, in the soles of the feet.
Numbness of the calves.
Coldness of the feet (after suppressed foot-sweat).
150. Sweat of the feet offensive, causing soreness between the toes.
Voluptuous tickling in the soles of the feet, driving to despair.
Ulceration of the big toe, with stinging pain.

Generalities.

Twitching of the limbs day and night.
Epileptic attacks (at night, during new moon).
155. The limbs go to sleep easily.
Great restlessness in the body when sitting long.
Soreness and lameness in the limbs, in the evening.
Stinging in the limbs at night.
Takes cold easily, especially when uncovering the head and feet.
160. Sensation of great debility and sleepiness during a thunderstorm.
Ebullitions and thirst from drinking small quantities of wine.
Great nervous debility; emaciation; fainting when lying on the side.
The child learns to walk.

Sleep.

Sleeplessness with sleepiness.
165. Sleeplessness from ebullitions of the blood; restlessness and heat in the head.
Frequent starting jerks, and twitches during sleep.
Night walking; gets up while asleep, walks about, and lies down again.

632 SILICEA.

Sleep disturbed by many unpleasant, anxious, fantastic dreams.
Awakens with erections and urging to urinate.
170. Snoring when asleep; nightmare.

Fever.

Pulse small, hard and rapid; frequently irregular and then slow.
The circulation is easily agitated.
Violent chill in the evening in bed, aggravated from uncovering oneself.
Great chilliness from every movement.
175. Continuous internal chilliness, with want of animal heat.
Chill in the evening, with sensation as if cold air were blowing around the waist; not relieved by wrapping up; followed by severe fever and perspiration.
Heat predominates.
Frequently during the day short flushes of heat, principally in the face.
Violent general heat, with violent thirst in the afternoon, evening and all night.
180. Periodically returning heat during the day, without any previous chill and followed by slight perspiration.
Debilitating perspiration at night, or only during the morning hours.
Perspiration from slight exercise; most profuse on the head and face.
Perspiration only on the head.
Night-sweat sour or offensive smelling.
185. The perspiration comes periodically; is worse 11 P. M., 6 A. M., or 3 to 5 P. M.
Intermittent fever, heat predominating.

Skin.

Painless swelling of the glands; they only cause very unpleasant itching.
Suppuration of the glands.
Lymphatic swellings, with suppuration.
190. Bones swollen, inflamed.
Caries.
Skin painful and sensitive.
Itching over the whole body.
Rose-colored blotches.
195. Suppurations; ulcers with good-and bad pus, especially in membranous parts.
The skin heals badly; a small injury suppurates much.

Ulcers of all kinds; also after the abuse of Mercury.
Ulcers smell very offensive.
Ulcers with proud flesh and putrid acrid ichor.
200. Ulcers with stinging, burning, pressing, itching, and smarting.
Painful, hard, high, and spongy edgers of the ulcers.
Panaritium; blood-boils; carbuncles; warts.
Cancerous ulcers; fistulous ulcers.

Conditions.

Aggravation; in the night; in the open air; from cold, upon single parts getting cold; from getting wet; after eating; from uncovering the head or feet; when lying on the painful side; from drinking wine; from external pressure; during sleep; during the new (and full) moon, and from change in the weather.
205. *Amelioration;* from wrapping the head up; in the room; from warmth; from wrapping oneself up warmly.
Especially suitable for scrofulous children, who have also worm diseases, and for children during dentition.
It is an antidote to Mercury when it has produced bad effects in large doses, but it does not follow well after Mercury, nor does Mercury follow well after Silicea.
Fluoric acid follows well after Silicea, and antidotes the bad results from too frequent repetition of Silicea.

SPIGELIA ANTHELMINTICA.

Mind and Disposition.

Restlessness, with anxiety and great solicitude for the future.
Difficulty of thinking and disinclination to mental exertion.
Weakness of memory.

Head.

Giddiness when looking downwards.
5. Vertigo, with nausea.
Boring headache, from within to without, in the forehead, vertex, or cerebellum.
Pressing headache, principally in the right temple; worse from the least motion, stooping, noise, and from opening the mouth; relieved while at rest and lying high with the head.

Sensation of soreness in the forehead and vertex.
Shaking in the brain; worse when moving the head or when stepping hard.
10. Tearing in the forehead in paroxysms, with fixed eyes.
Headache, beginning in the cerebellum (in the morning), spreading over the left side of the head, causing violent and pulsating pain in the left temple and over the left eye, with stitches in the left eye; returning periodically.
Stitches in the left side of the head and out of the left eye.
Painfulness of the cerebellum, with stiffness of the neck.
The headaches are aggravated from the least motion and exertion, from stooping, from the least noise, and are relieved when lying high with the head and from washing the head with cold water.
15. Periodical headaches
Tension of the scalp.
Sensitiveness of the scalp to the touch

Eyes.

Painfulness of the eyes, deep in the sockets, especially when moving them.
Sensation as if the eyes were too large.
20. Pressure in the balls of the eyes, especially when turning them.
Stitches in the eyes.
Dry heat and burning in the eyes; is compelled to close them.
Redness of the white of the eye; the vessels strongly injected.
Inflammation of the cornea.
25. The eyelids hang down, are hard and immovable.
Lachrymation; tears acrid.
Inflammation and ulceration of the eyelids.
Weakness of the eyes; in whatever direction they are turned they remain.
Great inclination to wink with the eyes.
30. Far-sightedness.

Ears.

Otalgia, with pressing pain, as from a plug.
The ears feel as if they were stuffed up. Periodical deafness.

Nose.

Tickling and itching in the nose.
Herpetic, sore, painful eruption on the nose.

SPIGELIA ANTHELMINTICA. 635

35. Secretion of large quantities of mucus through the posterior nares, the nose being dry.

Face.

Pale, bloated and distorted face, especially when awaking from sleep in the morning.
Yellow rings around the eyes.
Redness of the face; perspiration on the face.
Periodical faceache; pains burning and tensive, especially in the cheek-bones, above the eyebrows, in the eyeball, in the left side.

Mouth and Throat.

40. Toothache immediately after eating, or at night, driving one out of bed.
Twitching or pulsating toothache in decayed teeth; aggravated by cold water and from cold air.
Putrid, fetid breath.
Stinging dryness in the mouth on waking in the morning.
White or yellow mucus in the mouth or throat.
45. Blisters on the tongue and in the throat, burning.
Cracked tongue.

Stomach and Abdomen.

Loss of appetite, with violent thirst.
Ravenous hunger, with nausea and thirst.
Sensitiveness of the pit of the stomach to the touch.
50. Pressure in the stomach, as from a hard lump.
Nausea in the morning, fasting, as if something were rising in the throat from the stomach.
Pressing in the region of the navel, as from a hard lump.
Stitches in the abdomen.
Colic (cutting) pain in the abdomen (from worms).
55. Emission of fetid flatus.

Stool and Anus.

Frequent inefficient urging to stool.
Discharge of large lumps of mucus without feces.
Discharge of feces with worms.
Itching and tickling at the anus and in the rectum.
60. Lumbrici, ascarides.

Urinary Organs.

Frequent micturition, with profuse discharge.
Urine with whitish sediment.
Involuntary dripping of urine, with burning in the orifice of the urethra.

Sexual Organs.

Erections and voluptuous fancies, but without sexual desire.
65. Tingling around the corona glandis.
Swelling of one-half of the corona.

Respiratory Organs.

Catarrh with hoarseness; continuous coryza; dry heat without thirst; protruded eyes; violent headache and weeping.
Nightly catarrh with cough (Influenza).
Shortness of breath, especially when talking, with redness of the cheeks and lips.
70. Dyspnœa when moving in bed; can only lie on the right side, or lying very high with the head.
Dyspnœa and suffocating attacks on moving and raising the arms up; violent cough, with dyspnœa.
Constriction in the chest, with anxiety and difficulty of breathing.
Stitches in the chest worse from the least movement, or when breathing.
Sensation of tearing in the chest.
75. Trembling sensation in the chest; aggravated from the least movement.
Stitches in the diaphragm, with dyspnœa.
Violent (visible and audible) palpitation of the heart; aggravated when bending the chest forward.
Stitches in the heart. Organic diseases of the heart. (Rubbing, bellows sounds.)

Back.

Stitches in the back; also when breathing.

Extremities.

80. *Upper.* Stitches in the joints of the arms and hands.
Hard, burning-itching nodosities in the hands.
Lower. Stitches in the joints of the legs and feet and in the thigh.
Wart-like excrescences on the toes.

Generalities.

Stinging pain in the limbs and principally in the joints.
85. Heaviness and soreness in the body when rising from a seat.
Painful sensitiveness of the body to the touch with chilliness on the parts touched, or with tingling running through the whole body.

Sleep.

Great sleepiness during the day, even in the morning, with late going to sleep at night.
Restless, unrefreshing sleep at night and sleepiness in the morning.

Fever.

Pulse irregular, generally strong but slow.
90. Trembling pulse.
Chill, frequently returning at the same hour in the morning.
Chill alternating with heat or perspiration.
Chilliness on some part of the body, on others heat.
Chilliness from the least movement.
95. The chill extends from the chest.
Heat especially in the back.
Flushes of heat at night, with thirst for beer.
Heat in the face and on the hands, with chill in the back.
At night putrid perspiration with heat at the same time.
100. Clammy perspiration on the hands.
Cold perspiration.

Skin.

Painful glandular swellings.
Pale, wrinkled skin of the body.

Conditions.

Aggravation: after washing; after coition; on bending down; while inhaling; from the least movement; from noise; on rising from a seat; from touching the parts; when walking in the open air.

SPONGIA TOSTA.

Attacks of anxiety, with pain in the region of the heart.
Excessive mirth with irresistible desire to sing.

Head.

Vertigo; at night when waking, with nausea.
Congestion of blood to the head, with pressing, beating, and pulsation in the forehead, with redness of the face, anxious look, restless sleep, relieved in a horizontal position.

5. Pressing headache in the (right) frontal eminence, from within to without, worse when sitting, when entering a warm room, after walking in the open air, when looking intensely at any thing; better when lying on the back in a horizontal position.
Violent itching on the scalp.
Sensation as if the hair were standing on an end (on the vertex).

Eyes.

Pressing and stinging in the eyes.
On looking intensely on one spot lachrymation and headache.
10. Redness of the eyes with lachrymation and burning.
Pressing heaviness of the eyelids.
Double vision.

Ears.

Suppuration of the external ear.
Hardness of hearing.

Nose.

15. Bleeding of the nose, especially when blowing it (at dinner)
Eruptions on the tip of the nose.

Face.

Pale face with sunken eyes.
Redness of the face with anxious expression of the countenance; heat on one side of the face, renewed when thinking of it.
Swelling of the cheeks.
20. Itching and stinging on the cheeks.
Eruptions on the lips.
Tension in the articulation of the (left) jaw (when walking in the open air).
Swelling of the submaxillary glands with tension.

Mouth and Throat.

Mouth and tongue full of vesicles, with burning and stinging pains, on that account cannot eat any solid food.
25. Weak voice.
Salivation.
Burning and stinging in the throat.
Tongue brown, dry.
The teeth feel dull and loose when masticating.
30. Itching and stinging in the teeth.

Stomach and Abdomen.

Bitter taste, only in the throat.
Ravenous hunger; unquenchable thirst.
Nausea with acidity in the mouth.
Vomiting after drinking milk.
35. The pressure of tight clothes around the stomach is unbearable.
Stitches in the region of the stomach from the least pressure.
Swelling and inflammation of the (left) inguinal gland.
Rumbling in the abdomen, especially in the evening and in the morning.
Sensation as if the stomach were relaxed and not closed.

Stool and Anus.

40. Stool hard, insufficient.
During stool tenesmus.
Itching, biting, and soreness at the anus, discharge of ascarides.

Urinary Organs.

Incontinence of urine.
Frequent urging to urinate, with small discharges.
45. Urine frothy; sediment thick, grayish white or yellow.

Sexual Organs.

Men. Hard swelling of the testicles and spermatic cord, with pressure.
Women. Menstruation too early and too profuse.
Before the menstruation, pain in the back; later, palpitation of the heart.

Respiratory Organs.

Difficult respiration as from a plug in the larynx.
50. Dyspnœa relieved by bending the body forward.
Wheezing, anxious breathing (inhalation), with violent laboring of the abdominal muscles.
Constrictive spasmodic pain through the chest and larynx.
Burning in the chest; soreness in the chest.
Congestions in the chest from the least movement or exertion, with dyspnœa, nausea, and faintish weakness.
55. Stinging and pressing pain in the præcordial region.
Sensitiveness of the larynx to the touch and when turning the neck.
Dry, hollow, barking cough day and night.
Dry cough from burning-tickling in the larynx.

Cough day and night with burning in the chest, relieved by eating and drinking.
60. Hoarseness with cough and coryza.
Weak voice, giving out when singing or talking.
Pressure in the larynx when singing.
Inflammation of the larynx, trachea, and bronchus.
Croup.
65. Bronchitis.
Hooping-cough, deep, hollow, barking, caused by the sensation of a plug in the larynx, with expectoration only in the morning of small quantities of tough, yellow, hardened mucus, compelling one to swallow it again.
Aggravation of the cough in the evening till midnight; from cold air; from turning the head; from exercise; from lying low with the head; from talking and singing.
Palpitation of the heart (before menstruation), with suffocation, violent gasping respiration, pain in the heart.
Rheumatic affections of the valves of the heart (fibrous deposit upon the valves).
70. Violent palpitation of the heart, beats rapid (each beat was accompanied by a loud blowing, as of a bellows), awakens him after midnight, with a sense of suffocation, loud cough, great alarm, agitation, anxiety, and difficult respiration.

Back and Neck.

Painful stiffness of the muscles of the neck and throat.
Large goitre, with stinging, pressing and tingling pain.

Extremities.

Heaviness and trembling of the forearms and hands.
Swelling of the hands and stiffness of the fingers.
75. Redness and swelling of the joints of the fingers, with tension on bending them.
Numbness of the tips of the fingers.
Large vesicles on the forearm.
Lower. Stiffness of the legs.
The thighs are spasmodically drawn forward or backward.

Generalities.

80. Stiffness in the extremities.
Sensation of numbness in the lower part of the body.
The whole body feels heavy.

Sleep.

Sleeplessness, and when going to sleep delirium.

Awakens towards morning from a jerk upwards from the larynx, as if she would suffocate, must sit up, and raises sour, salty mucus.

Fever.

85. Pulse rapid, full and hard.

Chill with shaking, even near a warm stove, principally over the back.

Violent heat, soon after the chill, with dry, burning heat all over the body with the exception of the thighs; they remain numb and chilly.

Attacks of flushes of heat.

Anxious heat, with red face and weeping, inconsolable mood.

90. Cool perspiration on the face in the evening.

Morning sweat over the whole body.

Skin.

Swelling and induration of the glands.
Red, itching blotches on the skin.
Herpes.

Conditions.

95. *Aggravation;* when ascending; from smoking tobacco; in the room.

Amelioration; on descending.

All the symptoms, with the exception of those of the respiratory organs, are relieved when at rest and while lying in a horizontal position.

STANNUM.

Mind and Disposition.

Great anxiety and restlessness.
Irritable sadness, with aversion to men, and disinclination to talk; hopelessness.

Head.

Vertigo, it seems as if all the objects were too far distant.
Painful jerks through the (left) temple, forehead and cerebellum, leaving a dull pressure, worse during rest, better from motion.

41

5. Burning in the forehead with nausea, better in the open air.
Pulsation in the temples.

Eyes.

Dull, sunken eyes without lustre.
Nightly agglutination of the eyes.
Burning stitches in the eyelids.   Styes.
10. Fistula lachrymalis.

Ears.

Ulceration of the ring-hole in the lobule.
Screaming in the ears when blowing the nose.

Nose.

Dry coryza on one side, with soreness, swelling, and redness of the nostril.
The nose is stuffed up, high up.

Face.

15. Pale, sunken face, with deep, sunken eyes.
Drawing pain in the face, in the malar bone and orbits.

Mouth and Throat.

Fetid smell from the mouth.
Sensation of stinging dryness in the throat.
Hawking of mucus with soreness of the throat.
20. After hawking mucus the voice for singing is higher.
Difficult and weak voice from debility.

Stomach and Abdomen.

Increased appetite, he cannot eat sufficiently to satisfy his hunger.
All the food tastes bitter.
After eating, nausea followed by bitter vomiting.
25. Violent retching, followed by vomiting of undigested food.
Vomiting of blood.
Heavy pressure in the stomach, with soreness of it to the touch.
Colic with bitter eructations, sensation of hunger in the stomach, and diarrhœa.
Spasmodic colic above and below the navel.
30. Hysterical spasms in the abdomen.
Sensitiveness of the abdomen to the touch.
Sensation of emptiness in the abdomen.

Stool and Anus.

Constipation; stool hard, dry, knotty, or insufficient and green.
Diarrhœa consisting of mucus.

Urinary Organs.

35. Scanty secretion of urine.
 The urging to urinate is wanting, as if there were no sensation in the bladder; only a sensation of fulness indicates the necessity to urinate.

Sexual Organs.

Men. Increased sexual desire; violent voluptuous irritation to discharge the semen.
Women. Menstruation more profuse.
 Leucorrhœa, of transparent mucus or yellow with great debility.

Respiratory Organs.

40. Hoarseness and roughness of the larynx.
 Accumulation of great quantities of mucus in the trachea, easily thrown up by coughing. Bronchitis.
 Great dyspnœa with anxiety in the evening, compelling one to loosen the clothing.
 Oppressed breathing and want of breath from every movement, also when lying down; or in the evening.
 Drawing a long breath causes a pleasant sensation of lightness, for a short time.
45. Stitches in the left side of the chest when breathing or when lying on that side.
 Sensation of emptiness and weakness in the chest.
 Sensation of great soreness in the chest.
 Itching-tickling in the chest.
 Tension in the chest. (Hydrothorax.)
50. Dry cough in the evening in bed, till midnight.
 Cough during the day, with copious, greenish, salty expectoration; in the morning the expectoration is most profuse.
 Cough with expectoration of mucus, tasting putrid, sweet, or salty.
 After expectoration great soreness (or stitches) in the chest.
 Cough caused from talking, singing, or laughing, from lying on the (right) side, from drinking any thing warm.
55. Phthisis pituitosa.

Extremities.

The pains in the limbs increase gradually and decrease in the same manner.
Upper. Swelling of the hands and feet in the evening.
Weakness and trembling of the hands.
Paralytic heaviness in the arms.

60. Burning in the hands.   Chilblains on the hands.
Lower.   Paralytic heaviness and weakness in the legs.
Stiffness and tension in the bends of the knee.
Swelling of the ankles in the evening.
Burning of the feet.

Generalities.

65. Pain as if paralyzed in the extremities.
Paralysis of the arms and legs.
Emaciation; weakness; trembling, which is more felt when slowly exercising, or when talking.
Hysterical spasms, with pain in the abdomen and in the diaphragm.
Epileptic attacks; in the evening, in children during dentition.

Sleep.

70. Sleepiness during the day; goes to sleep late at night.
Nightly restlessness, with lamentations, weeping, and timid supplications while asleep.

Fever.

Pulse small and quick.
Chill in the evening, especially over the back, preceded by heat with perspiration.
Chill every forenoon, (10 A. M.)
75. Chill only on the head.
Slight chilliness with violent chattering of the teeth.
During the morning chill, numbness in the tips of the fingers.
Heat in the afternoon (4 to 5 P. M.) every afternoon, with perspiration at the same time.
Burning heat in the limbs, mostly in the hands, every evening.
80. Anxious sensation of heat from the least movement.
Predominating sensation of internal heat.
Very debilitating night-sweats, in the morning, principally on the neck.
Debilitating perspiration from the least exertion.
The perspiration smells mouldy.

Skin.

85. Chilblains.   Painful hang-nails.

Conditions.

The symptoms, with exception of the debility, are better while walking, and cease entirely, but return at once during rest.

The (pressing, drawing) pains increase and decrease slowly and very gradually.
Aggravation when lying on the (painless) side; after moving; from talking.
Amelioration when lying on the back; from loosening the garments.

STAPHYSAGRIA.

Mind and Disposition.

Anger and indignation, with pushing or throwing away of what one holds in his hand.
Justifiable ill-humor over what has happened or has been done by oneself; weeping and dejected over the supposed ill consequences of it.
Continuous grief and anxiety about the future.
Hypochondria and Hysteria after unmerited insults (or sexual excesses), with complaints of flatulence.
5. Weakness of memory.
Hypochondriacal indifference (after onanism).

Head.

Dull feeling of the head, with inability to perform any mental labor.
Pressing in the forehead, as from a very heavy lump which will not be shaken off; worse in the morning, from motion and from stooping; better when at rest, and when leaning the head against something.
Stupefying, pressing headache, as if the brain were compressed.
10. Sensation as if the head would burst, especially in the forehead and when stooping.
Humid, scalding-itching, fetid eruption on the back part of the head, the sides of the head, and behind the ears; when scratching, the itching changes the place, but makes it more humid.
Painful sensitiveness of the scalp; the skin peels off, with itching and biting; worse in the evening and from getting warm.

The hair falls off, mostly on the back part of the head and around the ears, with humid, fetid eruption, or dandruff on the scalp.

Pressing-stinging and tearing pains in the bones and in the periosteum on the cranium; swelling up and suppuration of the bones (caries), with putrid smelling perspiration day and night; worse from motion and contact.

15. Burning-stinging on the external head, mostly on the left temple; worse from the heat of the bed, when lying on it, and at 3 P. M.

Eyes.

Dryness of the eyeballs and lids.
Inflammation of the edges of the eyelids, with agglutination at night.
Styes. Nodosities in the eyelids.
Inflammation of the eyes, with pimples around them.

Ears.

20. Hardness of hearing with swelling of the tonsils, especially after the abuse of Mercury.

Nose.

Ulceration of the nostrils with scabs deep in the nose.
Violent coryza, one nostril is stuffed up, with much sneezing and lachrymation.

Face.

Countenance sunken, nose peaked, eyes sunken and blue margins around them.
Inflammation of the bones of the face.
25. Brown and blue color of face when getting angry.
Scurfy lips with burning pains.
Easy dislocation of the articulation of the jaw.
Painfulness of the submaxillary glands, with (or without) swelling.

Mouth and Throat.

Teeth become black and exfoliate.
30. The teeth are very sensitive to the touch and to cold drinks, but not when biting on them.
White, painful swelling and ulceration of the gums.
Excrescences and nodosities on the gums.
Painful excrescence on the inside of the cheek.
Stomacace: mouth and tongue full of blisters.
35. Throat dry and rough, with soreness when talking and swallowing.

Feeble voice from weakness of the vocal organs, after anger.
Nasal voice from stoppage of the posterior nares.
While talking she swallows continually.
Swelling of the tonsils, also after the misuse of Mercury.

Stomach and Abdomen.
40. Ravenous hunger even when the stomach is full.
Longing only for thin, fluid food (soup).
Great desire for brandy and tobacco.
All the food tastes bitter.
Bitter eructations after sour food.
45. Water-brash.
Spasmodic cutting in the abdomen after eating and drinking.
Sensation of weakness in the abdomen as if it should vanish.
Swollen abdomen (in children).
Colic with urging to urinate.
50. Painful swelling of the inguinal glands.
Flatulence smelling like rotten eggs.

Stool and Anus.
Constipation with urging to go to stool.
Retarded but soft feces.
Evacuations with much flatulence.
55. Dysenteric stools; with pressing and cutting in the abdomen before, during, and after stool.

Urinary Organs.
Frequent urging to urinate, with scanty discharge in a thin stream, or discharge of dark urine by drops.
Profuse discharge of watery, pale urine with much urging.
During and after micturition burning in the urethra, after micturition urging, as if the bladder were not emptied.

Sexual Organs.
Men. On and behind the corona glandis soft, humid excrescences. (Sycosis.)
60. Inflammation of the testicles (and ovaries) with burning, stinging, and pressing-drawing.
Sexual instinct excited.
Women. Painful sensitiveness of the sexual organs, especially when sitting.

Respiratory Organs.
Sensation of constriction and pressure in the throat-pit after anger, aggravated when swallowing.
Rawness in the larynx from talking.
65. Soreness and rawness in the chest, especially when coughing.

Dyspnœa with constriction and restlessness in the chest.
Hoarseness with much tenacious mucus in the larynx and chest.
Violent spasmodic cough with expectoration of yellow, tough, purulent mucus at night.
Palpitation of the heart from the least exertion, from mental exertion, from hearing music, and after the siesta.

Back and Neck.

70. Pain in the small of the back as after overlifting, worse at rest at night and in the morning, and when rising from a seat.
Violent stitches upwards in the back.
Suppurating swelling in the psoas muscle.
Painful swelling of the glands of the neck and under the arms.

Extremities.

Upper. Herpes with scabs on the elbows. Herpes on the hands.
75. Numbness in the tips of the fingers.
Arthritic nodosities on the fingers.
Lower. Pulsating pain in the hip-joint as from beginning suppuration.
Painful weakness of the legs, especially the knees.
Stitches in the knees and knee-joints.

Generalities.

80. Paralysis on one side from anger.
Twitches at night.
Stiffness and sensation of fatigue in all the joints in the morning.
The muscles are painful to the touch, and the joints on motion.
Bad effects from the abuse of Mercury.

Sleep.

85. Violent yawning and stretching, bringing the tears to the eyes.
Goes to sleep late, from crowding of ideas or because the herpes and ulcers burn and itch, or the calves pain violently.

Fever.

Pulse very fast but small and trembling.
Chilliness and coldness predominate.
Violent chill in the evening with heat in the face.
90. Chilliness 3 P. M.; better when exercising in the open air.
Chill ascending from the back over the head.
Chill running down the back.

External heat with thirst after midnight, followed by chill towards morning.
Burning heat at night, especially on the hands and feet, with desire to uncover oneself.
95. Profuse perspiration and disposed to perspire.
Night-sweats smelling like rotten eggs.
Cold perspiration on the forehead and on the feet.
Tertian fever with symptoms of scurvy, such as putrid taste in the mouth, bleeding gums, want of appetite, constipation.
The intermittent fever consists almost solely of a chilliness.
100. Before and after the paroxysms of intermittent fever, ravenous hunger.

Skin.

Painful swelling of the glands.
Swelling and suppuration of the bones and of the periosteum.
Itching herpes, burning after scratching.
Dry herpes with scabs on the joints.
105. Chronic herpes with nightly twitching.
The skin is hard to heal.
Mechanical injuries from sharp-cutting instruments.
Arthritic nodosities on the joints.

Conditions.

Aggravation from anger, grief, sorrow, mortification caused by offences; from loss of fluids; from masturbation; from sexual excesses; from touching the affected parts; from tobacco; from the abuse of Mercury.
110. Amelioration after breakfast.

STRAMONIUM.

Mind and Disposition.

Mental derangement, especially in drunkards.
Loquacious delirium and mania.
Attacks of rage with beating and striking persons.
Desire for company and light.

5. Very changeable disposition; alternate; anticipations of death and rage; laughable gestures and melancholy deportment; affected haughtiness and inconsolableness; loud laughing and groaning.
Mania-à-potu with clonic spasms, with consciousness and desire for light and company.
Insensibility to mental impressions.

Head.

Staggering vertigo with obscurations of vision, headache and red face, colicky pain and diarrhœa.
Stupefaction with vanishing of vision and hearing, and convulsive movements of the head.
10. Fainting with paleness of the face, dryness in the throat, and subsequent red face.
Congestion of blood to the head, with pulsation in the vertex, loss of sight and hearing, bloated turgid face, total loss of consciousness, and painlessness.
Inflammation of the brain, with heat and pulsation of the vertex, attacks of fainting, loss of sight and hearing, convulsive movements of the head, frequently raising the head up or bending it backward, better while lying still.
Hydrocephalus with convulsive motions of the head, sensation of lightness of the head, and frequently raising the head up.
Painful dark-red swelling of the highly-congested head and turgid face, with convulsive movements, delirium, and desire for light and company.

Eyes.

15. Red, inflamed, swollen eyes.
Staring, glistening eyes. Photomania.
Contortion of the eyes and eyelids.
Pupils dilated, insensible.
Blindness (at night), (periodical).
20. The objects appear blue.
Double vision, the objects appear oblique.

Ears.

Wind is rushing out of the ears.
Hardness of hearing; deafness.

Face.

Red, swollen, turgid face. Circumscribed redness of the face.
25. Stupid distorted countenance.
Anxiety and fear is expressed in the countenance.

STRAMONIUM. 651

Deep furrows and wrinkles in the face.
Distortion of the mouth.
A yellow stripe in the red part of the lip. Trembling of the lips.

Mouth and Throat.

30. Grinding of the teeth.
Dryness of the mouth; dry, sticky lips.
Violent thirst (for large quantities, drinking with avidity).
Fear of water and aversion to all fluids.
Bloody froth before the mouth.
35. Difficult deglutition from dryness and spasmodic constriction of the throat.
Swelling and paralysis of the tongue.
Stuttering with distortion of the face. Speechlessness.

Stomach and Abdomen.

The food tastes like sand or straw, or they have no taste at all.
Violent (spasmodic) hiccough.
40. Bitter taste in the mouth.
Vomiting of sour mucus or green bile.
Anxiety in the pit of the stomach with dyspnœa.
Abdomen hard, tympanitic.
Painfulness of the abdomen when moving and to the touch.
45. Pain in the abdomen as if the navel were pulled out.
Hysterical abdominal spasms.

Stool and Anus.

Constipation; unsuccessful urging to go to stool.
Putrid smelling diarrhœic stools.
Discharge of clotted blood through the anus.

Urinary Organs.

50. Suppressed secretion of urine (in typhus). Involuntary secretion of urine.
The urine is only discharged in drops with constant painful urging.

Sexual Organs.

Menstrual flow too profuse of black blood in large clots.
Metrorrhagia. Eclampsia.
During menstruation rank stench of the body.
55. Too profuse secretion of milk in nursing-women.

Respiratory Organs.

Difficult sighing breathing.
Spasms in the pectoral muscles.

Constriction of the chest with dyspnœa. Constrictions of the larynx.
Fine shrieking voice.
60. Periodically returning attacks of painless, barking, spasmodic cough, in fine shrieking tone, from constriction of the larynx and chest, without expectoration.

Back.

The back is drawn backwards.

Extremities.

Upper. Convulsive movement of the arms over the head.
Trembling of the hands.
The hands are closed to a fist.
65. The fingers go to sleep.
Lower. Twitching in the limbs.
Trembling of the feet.
The legs give way when he walks; he falls over his own legs.

Generalities.

Trembling of limbs (also in drunkards).
70. Tingling in the limbs; sensation as if the limbs were separated from the body.
Spasms and convulsions, caused whenever he is touched, or from light and glittering objects.
Cataleptic stiffness and immovability of the body.
The body is bent backwards with distorted countenance.
Convulsions (in children) with profuse perspiration, followed by sleep.
75. St. Vitus' dance; eclampsia. Epileptic convulsions with consciousness.
The movement of the muscles subject to the will is easier and increased.
Painlessness with most all ailments.
Suppression of all secretions and excretions.

Sleep.

Deep stupefied sleep with snoring.
80. He lies on his back with open staring eyes.
Sleep interrupted by screams.
Frightful visions during sleep.

Fever.

Pulse very irregular, generally full, hard and quick, or small and rapid, at times slow and scarcely perceptible, occasionally intermitting and trembling.

Chill and general coldness, with redness of the face and twitches.
85. General coldness in the afternoon after previous heat of the head and face, followed by general heat.
During the chill great sensitiveness to being uncovered.
Chill running down the back.
Heat over the whole body, with red face and perspiration.
Hot red face with cold hands and feet.
90. Anxious heat with vomiting.
Profuse perspiration already during the heat with violent thirst.
Greasy, oily, putrid-smelling perspiration.
Cold perspiration over the whole body.
Intermittent fever. Chill over the whole body without thirst, followed by heat with anguish; sleep during the hot stage, and violent thirst after waking up, which causes a stinging in the throat, until he drinks something.

Skin.

95. Suppressed eruptions and the consequences from it.

Conditions.

Aggravation after sleep (in the morning); during perspiration; from being touched; from looking at glistening objects; in the dark; when alone.
Amelioration from bright light.

STRONTIANA CARBONICA.

Mind and Disposition.

Ill-humor with inclination to anger and impetuosity.
Great forgetfulness.

Head.

Tension from the vertex to the upper jaw as if the head were expanded from within, and as if the scalp were too tight, worse in the evening when lying low with the head, slowly increasing and decreasing, better from heat.
Stitches in the head.

5. Burning in the forehead.
Chilliness over the scalp and upper part of the back, worse in the evening, at night, and in the cold air.
Tension on the head (externally and internally), worse in the evening, and from cold, better from warmth, especially in the heat of the sun.
Sensation of heat of the head and face, with red face, anxiety, and sleepiness.

Eyes.
Burning in the eyes.
10. Pressing pain on the upper surface of the eyes.
Pressing in the eyes after rubbing them, which causes one to see red and blue margins.
Green spots before the eyes in the dark.
Luminous vibrations before the eyes.

Nose.
Dark, bloody scabs are blown from the nose.

Face.
15. Face red, burning hot.
Tearing pain in the malar bone, cheeks, and lower jaw.
Violent boring pain in the (right) malar bone.

Mouth and Throat.
Sensation in the teeth as if screwed together.
Violent tearing in the teeth after previously increased saliva in the mouth.
20. Sensation of numbness in the mouth (early on waking).
Heat emanating from the mouth and nose, with thirst.
The fauces are inflamed and painful (stinging) during deglutition.

Stomach and Abdomen.
Hunger soon after dinner.
Violent thirst, especially for beer.
25. Taste in the mouth like earth.
Nausea, with burning heat in the face.
Pressure in the stomach, relieved by eating.
Colic with diarrhœa and chilliness.

Stool and Anus.
Stool retarded, compact and in large lumps; is expelled with great effort and violent pain in the anus.
30. After stool, contractive sensation in the rectum; burning at the anus.
Diarrhœa of yellow water.

Urinary Organs.
Urine pale, strongly smelling of ammonium.

Sexual Organs.
Women. Menstruation retarded, the discharge being serous at first, later clots of blood are passed.
Menses too early and of too short a duration.

Respiratory Organs.
35. Violent dry cough from irritation in the larynx at night.
Dyspnœa, with hot, red face while walking.

Back.
Sensations as if bruised in the back and sacrum, worse from stooping and when touched.

Sleep.
When going to sleep twitching and starting.

Generalities.
Rheumatic pains, especially in the joints, worse in the evening and at night in bed.
40. Great emaciation.
Immovability of the limbs (on one, the right, side of the body) like paralysis, in the evening.
Most of the symptoms can hardly be determined as to locality, but seem to be in the marrow of the bones.
One side of the body is generally only affected (right side).

Fever.
Pulse full and hard, with violent pulsation in the arteries.
45. Chill in the forenoon, descending from the sacrum to the posterior part of the thighs.
Chilliness from the head over the shoulder-blades.
Dry heat at night with thirst.
Heat which seems to stream from the mouth and nostrils.
Perspiration during the morning hours.
50. Perspiration at night, mostly on the affected parts, with increased pain when uncovering them.

Skin.
Tension of the skin on various parts in the evening in bed.
Itching which grows worse from scratching.

Conditions.
The rheumatic pains are worse in the evening and at night.
Trembling sensation in the body, and debility worse in the evening (and morning).

55. The pains and ailments increase gradually and decrease in the same manner.
When the pains cease, the itching begins, and vice versa.
Aggravation; in the evening and at night; from cold; from denudation; from water and washing.
Amelioration; in the open air, especially in the heat of the sun; from warmth in general.

SULPHUR.

Mind and Disposition.

Peevishness; irritability; restless, quick temperament.
Melancholy, with great inclination to philosophical and religious speculations; with anxiety about the salvation of one's soul, and great indifference to the welfare of others.
Hypochondriac mood (through the day, in the evening he is inclined to be merry).
Dulness: difficulty of thinking; misplaces, or cannot find the proper words when he speaks.
5. Fantastic illusions.

Head.

Vertigo when sitting; with bleeding of the nose; when stooping; when rising from the bed; in the morning; with nausea; with inclination to fall to the left side; with vanishing of sight.
Congestion of blood to the head with heat in it; the blood rising up to the head from the chest; better in the room.
Heaviness and fulness in the forehead, worse when raising the head and after sleeping and talking, better when sitting or when lying high with the head.
Tearing or stitches in the forehead or temples, from within to without, worse from eating or stooping, better when pressing the head together, or when moving about.
10. Sensation of emptiness in the back part of the head, worse in the open air and when talking, better in the room.
Pulsation in the head with heat in the brain, pulsation of the carotid arteries and of the heart, worse on waking in the morning, when moving about, on stooping, when talking, in the open air; better when at rest and in the warm room.

Painful tingling on the vertex and in the temples.
Tension in the forehead and in the eyes on exercising the brain; worse when lifting up the eyes, after sleeping; better when sitting and in the room.
He feels every step painful in the head.
15. Headache generally worse in the open air, better in the room.
Sensitiveness of the vertex, pressing pain when touching it, worse from the heat of the bed, in the morning when waking, on scratching it, it bites and burns.
Feeling of coldness about the head.
The roots of the hair are painful, especially when touched.
Dry (seldom humid) offensive, scabby, easily bleeding, burning, and sore paining eruption on the back part of the head and behind the ears, with cracks, better from scratching (Tinea capitis).
20. Contractive pain as from a band around the cranium, with the sensation as if the flesh were loose around it, followed by inflammation and swelling of the bones and caries; worse in wet, cold weather and when at rest; better from motion.
Falling off of the hair, with great dryness of the hair, painfulness of the scalp to the touch and violent itching in the evening when getting warm in bed, with swelling of the glands on the neck (also in lying-in women).
Fontanelles remain open too long,
Exanthema and itching on the forehead.

Eyes.

Dryness of the eyes in the room, lachrymation in the open air.
25. Running of the eyes.
Photophobia with stitches, worse in sultry weather.
Specks or ulcers on the cornea.
Obscuration of sight; blindness; dim-sightedness, cataract.
Like gauze before the eyes.
30. Halo around the candle.
Inflammation of the eyes or of the eyelids.
Stinging in the eyes, especially in the sunshine and from the light of a candle, or burning in the eyes.
Painful inflammation of the eye from a foreign body coming into the eye.
Eyelids burning; twitching (lower), itching.
35. Ulceration of the margins of the eyelids.
Itching of the eyebrows.

Ears.

Stinging in the ear (left).
Wabbling in the ears as if water was in them.
Otorrhœa; discharge of pus from the ear.
40. Humming of the ears.
Hardness of hearing; over-sensitiveness of hearing.
Itching in the external ear.

Nose.

Blood comes from the nose whenever blowing it.
Bleeding of the nose (3 P. M. or with vertigo), afterwards it feels sore when touched.
45. Swelling and inflammation of the nose.
Dry ulcers or scabs in the nose.
Smell before the nose as from an old catarrh.
Freckles and black pores on the nose.
Herpes across the nose, like a saddle.
50. Burning coryza in the open air, obstructions of the nose in the room.
Dryness of the nose.

Face.

Face pale, yellow color of the face.
Circumscribed red spots on the cheeks.
Red blotches on the face.
55. Erysipelas of the face (beginning on the right ear and spreading over the face).
Freckles on the face; red roughness of the face.
Exanthema on the upper lip. Tinea faciei. Crusta lactea.
Sunken eyes with blue margins.
Swelling of the (upper) lips. Yellow spots on the upper lip.
60. Red lips. Lips dry, rough, and cracked. Burning of the lips. Trembling and twitching of the lips.
Cancer of the lips.
Cold perspiration on the face.
Painful eruptions around the chin.
Herpes on the corners of the mouth.

Mouth and Throat.

65. Great sensitiveness of the points of the teeth.
Aching in sound and carious teeth.
The teeth feel as if they were too long.
Tearing toothache on the left side.
Pulsation and boring in the teeth, worse from heat.
70. Teeth feel as if they were loose.

Toothache in the open air, from the least draught of air, at night in bed, from washing with cold water; with congestions to the head, or stitches in the ears.
Swelling of the gums, with heating pain in them.
Bleeding of the gums.
Fistula dentalis.
75. Stomacace. (Blisters and vesicles in the mouth.) Aphthæ.
Ptyalism from the abuse of Mercury or during a fever.
Saliva tastes salt, sour or bitter, or is mixed with blood.
Breath offensive (after meals).
Tongue white, with red tip and red borders, or dry (in the morning), or brown and dry; burns, or red and cracked, or coated white.
80. Long-continued sensation of a lump in the throat.
Sensation as if swallowing a piece of meat during empty deglutition.
Dryness of the throat.
Stitches in the throat on swallowing.
Sensation of contraction in the throat, when swallowing.
85. Burning in the throat, as from sour eructations.
Elongation of the palate; swelling of the palate and tonsils.
Sensation of a hair in the throat.
Angina gangrenosa.

Stomach and Abdomen.

Sour taste in the mouth all day.
90. Bitter taste in the morning; putrid taste in the morning.
No appetite, but constant thirst; or canine hunger.
Disgust for drinking wine; violent thirst for beer and longing for brandy.
The food tastes too salt.
Milk disagrees, causing sour taste and sour eructations.
95. Aversion to meat.
After eating but little he feels full in the stomach.
Water-brash.
The food rises into the throat.
Loud eructations as soon as he presses on the stomach; or empty eructations.
100. Qualmishness; nausea (in the morning).
Vomiting: first of water, later of solid food, or sour; of the ingesta, sour or bitter, with cold perspirations in the face, or of blood.
The region of the stomach becomes very painful when pressing upon it,—even the bed-cover causes pain.

Burning in the stomach.
Spasms in the stomach immediately after a meal.
105. Stitches or pressing pain in the region of the liver.
Stitches in the spleen, worse when taking a deep inspiration and when walking.
Inflammation, swelling, and induration of the liver.
Stitches in the left side of the abdomen when coughing.
Painful sensitiveness of the abdomen, as if all the parts in it were raw and sore.
110. Rolling and rumbling in the abdomen.
Incarcerated flatulence in the left side of the abdomen, with constipation.
Colic; (hæmorrhoidal) after drinking or eating, obliging one to bend double.
Flatus stinking, and frequent discharges of it.
Incarcerated hernia.
115. Dropsy.
Movements in the abdomen as from a fist of a fœtus.

Stool and Anus.

Constipation; frequent unsuccessful desire for stool; stool hard, knotty, insufficient.
Diarrhœa; painless; in the morning compelling one to rise from his bed; watery, of white mucus, smelling sour, undigested, involuntary.
Diarrhœa in children, green, of bloody mucus, with crying and weeping.
120. Dysenteric stools at night, with colic and violent tenesmus.
Colic before every loose evacuation.
Stools with ascarides, lumbrici, or tape-worm.
During stool, discharge of blood; pain in the small of the back; palpitation of the heart; congestion of the head; prolapsus recti, especially during a hard stool; itching, burning, and stinging at the anus and in the rectum.
After stool tenesmus, constriction at the anus.
125. Hæmorrhoids. oozing or bleeding.
Swelling of the anus. Soreness of the anus. Stitching at the anus.

Urinary Organs.

Retention of urine.
Frequent micturition, especially at night.
Discharge of urine only by drops.
130. Involuntary discharge of urine (and stool) at night, (wetting the bed).
Burning in the orifice of the urethra during micturition.

Fetid urine; greasy pellicle on the urine.
Hemorrhage from the urethra.
Stitches in the bladder.
135. Cutting pain in the urethra when urinating.
Redness and inflammation of the orifice of the urethra.
Discharge of (white) mucus from the urethra. (Secondary gonorrhœa.)

Sexual Organs.

Men. Involuntary discharge of semen, with burning in the urethra.
Too quick discharge of semen during coition.
140. Coldness of the penis (prepuce); weak sexual powers; impotence.
Inflammation, swelling, and phymosis of the prepuce, with deep rhagades, burning, and redness.
Deep suppurating ulcer on the glans and prepuce, with puffed edges.
Discharge of prostatic fluid, also after micturition.
Phymosis, with discharge of fetid pus.
145. Stitches in the penis.
The testicles hang down loosely.
Hydrocele.
Offensive perspiration around the genitals.
Soreness and moisture of the scrotum.
150. Soreness between the thighs when walking.
Women. Menstruation too late, of too short duration, too scanty, or suppressed; first menses delaying, or too profuse and too early.
Menstrual blood acrid, corroding the thighs, smelling sour, or else too pale.
Before menstruation, headache; bleeding from the nose; itching on the genitals.
During menstruation, bleeding from the nose; congestion of blood to the head; spasms in the abdomen.
155. Bearing-down in the pelvis; congestion to the uterus.
Sterility, with too early and profuse menstruation.
Leucorrhœa, of yellow mucus, corroding, preceded by pains in the abdomen.

Respiratory Organs.

Hoarseness and roughness in the throat, with much mucus on the chest.
Deep, rough voice—aphonia.

160. Coldness in the throat during an inspiration.
Dry cough day and night, with spasmodic constriction of the chest.
Cough, with expectoration during the day, without expectoration at night.
Short, dry cough, with stitches in the chest, or stitches in the (left) shoulder-blade.
When coughing, pain in the head and in the abdomen.
165. Cough after a meal, or only when walking in the open air.
Spasmodic hooping-cough in successive double attacks, shortly following one another, from tickling in the larynx, as from dust; only with expectoration during the day, of either dark blood or yellow-greenish purulent matter, or of cold, milk-white mucus, generally tasting sour, or putrid, or salty, or like old catarrh.
Congestion of blood to the chest, with sensation of fulness in it.
Heaviness in the chest (when walking).
Stitches through the chest, extending into the left shoulder-blade; worse when lying down on the back, during the least motion, when drawing a deep breath, when lifting up the arms (over the head).
170. Pain in the chest from overlifting or after inflammation of the lungs.
Sensation as if the lungs were touching the back.
Burning in the chest, up to the face.
Sensation of coldness in the chest.
Sensation of weakness in the chest when talking.
175. Dyspnœa; shortness of breath and oppression of breathing on bending the arms backwards.
Asthma at night.
Palpitation of the heart; anxious, and visible (when ascending).
Sensation as if the heart were enlarged.
Swelling of the mammæ.
180. Nodosites in the mammæ.
Nipples cracking, stinging, and burning.

Back.

Cracking in the vertebræ of the neck, especially on bending backwards.
Stiffness in the neck.
Drawing in the back.
185. Pain in the small of the back on rising from a seat.
Gnawing pain in the small of the back.

SULPHUR.

Pain as if sprained, or as if bruised in the left shoulder.
Stitches in the shoulder-blades.
Pain in the small of the back, not permitting one to stand erect.
190. Curvature of the vertebræ.

Extremities.

Upper. Tearing in the joints of the arms, hands and fingers.
Rheumatic pain in the shoulders, especially the left.
Erysipelatous swelling on the fingers, numbness of the fingers.
Offensive perspiration in the arm-pit.
195. Perspiration of the hands; in the palms of the hands.
Trembling of the hands when writing. Cold trembling hands.
Rhagades on the hands, especially between the fingers, on the joints of the fingers, in the palms of the hands.
Hang-nails. Panaritium.
Lower. Heaviness of the legs.
200. Swelling of the knee (white, or shining).
Erysipelas of the legs. Phlegmasia alba dolens.
Stiffness of the knee and ankle-joint.
Cramps; in the legs (calves) at night; in the soles of the feet at every step.
Cold sweat on the feet.
205. Burning of the soles of the feet.
Red, shining swelling of the toes.
Corns paining, pressing and stinging.
Cold feet and hands; cold soles of the feet.
Itching in the toes that had been formerly frozen.
210. Ulcer on the instep.

Sleep.

Great drowsiness and sleepiness in day-time, especially in the afternoon and after sunset.
Goes to sleep late. Long but unrefreshing morning sleep.
Sleep with his eyes half open. Talks loudly while asleep.
Jerks and twitches in the body during asleep.
215. He has to lie on his back.
Anxious dreams. Nightmare. Nightly delirium.

Generalities.

Tearing in the limbs, in outer parts, in the muscles and joints, from above downward.
Arthritic swelling and heat.
Bruised pain in outer parts.

220. Burning pain of external and internal parts.
Cutting pain in the inner parts.
Stinging pain; in outer and inner parts; in the muscles; in the joints; from within outwards.
Biting (pungent) pain.
Inflammatory swelling of the affected parts.
225. Sprained pains in outer parts and in the joints.
Sensation of tension in outer parts and especially the joints.
Sensation of roughness in inner parts.
Sensation of heaviness in inner parts.
Sensation of fulness in inner parts.
230. Sensation of a band (hoop) on and around parts.
Contraction of inner parts.
Trembling and shaking of outer parts.
Weakness of the joints.
Knocking in outer parts.
235. Humming and buzzing in the head; vibration like dull tingling in the body.
Congestion of blood to single parts (eyes, nose, chest, abdomen, arms, legs).
Dropsy of inner parts.
The limbs go to sleep.
Paralysis of the limbs (right side).
240. Great debility and trembling; talking fatigues.
Jerks in the muscles and single twitches in the limbs.
Epilepsy (it comes running from the arms and out of the back like a mouse).
Stooping gait (his head and shoulders are stooped when he walks).
Aversion to washing.

Fever.

245. Pulse full, hard and quick, at times intermitting.
Swollen veins.
Chilliness from want of natural heat.
Chilliness every evening in bed, followed by heat and profuse perspiration.
Chilliness in the forenoon; heat with cold feet in the afternoon.
250. Chilliness externally with internal heat and a red face.
Chilliness, beginning in the toes.
Slight chill, 10 A. M., continues till 3 P. M., followed by heat lasting two hours, mostly in the head and hands, with desire for beer.
Cold nose, hands and feet.

Dry heat, with thirst.
255. Heat at night, with headache, and burning of the hands and feet.
Heat at night without thirst, preceded by chilliness, with thirst.
Dry heat in the afternoon and evening, with dry skin, and much thirst, alternating with chilliness.
Flushes of heat.
Want of perspiration, or great inclination to perspire.
260. Perspiration from the least exertion.
Perspiration in the evening, mostly in the hands.
Perspiration with anxiety, very debilitating, pungent acid smell; very seldom offensive, at times cold.
Perspiration (only on one side of the body), only on the back part of the body; worse at night and in the morning.

Skin.

Swelling of the bones.
265. On the bones sensation of constriction, or as if a band were around them.
Skin cold, pale, dry.
Chapped exanthema.
Itch. Voluptuous itching and tingling, with burning after scratching, or with soreness after scratching.
Itching worse from the heat of the bed.
270. Liver, or scarlet-colored or yellow spots on the body.
Freckles.
Rhagades, after washing.
The nails crumble off.
Soreness in children; soreness in the folds of the skin.
275. Dropsical, burning swelling of external parts.
Herpes, scabby and scurfy.
Ulcers: cancerous; crusty; pricking; pulsating, swollen, tearing, with tension; pus from them offensive.
Warts.

Conditions.

Complaints arising from the abuse of Mercury or China.
280. Aggravation in the evening or after midnight; during the full moon; periodically (headache every seven days); during sleep; on waking; on getting warm in bed; on rising; from exertion of the body; on walking quickly; from talking; while at rest; when standing; from milk after eating; from suppressed perspiration; from wet poultices; from touching the affected parts; when swallowing food; from water and washing.

Amelioration. From drawing up the limbs; during motion; while lying on the right side; by heat; in dry weather; after rising.

Sulphur follows well after Pulsatilla, which also is often the antidote to it when it has been administered in too large doses. It is most suitable for lean persons, especially if they walk stooped; it will often serve to rouse the slumbering vitality if the proper medicines have failed to produce a favorable effect, especially in acute diseases.

SULPHURIC ACID.

Mind and Disposition.

Restlessness and irritability.
Changeable disposition; from seriousness he changes to great hilarity.
Inclination to weep.

Head.

Sensation as if the brain were loose in the forehead, and was falling from one side to the other; worse when walking in the open air; better when sitting quiet in the room.
5. Painful shocks in the forehead and temples, worse in the forenoon and evening.
Headache as if a plug was thrust quickly by increasingly severe blows in the head.
Gradually increasing and suddenly ceasing headache.

Eyes.

Lachrymation when reading.
Tension in the eyelids in the morning; it is difficult to open them.

Ears.

10. Hardness of hearing; it feels as if a leaf were lying before the ear.

Nose.

Bleeding of the nose in the evening.

Face.

Paleness of the face.
The face feels swollen, as if the white of an egg had dried on the face.
The lips peel off.

Mouth and Throat.

15. Dulness of the teeth.
Toothache worse in the evening in bed, aggravated by cold, relieved by heat.
Aphthæ (in children).
Sensation of dryness in the mouth.   Ptyalism.
Roughness in the throat.
20. Tongue dry.
Spitting of blood.

Stomach and Abdomen.

Desire for fresh fruit.
Sour eructations, violent heartburn.
Nausea in the stomach with chilliness.
25. Vomiting, first of water and then of food.
The water causes cold of the stomach, if not mixed with some alcoholic liquor.
Stitches in the liver and spleen.
Pain in the abdomen like labor, extending to the hips and back.
Flatulence in the abdomen, with the sensation as if a hernia should protrude.
30. Violent protrusion of an inguinal hernia.

Stool and Anus.

Ineffectual urging to go to stool.
Stool retarded, compact, hard, knotty, and black.
Stools chopped (in children).
Watery diarrhœa, very offensive.

Urinary Organs.

35. Diminished secretion of brown urine, which becomes turbid on standing, like loam water.
Sediment like blood and a cuticle on the urine.
Pain in the bladder if the call to urinate is postponed.

Sexual Organs.

Women.   Menstruation too early and too profuse.
Impotence, with too early and too profuse menstruation.
40. Leucorrhœa acrid or burning, or like milk.

Respiratory Organs.

Hoarseness, with dryness and roughness in the throat and larynx.
The larynx is painful; the parts feel deprived of elasticity, which causes a difficulty in talking.
Long-continued hæmoptysis.
Cough in the open air, from walking, riding, cold water, and when smelling coffee.
45. Cough from irritation in the chest, with expectoration in the morning of dark blood, or of a thin, yellow, blood-streaked mucus, generally of a sourish taste.
After the cough, eructations.
Stitches; in the chest; about the heart.
Sensation of great weakness in the chest.
Palpitation of the heart, with or without anxiety.

Back.

50. Stiffness in the back on rising in the morning.
Blood-boils on the back.

Extremities.

Upper. Stitches in the shoulder-joints on lifting up the arms.
Tension in the elbow-joint.
Stitches in the joints of the fingers.
55. Chilblains on the hands.
Lower. Painful weakness of the knees.
Red itching spots on the tibia.
Cold feet. Stitches in the corns.

Sleep.

Goes to sleep late and wakens early.
60. During sleep twitches, especially of the fingers.

Generalities.

Stitches in the joints. Tearing in the whole body, also in the face.
Slowly increasing but suddenly ceasing pain, as if a blunt instrument were pressed against the part.
Sensation of soreness, as if bruised over the whole body.
The left side is principally affected.
65. Weakness of the whole body, with the sensation of trembling.

Fever.

Pulse small, feeble, and accelerated.
Chilliness during the day, mostly in the room, better when exercising in the open air.

Frequent chills running down the body.
Heat in the evening and after lying down in bed.
70. In the evening frequent flushes of heat, especially when exercising.
Flushes of heat with perspiration (in climacteric years).
Much perspiration, principally on the upper part of the body.
Profuse morning sweat.
Perspiration from the least exercise, which continues for a long time after sitting down.
75. Cold perspiration as soon as one eats warm food.

Skin.

Bad effects from mechanical injuries, as from bruises, falling, knocking, pressure of blunt instruments, and contusions (especially in old women).
Blue spots as from suggillation.
Red, itching blotches on the skin.
Soreness of the skin; also with gangrenous ulceration; becomes easily chafed when walking or riding.
80. Painful sensitiveness of the glands.
Eating pain in the ulcers.
Most of the complaints are worse in the forenoon and evening.
Aggravation; in the open air; from smelling coffee.

SYMPHYTUM OFFICINALE.

Mechanical injuries, bad effects from blows, bruises, thrusts on the eye. Pain from fractured bones.

TABACUM.

Mind and Disposition.

Cheerful, merry, loquacious.
Great restlessness, anguish, melancholy.

Head.

Vertigo, with qualmishness of the stomach.

Face.

Death-like paleness of the face, with sick stomach.
5. Heat and redness of the left cheek (towards evening).
The right cheek glowing, the other pale.
Violent tearing in the (right) facial bones and teeth.

Stomach and Abdomen.

Qualmishness, nausea, vomiting, as soon as he begins to move.
Feeling of coldness in the stomach, with nausea.
10. Painful retraction of the navel; contraction of the abdominal muscles.
Pressure, heaviness, or stitches in the liver.

Stool and Anus.

Shifting of flatulence, formed by sudden, papescent, yellow-green or greenish, slimy stools, with tenesmus.

Respiratory Organs.

Cough and hiccough at the same time; or hiccough after every paroxysm of hooping-cough.

Extremities.

Upper. Coldness and trembling of the limbs.
15. Cramps in the hands and arms.
Lower. Cramps from the toes to the knee.

Fever.

Pulse full, hard, and rapid, or small, imperceptible, intermittent, slow.
Icy coldness of the legs from the knees to the toes.
Icy coldness of the legs with heat to the body.
20. Viscid cold sweat, with intermitting pulse.
Cold sweat, in the hands, on the forehead and face.

TANACETUM VULGARE.

Great mobility; extraordinary motion, and strange gesticulations. St. Vitus's dance.

TARAXACUM.

Mind and Disposition.
Irresoluteness. Inclined to talk, to laugh, and to be merry.

Head.
Sensation as if the brain were expanded or constricted.
The headache is felt only when standing (or walking).

Eyes.
Aversion to light; stinging-burning in the eyes.

Face.
5. Red, hot face. Pimples on the cheeks, wings of the nose, and corners of the mouth.
The upper lip is cracked.

Mouth and Throat.
Sour blood is drawn from the decayed teeth.
The teeth feel dull.
Dryness in the throat.
10. Hawking up of sour mucus, causing the teeth to feel dull.
Accumulation of sour water in the mouth.
The tongue is thickly coated, while it cleans off in patches, and they are very sensitive.

Stomach and Abdomen.
Bitter taste in the mouth before eating.
Saltish-sour taste of the food, especially butter and meat.
15. Nausea with headache and anxiety.
Nausea and vomiting after eating fat food.
Bitter eructations and hiccough.
Sudden sensation in the abdomen as if bubbles were bursting in it.
Stinging pain in the abdomen, especially in the sides.

Stool and Anus.
20. Inefficient urging to go to stool.
The stool is passed with difficulty, even if it is not hard.
Voluptuous itching on the perinæum, compelling one to scratch.

Urinary Organs.
Frequent urging to urinate, with copious secretion.
Diabetes.

Respiratory Organs.

25. Sensation as if the larynx were pressed together.
Stitches in the chest.
Twitching in the intercostal muscles.

Back and Neck.

Twitching and stinging in the muscles of the throat and neck.
Tearing from the ear downward to the neck.
30. Pressing-stinging in the spine and sacrum, with dyspnœa.
Rumbling and bubbling in the shoulder-blades, with chilliness over the whole body.

Extremities.

Upper. Twitching in the muscles of the arm.
Icy-cold tips of the fingers.
Lower. Stitches in the thighs, calves, and soles of the feet.
35. Burning in the knees, lower legs, and toes.

Generalities.

The limbs are movable, but it feels as if the power to move them were impeded.
All the limbs are painful to the touch, and if a wrong position.

Sleep.

Sleepiness, and going to sleep while listening to a scientific discourse.
Sleepiness in day-time, and yawning while sitting.

Fever.

40. Chilliness, especially after eating and drinking.
Chilliness all over, with headache.
Chill in the open air.
Heat at night on waking, especially on the face and hands.
Violent night-sweats, mostly before midnight, during the first sleep.
45. Very debilitating perspiration, causing biting on the skin.

Conditions.

Most complaints arise while sitting or standing, and disappear on walking.

TARTARUS STIBIATUS.

Mind and Disposition.
During the day hilarity, in the evening anxious and timid.
Despair and hopelessness, with lethargy.

Head.
Numbness of the head, with stupefaction and somnolency.
Pressing headache, as if the brain were compressed, with stupefaction and lethargy; worse in the evening, at night, and while at rest; better when exercising and washing the head.
5. Pulsation in the right side of the forehead; worse in the evening, when sitting stooped, and from heat; better from sitting erect, and in the cold air.
Stitches in the head.
Trembling with the head, especially when coughing, with an internal sensation of trembling, chattering of the teeth, and an irresistible somnolency; worse in the evening and from heat.
Trembling with the head and hands, with great debility; worse when lying and getting warm in bed, better when sitting up erect and in the cold.

Eyes.
Desire to close the eyes, as from sleepiness.
10. Obscuration of sight, with flickering of light before the eyes.

Face.
Face pale and sunken.
Twitching in the muscles of the face.
Lips dry and scaly or cracked.

Stomach and Abdomen.
Longing for acids and fruits; for cold drinks, or thirstlessness.
15. Aversion to milk.
Fatty taste in the mouth.
Empty eructations; at night eructations as from rotten eggs.
Continuous anxious nausea.
Violent straining to vomit, with perspiration on the forehead.
20. Continuous nausea, vomiting, and diarrhœa.

43

Vomiting of food with great effort, followed by debility, chilliness, and sleepiness.
Vomiting of mucus and mucous diarrhœa.
Pain in the stomach, as from overloading the stomach.
Pulsation in the pit of the stomach.
25. Beating and pulsation in the abdomen.
When sitting bent forward, a sensation as if stones were pressing in the abdomen.
Cutting flatulent colic; worse when sitting bent forward.

Stool and Anus.

Watery diarrhœa, preceded by colic.
Stools papescent, slimy or bloody.
30. Violent tension in the perinæum.

Urinary Organs.

Violent, painful urging to urinate, with scanty, frequently finally bloody discharge.
Dark, brown-red urine.
Stitches in the neck of the bladder and in the urethra.
Burning in the urethra after micturition.

Respiratory Organs.

35. Dyspnœa, compelling one to sit up.
Shortness of breathing from suppressed expectoration.
Suffocating attacks, with the sensation of heat at the heart.
Velvet feeling in the chest.
Inflammation of the lungs; paralysis of the lungs.
40. Cough with suffocating attacks.
Rattling, hollow cough.
Cough, with vomiting of food and perspiration on the forehead.
Nightly cough, with expectoration of mucus.
Hooping-cough, preceded by the child crying, or after eating or drinking, or when getting warm in bed; after the attack somnolency.
45. Accumulation and rattling of mucus in the trachea and chest.
Visible palpitation of the heart, without anxiety.

Extremities.

Upper. Twitches of the muscles on the arms and hands.
Trembling of the hands.
The tips of the fingers feel cold and as if dead.
50. *Lower.* Tension in the bend of the knee and on the instep.
The feet go to sleep, as soon as one sits down.

Sleep.

Great sleepiness in the day-time, with much yawning and stretching.
Irresistible somnolency, with heavy, stupefied sleep. Lethargy.
Shocks and twitches during sleep, which jerk up single limbs or the whole body.

Generalities.

55. Attacks of fainting.
Internal trembling.
Convulsive twitches. Convulsions.
Great heaviness in all the limbs and great debility.
Rheumatic pains (fever) with perspiration, which does not relieve.
60. Inflammation of internal organs. Gastric and bilious complaints.
The child wants to be carried, and cries if any one touches it.
Pulsation in all the blood-vessels.

Fever.

Pulse full, hard and accelerated; at times trembling.
The fever ceasing, the pulse becomes often slow and imperceptible.
65. The least exertion accelerates the pulse.
Chill with external coldness predominates at all times of the day, with sleepiness and often with trembling.
Violent but not long-continuing heat, preceded by a long-lasting chill; worse from every exertion; or long-continued heat, with lethargy and perspiration on the forehead, following a short-lasting chill.
Perspiration on the whole body; also at night.
Perspiration frequently cold and clammy.
70. The affected parts perspire most.
Intermittent fevers, with lethargic condition.

Skin.

Eruptions of pustules as large as peas, filled with pus, with a red areola (like small-pox) forming a scab and leaving a cicatrix.

Conditions.

Aggravation in the evening and when sitting; when sitting crooked (stooped); from warmth.
Amelioration from eructation; in the open, cold air.

TELLURIUM.

Mind and Disposition.
Quiet disposition.

Head.
Vertigo, in the morning, after rising from the bed; worse when walking, when sitting up, when turning the head; with accelerated pulse, nausea and vomiting of food; better when lying perfectly quiet.
Vertigo while going to sleep.
Heaviness and fulness in the head in the morning.
5. Violent (linear) pain in a small spot over the left eye.

Eyes.
Deposit of a chalky, white mass on the anterior surface of the lens. (Cataract.)

Ears.
Itching and swelling (left ear), with painful throbbing in the external meatus; after three or four days, a discharge of a watery fluid, smelling like fish pickle, which causes a vesicular eruption upon the external ear and the neck wherever it touches the skin; the ear bluish-red, as if infiltrated with water; hearing impaired.

Nose.
Coryza with hoarseness, while walking in the open air.

Face.
Sudden flushes of redness over the face.

Mouth and Throat.
10. Profuse bleeding of the gums.
Sore throat and sensation of dryness of the fauces, always removed by eating and drinking.
Sensation of weakness (like faintness) in the stomach after local congestion of blood in the head and nape.
Passage of very offensive flatus.

Stool and Anus.
Stools colored black through and through.

Urinary Organs.
15. Urine highly colored, acid.

Respiratory Organs.

Breath smells of garlic.
Dull pain in the region of the heart when sleeping on the left side; relieved when lying on the back.
Palpitation of the heart, with throbbing through the whole body and full pulse, followed by perspiration.

Back.

Painful sensitiveness of the spine, from the last cervical to the fifth dorsal vertebra; sensitive to pressure and touching.
20. Pain in the sacrum, passing into the right thigh; worse when pressing at stool, when coughing and laughing; it extends from the sacral plexus through the great sciatic foramen, along the sciatic nerve, down in the thigh (especially on the right side). Sciatica.

Fever.

Chilliness with the pains.
Perspiration at the face.
The spots which perspire itch more.

Skin.

Ringworms cover the whole body; red, elevated rings, very distinctly marked, especially on the lower extremities.
25. Ringworms on the abdomen, head, above the wrist, on the forearm.

TEREBINTHINA.

Head.

Sudden vertigo, with obscuration of sight.
Dull headache, with colic.

Ears.

Sensation in the ears as of the striking of a clock.

Face.

Face pale and sunken.

Nose.

5. Violent bleeding at the nose.

Abdomen.

Distended abdomen; frequent colic; constipation.
Burning in the right hypochondrium.

Stool and Anus.

Stools consisting of mucus and water.
Violent burning in the rectum and at the anus after stool.
10. Burning and tingling at the anus, with the sensation as if ascarides would crawl out.

Urinary Organs.

Pressure in the kidneys when sitting, going off during motion.
Sensation of heaviness and pain in the region of the kidneys.
Violent burning, drawing pains in the region of the kidneys.
Burning in the bladder and in the urethra.
15. Difficult micturition, the urine smells of violets; deposit of mucus, or thick, muddy deposit.
Suppression of urine. Strangury.
Hæmaturia.

Respiratory Organs.

Dryness of the mucous membranes of the air-passages.
Burning in the chest; along the sternum.

THEA SINENSIS.

Stomach and Abdomen.

Sensation of complete relaxation of the stomach, with qualmishness and nausea, and discharge of water from the mouth; her stomach felt as if hanging down like an empty bag, and heavy.

THERIDION CURRASSAVICUM.

Mind and Disposition.

Talkative, inclined to mental exertions; hilarity.
Disinclination to occupy oneself in any manner.
The time passes too quick.

Head.

Vertigo with nausea, worse on stooping; from the least movement; on closing the eyes; from any noise; with cold perspiration.

5. The head feels thick, with nausea and vomiting from the least movement, and especially on closing the eyes.
Headache as if it were behind the eyes.
Sensation of heat in the head; it feels heavy.
Headache when he begins to move.
Heavy, dull pressure behind the eyes.

10. Violent pain deep in the brain, which compels him to sit or walk; cannot lie down.
The headache is aggravated if others walk over the floor, and from the least movement of the head.
Sunstroke.

Eyes.

Luminous vibrations before the eyes, (in hysterical persons).
Sensitiveness to the light; if looking into the light, dark vibrations; and double vision.

Ears.

15. Roaring in the ears, as from a waterfall.
Every sound or shrill noise penetrates through the whole body, especially into the teeth, causes vertigo, which produces nausea.
Itching behind the ears, wants to scratch them off.

Nose.

Much sneezing, with blowing of the nose.

Mouth and Throat.

Foam at the mouth during the chill.

20. Toothache from shrill noise; cold water causes a sensation as if cold penetrated the teeth.
Mouth and nose feel too dry.
Salty taste in the mouth, and hawking of salty mucus.

Stomach and Abdomen.

Desire for wine, brandy and tobacco.
Longing for a variety of things, but does not know for what.
25. Much thirst.
Nausea and vomiting when the eyes are closed.
Burning in the region of the liver; contact increases the pain.
Pain in the groins, when moving, when drawing the leg up.

Stool and Anus.

Constipation, the soft stool is expelled with difficulty.
30. Prolapsus ani, especially painful when he sits down.
Spasmodic constriction of the rectum.
Heaviness in the peritoneum.

Sexual Organs.

Women. Hysterical complaints in the years of puberty, and in the climacteric period, and thus also violent headache.

Respiratory Organs.

Violent stitches in the upper part of the chest, below the left shoulder-blade, extending through to the neck.
35. Anxious feeling on the heart.

Sleep.

Sleepiness even in the morning; all day; before the chill.
During sleep biting in the tip of the tongue.
Wakens during the night with vertigo, in the morning with stiffness of the jaws.

Fever.

Pulse slow (with vertigo).
40. Pain in all the bones, as if they would fall to pieces, or as if they were broken from head to foot; then violent chill without thirst.
Icy-cold perspiration over the whole body, with faintish vertigo.

Conditions.

The least noise or shrill sounds cause an aggravation.
Motion aggravates the vertigo and nausea.

THLASPI BURSA PASTORIS.

Profuse hemorrhages from all parts of the body.

THROMBIDIUM.

Stool and Anus.

Griping pain in the abdomen, followed by stool; first, feces; later, they are mixed with mucus; worse after eating; stool with tenesmus and prolapsus ani, shivering in the back, perspiration. Dysentery.

THUJA OCCIDENTALIS.

Mind and Disposition.

Fixed ideas; as if a strange person were at his side; as if the soul were separated from the body; as if the body, especially the limbs, were of glass and would break easily; as if a living animal were in the abdomen.
In reading and writing he uses wrong expressions.
Talks hastily, and swallows words.
Thoughtlessness; forgetfulness.
5. Over-excited, becomes easily angry over trifles.
Music causes him to weep, with trembling of the feet.

Head.

Vertigo on closing the eyes, disappears as soon as he opens them; or on stooping; or on looking upwards or sideways.
Pressing headache in the vertex, as if a nail were driven into it (P. M. and 3 A. M.); worse when at rest. better after perspiration.
Heaviness in the cerebellum, with ill-humor and aversion to conversation.

10. The headache is relieved from exercising in the open air, from looking upwards, and when turning the head backwards.

The scalp is very painful to the touch, and the parts on which one lies.

He wants to have the head (and face) wrapped up warm.

Dry herpes on the head, extending to the eyebrows. Dandruff.

White, scaly, peeling-off eruption over the scalp, extending over the forehead, temples, ears, and neck.

15. Tingling-biting, stinging-itching on the scalp, relieved by scratching.

Perspiration, smelling of honey (sweetish), on the uncovered parts of the head (face and hands), with dryness of the covered parts, and of those on which one lies, mostly when first going to sleep; better after rising.

Eyes.

The eye must be warmly covered, when uncovered it pains at once, and it feels as if cold air were streaming out of the head through the eye.

Lachrymation, especially in the open air; the tears do not run off, but remain standing in the eye.

The whites of the eye are blood-red.

20. Inflammatory softening of the inner surface of the eyelids..

Inflammatory swelling of the eyelids, with hardness.

Weakness of the eyes; obscure sight.

Small, black spots float before the eyes.

Double vision.

25. In the dark it seems as if falling down of luminous lights or sparks alongside of the eye, during the day and in the light it is as if dark drops were falling down.

The objects appear smaller (before the right eye).

Ears.

Noise in the ear as from boiling water.

Stitches into the ear from the neck.

Sensation as if the inner ear were swollen, with increased hardness of hearing.

30. Oozing from the right ear, smelling like putrid meat.

Nose.

Nose red and hot.

Red eruption on the nose, at times humid.

Blowing from the nose of a large quantity of thick, green mucus, mixed with pus and blood; later of dry, brown scales, with mucus, which comes from the frontal sinuses and firmly adheres to the swollen upper portion of the nostrils.
Painful scabs in the nostrils.
35. Eruptions on the wings of the nose.
Accumulation of mucus in the posterior nares.
Swelling and induration of the wings of the nose.
Warts on the nose.
Smell in the nose as from brine of fish, or of fermenting beer.
40. Fluent coryza in the open air, and dry coryza in the room.

Face.

Heat and redness of the whole face, with fine nets of veins, as if marbled.
Circumscribed burning redness of the cheeks.
The skin of the face is red-hot, peeling off continually; when washing it feels sore and raw.
Dropsically-bloated face.
45. Œdematous erysipelas of the face.
Greasy skin of the face.
Light-brown blotches (freckles) on the face.
Eruptions on the face, leaving livid spots.
Swelling of the temporal arteries.
50. Faceache, originating in the left cheek-bone near the ear, extending through the teeth to the nose, through the eyes to the temples into the head; the painful spots burn like fire, and are very sensitive to the rays of the sun.
Perspiration of the face, especially on the side on which he does not lie.

Mouth and Throat.

Flat, white ulcers on the inside of the lips, and on the corners of the mouth.
Lips pale; swollen; peeling off.
Cracking of the articulation of the jaw.
55. The roots of the teeth become carious; or the teeth become carious from the side; the crown of the tooth remains sound.
The teeth crumble off.
Dirty-yellow teeth
Toothache from drinking tea.
Gums swollen, inflamed, with dark-red streaks on them.

60. Tongue swollen, especially on the right side; he bites himself on the tongue frequently.
Aphthæ in the mouth.
Blue swelling under the tongue; ranula.
Taste in the mouth sweet as sugar, with gonorrhœa.
Accumulation of a large quantity of mucus in the throat, which is hawked up with difficulty.
65. Painful swallowing, especially empty swallowing, or that of saliva.
Throat feels raw, dry, as from a plug, or as if it were constricted when swallowing.

Stomach and Abdomen.

The food tastes as if it were not salt enough.
Bread tastes dry and bitter.
Longing for cold food and drink.
70. Bad effects from fat things and onions.
Violent thirst, especially at night and early in the morning.
While masticating the food becomes very dry.
Eructations rancid or acid.
Gulping up of large quantities of acids from the stomach.
75. Taste of putrid eggs in the mouth in the morning.
Continuous eructations of air while eating.
Vomiting of mucus, or of greasy substances.
Induration of the stomach. Indurations in the abdomen.
The fluid which he drinks falls with a noise in the stomach.
80. The upper part of the abdomen is drawn in.
Soreness of the navel.
Swelling of the pit of the stomach.
Movement in the abdomen as of something alive, as if the abdominal muscles were pushed outward by the arm of a fœtus, but painless.
Painful swelling of the inguinal glands.
85. Intussusception of the intestines.
Yellow or brownish spots on the abdomen. Zona.
Flatulence, as if an animal were crying in the abdomen.

Stool and Anus.

Ineffectual urging to stool, with erections.
Obstinate constipation, as from inactivity, or from intussusception of the intestines.
90. Stool in hard balls.
Discharge of blood with the stool.
Diarrhœa; pale-yellow water is forcibly expelled, with much noisy discharge of wind.
In the morning (after breakfast), or in the morning, periodically returning diarrhœa, always at the same hour.

THUJA OCCIDENTALIS.   685

Stools oily or greasy.
95. Painful constriction of the anus during the stool.
Hæmorrhoidal tumors swollen, paining worse while sitting.
Offensive perspiration at the anus and in the perinæum.
Sycotic excrescences at the anus.
Fistula in ano.

Urinary Organs.

100. Frequent urging to urinate, and profuse secretion of urine, especially towards and in the evening.
The urine foams; the foam remains long on the urine.
Involuntary secretion of urine; at night; when coughing; in drops after having urinated.
The bladder (and rectum) feels paralyzed, having no power to expel.
Sediment of brown mucus.
105. Urethra burning, biting-itching.
The urine contains sugar.
Bloody urine.

Sexual Organs.

Men. Swelling of the prepuce; inflammation of the glands.
Sycotic excrescences on the frænulum and on the glands; they ooze, especially during the new moon.
110. Watery, copious discharge from the urethra (gonorrhœa).
Stitches in the urethra, with urging to urinate.
Sensation as if a drop were running through the urethra.
Nightly painful erections.
Impotence after gonorrhœa.
115. Profuse perspiration, smelling sweet like honey, on the genitals.
Women. Profuse perspiration before menstruation.
Abortion in the third month.

Respiratory Organs.

Voice low.
Dyspnœa, as from adhesion of the lungs.
120. Shortness of breath, from mucus in the trachea.
Shortness of breathing from fulness and constriction in the hypochondria and upper abdomen.
Cough only during the day, or in the morning after rising, and in the evening after lying down.
Cough as soon as one eats.
During the evening cough after lying down, the expectoration becomes loose; easier when he turns from the left to the right side.

125. Stitches in the chest after drinking any thing cold.
Violent congestions to the chest, with strong, audible palpitation of the heart.
Anxious palpitation of the heart when waking in the morning.
Blue color of the skin on the clavicle.
The expectoration tastes like old cheese.
130. Sensation as of a skin in the larynx.
Brown spots on the chest.

Back and Neck.

Greasy, brown skin on the neck.
Burning extending from the small of the back to between the shoulder-blades.
Beating and pulsating in the back,
135. Blood-boils on the back.
Pressing pain in the region of the kidneys.

Extremities.

Upper. Herpes on the elbow.
Brown color on the back of the hand.
White scaly herpes on the back of the hand and on the finger.
140. Cold perspiration on the hands.
Erysipelatous swelling of the tips of the fingers, with tingling in them.
Nails are crippled, discolored, crumbling off.
Twitching of the muscles of the arms.
Coldness and sensation of deadness of the fingers and tips of the fingers.
145. Stinging pains in the arms and the joints.
Lower. The hip-joint feels as if it were relaxed.
When walking the limbs feel as if they were made of wood.
Hip-ache, the leg becomes elongated.
Brown skin on the legs, especially on the inside of the thigh.
150. Nets of veins, as if marbled, on the soles of the feet.
Red swelling of the tips of the toes.
Toe-nails crippled, brittle.
Fetid sweat on the toes.
Suppressed foot-sweat.

Generalities.

155. Emaciation and deadness of the affected parts.
Jerking up of the upper part of the body.
The flesh feels as if it were beaten off the bones.
Sensation of lightness of the body when walking.

THUJA OCCIDENTALIS. 687

Cracking of the joints on stretching them out.
160. Bad effects from beer, fat food, acids, sweets, tobacco, tea, wine and onions; from the abuse of Sulphur and Mercury.
Stitches in the limbs and joints.
The limbs go to sleep.
One-sided complaints—paralysis.
St. Vitus' dance.

Sleep.

165. Continuous sleeplessness, with painfulness of the parts on which one lies.
Sleeplessness, with apparitions as soon as he closes his eyes; they disappear as soon as he opens them.
Goes to sleep late on account of heat and restlessness.
Anxious dreams if he lies on the left side.

Fever.

Pulse slow and weak in the morning, in the evening accelerated and full.
170. In the evening violent pulsations.
Swelling of the veins.
Chill in attacks at various times in the day, but mostly in the evening.
Chilliness on the left side, which feels cold to the touch.
Chill without thirst after midnight and in the morning.
175. Internal chilliness, with external heat and violent thirst.
Heat in the evening, especially on the face.
Burning in the face without redness.
Dry heat of the covered parts.
Perspiration when first going to sleep.
180. Perspiration on the parts of the body which are uncovered, with dry heat of the covered parts.
Anxious, at times cold sweat.
Perspiration after the chill, without any intervening heat.
Perspiration, at times oily or fetid, or smelling sweet like honey.
General perspiration, but not on the head.
185. When walking in the morning profuse perspiration; the most profuse on the head.
Perspiration only during sleep, disappearing at once as soon as he awakens.
Rachitis.

Skin.

Dirty-brownish color of the skin.
Brownish, or brown-red, or brown-white spots on the skin.

190. Pustules. Small-pox.
Eruptions only on the covered parts.
The eruptions burn violently after scratching.
Sycotic excrescences, smelling like old cheese, or like the brine of fish.
White, scaly, dry, mealy herpes.
195. Condylomata, large, seedy, frequently on a pedicle.
Flat ulcers, with a bluish-white bottom.
Zona.
Corns burning.
Crippled nails on the fingers and toes.

Conditions.

200. *Aggravation* in the evening and at night; the debility is worse in the morning; some complaints are aggravated at 3 A. M. and 3 P. M.; from cold wet; from the heat of the bed.
Amelioration; from warm wet; from eructations; from a development of coryza, with sneezing; and from turning from the left to the right side.

TILIA EUROPÆA.

Mind and Disposition.
Melancholy, disposed to weep.

Head.
Vertigo, with staggering, and like gauze before the eyes.
Stinging pain in the forehead, with heat in the head and face.

Ears.
Stinging in the ears.

Nose.
5. Bleeding from the nose; the blood is thin and pale, but coagulates quickly.

Mouth and Throat.
Shifting pain in all the teeth, aggravated by cold water.
Burning in the throat.
Sensation of swelling of the palate, with desire to swallow, and hoarse voice.

Stomach and Abdomen.

Putrid eructations.
10. Bloated abdomen; pain as from incarcerated flatulence; repeated noisy discharges of it, with much relief.
Abdomen painful when touched, especially around the navel.
Sensitiveness, soreness, and sensation of subcutaneous ulceration in the upper part of the abdomen.
Stitches suddenly appearing in the abdomen, extending into the pelvis, and impeding breathing.

Sexual Organs.

Women. Frequent pressing on the uterus, as if every thing would fall out of the pelvis.
15. Spasmodic labor-like drawing from the abdomen down the small of the back, as if the catamenia would set in.
Great sensitiveness and soreness of the whole uterus, as after parturition.
Redness, soreness, and burning of the external parts.
Menstruation too late and very scanty (blood pale).

Sleep.

Sleeplessness, with restlessness; the bed seems to be too hard to him.

Fever.

20. Pulse full, hard, and quick.
Chilliness in the evening.
Heat all over, but most in the head and cheeks.
Night-sweat.

Conditions.

Especially suitable for women after parturition, and for children during dentition.
25. The left side of the body is most affected.
Aggravation; in the afternoon and evening; in the warm room; in the heat of the bed (skin symptoms); during motion (the rheumatic symptoms).
Amelioration; in the cool room, and from motion.

URTICA URENS.

Hæmoptysis, from violent exertion of the lungs.
Dysentery.
Insufficiency, or entire want of secretion of milk after parturition.
Nettle-rash. Burns.

UVA URSI.

Painful micturition, with burning.
Hæmaturia; slimy, purulent urine.

VALERIANA OFFICINALIS.

Mind and Disposition.
Hypochondriacal restlessness.
Very changeable disposition; hypocondriacal anxiety, or trembling excitability.
Fear, especially in the evening in the dark.
Hysteria, with nervous over-excitability of the nerves, and very changeable disposition and ideas.

Head.
5. Headaches appearing suddenly, or only in jerks.
Pressing in the head, as from a stupefying constriction in the forehead, drawing into the orbits, with paleness of the face; worse in the evening, when at rest, and in the open air; better from movement, in the room, and when changing the position.
Sensation of coldness in the upper part of the head when covering it with the hat.
One-sided, drawing headache, from draught of air.
Headache in the sunshine.
10. Stinging or pressing in the forehead, extending to the orbits.

Eyes.

Inflammation of the edges of the eyelids, with biting and stinging.

In the evening, in the dark, luminous appearance before the eyes, as if one could see the objects.

Face.

Redness and heat of the cheeks, especially in the open air.

White blisters on the cheeks and the upper lip, painful to the touch.

15. Stinging pain in the teeth.

Stomach and Abdomen.

Taste in the mouth (and smell before the nose) like putrid tallow.

Voracious hunger with nausea.

Eructations as from putrid eggs (in the morning on waking).

Nausea, as if a string were hanging down the stomach, with profuse ptyalism.

20. Nausea, with white lips, vertigo and coldness of the body.

Abdomen swollen and hard.

Spasms in the abdomen (hysterical), most frequently in the evening in bed, or after dinner; not relieved in any position.

Colic; from hæmorrhoids; from worms.

Stool and Anus.

Stools papescent, greenish, with blood.

25. Discharge of blood from the rectum.

Discharge of ascarides.

Urinary Organs.

Urinary discharge frequent and profuse.

Respiratory Organs.

Frequent jerks and stitches in the chest, with the sensation as if something were pressed out.

Stitches in the left side of the chest (region of the heart).

Back.

30. Pain in the loins, as if from cold, or from overlifting.

Rheumatic pain in the shoulder-blades.

Generalities.

Rheumatic pains in the limbs (rarely in the joints); worse during rest after previous exertions; better from movements.

Twitching, suddenly appearing pains, relieved by a change of position.
Over-sensitiveness of all the senses.
35. Hysterical complaints.

Sleep.

Sleeplessness, with great restlessness and tossing about.

Fever.

Pulse irregular; generally rapid and somewhat tense, sometimes small and weak.
Attacks of chilliness, lasting but a short time and followed by continuous heat.
The chilliness generally begins in the neck, and runs down the back.
40. Predominating, long-continued, and general heat, frequently with perspiration in the face.
Heat with thirst predominates.
Heat worse in the evening and when eating.
Profuse perspiration, especially at night, and from exertion, with violent heat.
Frequent sudden attacks of perspiration, especially on the face and on the forehead, which again disappear suddenly.

Conditions.

45. Periodical attacks every two or three months.
Aggravation at noon and during the first hours of the forenoon, or towards evening, till midnight; when bending down; while reposing; while standing; in the sun.
Amelioration; in the light; from moving; when walking.
Bad effects from the abuse of Mercury.
Especially suitable for women.

VERATRUM ALBUM.

Mind and Disposition.

Insanity, he wants to cut up every thing.
Melancholy, depressed, the head hangs down, he sits down thoughtlessly.
Great despair and hopelessness of life.
Mental anxiety and pangs of conscience, as if he had done something sinful.

5. Restlessness, much occupied.
Persevering refusal to talk; if he does he scolds, and the voice is weak and scarcely audible.
Loquaciousness, he talks rapidly.
Attacks of rage, with swearing, inclination to run away, tearing things.
Delirium, religious or exalted.
10. Imaginary diseases; thinks herself pregnant, or that she will be delivered soon.
Mental disorders, with lechery and obscene talk.

Head.

Vertigo, with cold perspiration on the forehead.
Coldness in and on the vertex, as if ice were lying on it, with icy-cold feet and nausea; worse when rising from the bed; better from external pressure, and when bending the head backwards.
Sensation of soreness of the head, with nausea.
15. Heaviness of the whole head.
Headache, with stiffness of the neck and profuse micturition.
Headache, with nausea and vomiting.
Great sensitiveness of the hair.
Cold perspiration of the forehead.

Eyes.

20. Eyes fixed, watery, sunken, with loss of lustre.
The eyeballs are turned upwards.
Pressing in the eyes.
Heat in the eyes.
Lachrymation, with dryness in the eyes and of the lids.
25. The eyes look yellow or blue.
Blindness at night.
Trembling of the upper eyelids.
Paralysis of the eyelids.

Ears.

Hardness of hearing; as if the ears were stopped up.

Nose.

30. Icy coldness of the nose.
Smell before the nose as from manure, or from smoke.
Painful sensation of dryness in the nose.
Frequent sneezing.

Face.

Face pale, bluish, cold, disfigured, death-like.
35. Blue or green circles around the eyes.

The face is red while lying in bed, but becomes pale as soon as he rises.
Cold perspiration on the face, especially on the forehead.
Spasms of muscles when masticating.
Lock-jaw.
40. Lips wrinkled, pale or black, and cracked.
Grinding of the teeth.

Mouth and Throat.

Toothache, with pain in the head and red, swollen face.
Burning in the mouth and throat.
Dryness and stickiness in the mouth.
45. Salivation, with nausea and sharp, salty taste.
Tongue red and swollen; or dry, black and cracked; or coated yellow; or cold and withered.
Stuttering; speechlessness.
Froth before the mouth.
The throat feels constricted, as by a pressing swelling.
50. Sensation of coldness or burning in the throat.
Dryness in the throat, not relieved by drinking.

Stomach and Abdomen.

Violent, unquenchable thirst, especially for cold water.
Voracious appetite; appetite and hunger between the paroxysms of vomiting.
Strong desire for acids and refreshing things.
55. Aversion to warm food.
Bitter taste in the mouth.
Cool sensation in the mouth, as from peppermint.
After the least food, vomiting and diarrhœa.
Violent empty eructations; sour or bitter eructations.
60. Nausea, with sensation of fainting generally, with violent thirst.
Violent vomiting with continuous nausea; great prostration.
Vomiting of food, of acid, bitter, foamy, white, or yellow-green mucus.
Vomiting of black bile and blood.
Vomiting, with diarrhœa and pressure in the pit of the stomach.
65. While vomiting the abdomen is painfully contracted.
Vomiting whenever he moves or drinks.
Nausea, with violent thirst, salivation and increasd flow of urine.
Great sensitiveness of the stomach and pit of the stomach.
Burning in the pit of the stomach.
70. Great sensitiveness of the abdomen to the touch.

VERATRUM ALBUM.

Cutting in the abdomen, as with knives.
Burning in the abdomen, as from hot coals.
Bloated, hard abdomen.
Flatulent colic with loud rumbling in the abdomen.
75. Inguinal hernia.

Stool and Anus.
Constipation, as from inactivity of the rectum; stool hard, of too large a size.
Unsuccessful urging to stool.
Watery, greenish diarrhœa, mixed with flakes.
Blackish diarrhœa.
80. Insensible discharge of thin stool (while passing flatulence).
Fainting during stool.
During stool, paleness of the face, cold sweat on the forehead, burning at the anus.

Urinary Organs.
Suppressed urinary secretion.
Continuous urging to urinate.
85. Involuntary flow of urine.
Dark-red urine, discharged frequently, but in small quantities.
Green urine.
Frequent micturition, with violent thirst and hunger, headache, nausea, colic, constipation and coryza.

Sexual Organs.
Women. Menstruation too early and too profuse.
90. Suppressed menstruation.
On the appearance of the menstruation, diarrhœa, nausea and chilliness.
Before the menstruation, headache, vertigo, bleeding of the nose and night-sweat.
During the menstruation, morning headaches, nausea, ringing in the ears, thirst and pain in all the limbs.
At the end of the menstruation, grinding of the teeth and bluish face.
95. Suppressed lochia (and secretion of milk), with delirium.
Nymphomania of lying-in women.

Respiratory Organs.
Cold breath.
Difficult respiration; dyspnœa.
Suffocative attacks, caused by a constriction in the larynx, or in the chest.
100. Painful spasmodic constriction of the chest.

Hoarseness.
Dry cough, from tickling in lower bronchia.
Deep, hollow cough, as from the abdomen, with cutting pain in the stomach; expectoration yellow, tough, bitter or salt only during the day. Hooping-cough.
Stitches in the sides of the chest, worse when coughing.
105. Attacks of cough are worse in the morning, or in the evening till midnight; when entering a warm room from the cold air; in the warm room; when getting warm in bed; from eating and drinking, especially cold things (water); when the child cries; in the spring (or fall).
Violent, visible, anxious palpitation of the heart.

Back and Neck.

Paralytic weakness of the muscles of the neck, they will not support the head.
Back and small of the back feel sore and bruised.
Tension, like cramp, below the shoulder-blades.

Extremities.

110. *Upper.* Sensation of coldness and fulness, with heaviness in the arms.
Tingling in the hands and fingers.
The hands go to sleep and feel like dead.
Icy coldness and blueness of the hands.
Lower. Cramps in the calves.
115. Painful heaviness in the knees and lower legs.
Sudden swelling of the feet.
Trembling of the feet, with coldness, as if of cold water running in them.
Stitches in the (big) toes.

Generalities.

Sudden sinking of strength.
120. Continuous weakness and trembling.
Numbness and tingling in the extremities.
Paralytic pains in the limbs.
Rheumatic pains, worse from the heat of the bed; better after rising, and entirely disappearing on walking about.
Attacks of fainting from the least exertion.
125. Inflammation of inner organs, especially those of digestion.
Shocks in the limbs, as from electric sparks.
Spasms, with convulsive motions of the limbs.
Violent tonic spasms; the palms of the hands and soles of the feet are spasmodically drawn inward.

Tetanic stiffness of the body.
130. Sporadic and Asiatic cholera.

Sleep.

Somnolency, with half consciousness (coma vigil).
Long, uninterrupted, heavy sleep.
Sleep with thirst and diuresis.
Nightly anxiety and sleeplessness.

Fever.

135. Pulse irregular, generally small, thread-like, weak, and slow; often it cannot be felt at all.
The blood runs like cold water through the veins.
Chilliness and coldness, mostly externally, with internal heat and cold, clammy perspiration.
Shaking chill with perspiration, soon changing to general coldness.
Chilliness and coldness predominate, and run from below upwards.
140. Chill aggravated by drinking.
Icy coldness of the whole body.
Heat only internal, with thirst, but without desire to drink.
Heat in the evening, with perspiration
Heat suddenly alternating with chilliness.
145. Violent perspiration in the morning, in the evening, or all night, as well as during every stool.
Cold, sour cr putrid perspiration, sometimes coloring the linen yellow, always with deathly paleness of the face.
Cold perspiration over the whole body, mostly on the forehead.
Perspires easily during the day from slight exertion.
Intermittent Fever. External coldness, with dark urine and cold perspiration, desire for cold drinks, and chill with nausea; afterwards heat with unquenchable thirst, delirium, redness of the face, constant slumber; finally perspiration without thirst, and very pale countenance.

Skin.

150. Color of the skin blue, purple color, and cold.
The elasticity of the skin is lost, the folds remain in the state into which the skin has been pressed.
Dry eruptions, like itch.
Desquamation of indurated or thickened portions of the skin.
Pyæmia.

Conditions.

155. The attacks of pain cause for a short time delirium and mania.

The pains in the limbs are aggravated by the heat of the bed, by wet-cold weather, and are relieved by rising and walking about.

After fright, involuntary stools with icy coldness of the body.

Aggravation; after drinking; during perspiration; after sleep; before and during stool; from wrapping oneself up warmly.

Amelioration; from uncovering the head; after perspiration.

VERBASCUM THAPSUS.

Mind and Disposition.

Unusual hilarity, with continuous flow of ideas.

Head.

Vertigo, when leaning the left cheek on the hand.

Pressing, stupefying headache when entering a warm room from the cold air, and vice versa.

Deep, stupefying stitches in the brain.

Eyes.

5. Pain in the eyes, with the sensation as if the orbits were drawn together, with heat in the eyes.

Ears.

Hardness of hearing, as from an obstruction of the ear.

Sensation as if the ear (nose and larynx) were stopped up when reading aloud.

Face.

Violent pressure in the (left) malar bone, and zygoma.

Faceache; dull pressure and stupefying tension in the whole cheek, beginning in the malar bone and articulation of the jaw, especially caused and aggravated by a change of temperature.

Mouth and Throat.

10. Tongue coated yellow in the morning.

Stomach and Abdomen.

Pressing pain on the navel, aggravated by bending forward.
Constriction in the lower abdomen and navel.
Stinging pain in the abdomen.

Stool and Anus.

Stool retarded; by very hard pressing he passes stool like sheep dung, in small, hard balls.

Urinary Organs.

15. Frequent micturition, with profuse secretion.

Respiratory Organs.

Hoarseness from reading aloud.   Deep voice.
Stupefying, periodical stitches in the chest.
Tension over the chest, with stitches in the region of the heart; in the evening after lying down.
Frequent attacks of a deep, hollow, hoarse cough, with the sound like a trumpet, caused by a tickling in the larynx and chest.

Generalities.

20. Stinging pains in the limbs.
Tearing, stinging pain in various parts, going downwards.
Benumbing sensation with most all the pain.

Sleep.

Great sleepiness after eating.
Awakens early in the morning, (4 A. M.)

Fever.

25. External and internal sensation of coldness over the whole body.
Coldness and chill predominate.
Shuddering on one side of the body, as if cold water were poured over him.

Conditions.

The ailments are caused and aggravated by change of temperature, especially when entering the room from the open air, and vice versa.
Aggravation, while sitting.
30. Amelioration, after rising from a seat.

VINCA MINOR.

Head.
Corrosive itching on the hairy scalp.
Badly-smelling eruptions on the head, in the face and behind the ears.
The hairs are entangled, as in plica polonica.
Humid eruptions on the head, with much vermin, and nightly itching, with burning after scratching.

Nose.
5. The tip of the nose becomes red on getting the least angry.

Face.
Bloated face, with pimples.
Dry lips.
Swelling of the upper lip and the corner of the mouth.

Mouth and Throat.
Aphthæ in the mouth.
10. Ulcers in the throat.

Sexual Organs.
Women. Excessive, profuse menses, flowing like a stream, with great debility.

Fever.
Pulse full and hard.
Sensation of tremor in every blood-vessel.

VIOLA ODORATA.

Mind and Disposition.
The intellect predominates over the mind (emotions).
Increased activity of the intellect.
Hysteric mood. with constant weeping.
Weakness of memory.
5. Excessive flow of ideas.

VIOLA ODORATA.

Head.

Vertigo while sitting.
Congestion of blood to the head, with pricking in the forehead.
The head feels heavy and sinks forward.
Tension in the scalp, which extends to the upper part of the face.

Eyes.

10. The eyelids are drawn down, as from sleepiness.

Ears.

Stitches in and around the ears.
Aversion to music, especially to the violin.

Nose.

Numbness of the tip of the nose.

Face.

Hot forehead.
15. Tension below the eyes and above the nose, extending to the temples.

Respiratory Organs.

Shortness of breathing and violent dyspnœa, as if a stone were lying on the chest.
Difficulty of breathing, with painful exhalation, anxiety and palpitation of the heart.

Extremities.

Aching pain in the (left) wrist.
Drawing pain in the elbow joint and dorsum of the hand.

Generalities.

20. Passing burning, here and there, as if it concentrated there and burned there with a small flame.
Trembling of the limbs.
Relaxation of all the muscles.
Great nervous debility.
Hypochondriacal and hysterical complaints.

VIOLA TRICOLOR.

Mind and Disposition.

Great dulness of the intellect.
Low spirited about domestic affairs.
Bad, morose humor, with disinclination to talk.
Very sensitive and inclined to scold.

Head.

5. Vertigo when walking.
Heaviness of the head when raising it, which disappears by stooping.
Burning stitches in the scalp, especially in the forehead and temples.

Eyes.

Biting in the eyes.
The eyelids sink down as from sleepiness.

Face.

10. Induration of the skin of the face.
Milk-crust, burning and itching, especially at night, with discharge of tough yellow pus.
Heat and perspiration of the face after eating.
Heat of the side of the face on which he does not lie, in the evening in bed.

Mouth and Throat.

Tongue coated with white mucus and bitter taste.
15. Sensation of dryness in the mouth, with much saliva.

Stomach and Abdomen.

Stitches and cutting pain in the abdomen, with urging to stool and crying and lamentations, followed by discharge of lumps of mucus and flatulence.
Pressing-stinging in the diaphragm.

Stool and Anus.

Chopped soft stools.
Stool with mucus and much flatulence.

Urinary Organs.

20. Urging to urinate, with profuse discharge of urine.
Fetid urine; it smells like the urine of cats.
Very turbid urine.
Stitches in the uretha.

Sexual Organs.

Swelling of the prepuce with itching.
25. Stitches in the penis or pressing in the glans; burning of the glans.
Itching stitches in the scrotum.
Involuntary seminal discharges, with lewd dreams.

Respiratory Organs.

Stitches in the chest, on the ribs, sternum and intercostal muscles.
Oppression and stitches in the heart, on bending the chest forward when sitting.
30. Anxiety about the heart while lying, with beating like waves.

Back.

Tension between the shoulder-blades, with cutting and tingling in the skin.

Extremities.

Upper. Stitches in the shoulder-joints, elbows, forearms and fingers.
Lower. Stitches in the patella, tibia and feet.

Sleep.

Goes to sleep late on account of ideas crowding his mind.
35. Awakens frequently from vigilance.
The child twitches with his hands in his sleep, with clenched thumbs, general dry heat and red face.

Fever.

General heat, especially in the face, with anxiety; dyspnœa immediately after eating.

Skin.

Stinging-biting rash.
Dry scabs over the whole body; when they are scratched, they exude yellow water.

ZINCUM METALLICUM.

Mind and Disposition.

Very variable mood: at noon, low-spirited; and in the evening, hilarity, or vice versa.
Morose and indisposed to converse (especially in the evening).
Great sensitiveness to the talking of others and to all noise.
Aversion to work and to walk.
5. Weakness of the memory.
Thoughtlessness and dulness of the intellect.

Head.

Vertigo in the cerebellum (when he walks, he feels as if he should fall to the left side).
Sharp pressure on a small spot in the forehead (evening).
Tearing and stinging pains in the sides of the head; worse after dinner.
10. Pressure on the root of the nose, as if it would be pressed into the head.
Sensation of soreness in the head.
Stupefying headache; every thing gets black before the eyes; worse in the morning in the warm room and after eating; better in the open air.
Sensitiveness of the vertex, as from soreness or ulceration, without regard to touch; worse in the evening in bed and after eating; better after scratching.
The hair falls off from the vertex, causing complete baldness, with sensation of soreness of the scalp.
15. Hydrocephalus.
Headache from drinking even small quantities of wine.
The headaches are worse in the room, better in the open air.

Eyes.

Pressure on the eyes; they feel as if they were pressed into the head.
Itching, biting, pricking, and sensation of soreness of the eyes, lids and inner angle of the eyes. (Pterygium.)
20. The upper eyelids fall down, as if paralyzed.
When lifting up the eyes he sees luminous flakes.

Ears.

Otalgia, with tearing stitches and external swelling (especially with children).
Discharge of fetid pus from the ear.

Nose.

The nose feels sore internally.
Swelling (of one side) of the nose, with loss of smell.
25. Coryza, with hoarseness and burning in the chest.

Face.

Paleness of the face.
Tearing and sore pain in the facial bones.
Lips and corners of the mouth cracked, with ulceration of the inside of them.
Thick, viscid, tasteless humor on the lips.
30. Redness and itching eruption on the chin.

Mouth and Throat.

Sensation of soreness of the teeth.
Looseness of the teeth.
The teeth and gums bleed.
The gums are swollen, white, sore and ulcerated.
35. Small yellow ulcers on the inside of the cheek (and in the throat).
Tingling on the inside of the cheek, with ptyalism of metallic taste.
Blisters on the tongue.
Sensation of soreness in the throat.
Sensation of constriction and spasm in the œsophagus.
40. Accumulation of mucus in the throat, which frequently enters the mouth through the posterior nares.
Bluish herpes in the throat after suppressed gonorrhœa.

Stomach and Abdomen.

Saltish taste in the mouth.
Taste in the mouth as from blood.
Voracious appetite and insatiable hunger.
45. Aversion to meat, fish, and cooked or warm food and sweet things.
Sour eructations, especially after drinking milk.
Heartburn after eating sweet things.
Nausea, with retching and vomiting of bitter mucus; renewed by the least motion.
Hiccough, especially after breakfast.
50. Vomiting of blood.
Burning in the stomach.
Disagreeable sensation (of heat) in the upper orifice of the stomach, extending to the œsophagus.
Pain in the hypochondria, like a spasm, alternating with dyspnœa.

Pressure under the short ribs, after eating, with depression of spirits.
55. Stitches in the spleen.
Pressure and tension in the abdomen.
Flatulent colic, especially in the evening.
Expulsion of hot, fetid flatus.
Inguinal hernia.

Stool and Anus.

60. Constipation; stool hard and dry; insufficient; frequently only expelled by hard pressing.
Soft, papescent, or thin diarrhœic stools, frequently with discharge of pale blood.
Involuntary stools.
Sensation of soreness, and violent itching at the anus.
Tingling at the anus, as from ascarides.

Urinary Organs.

65. Pressing, stinging and soreness in the kidneys.
Violent pressure of urine on the bladder.
Retention of urine when beginning to urinate.
Can only pass urine (which she must do every hour) while in a sitting posture.
Excessive desire to urinate, also at night.
70. Urine turbid, loam colored in the morning.
Frequent micturition of pale-yellow urine, which later deposits a white flaky sediment.
Discharge of blood from the urethra after painful micturition.
Burning during and after micturition.
Cutting pain in the orifice of the urethra.
75. Involuntary discharge of urine when walking, coughing and sneezing.
Stones (Gravel) of the kidneys and bladder.

Sexual Organs.

Men. Painfully swelled (sore) testicles. One or the other testicle is drawn up.
Drawing in the testicles, extending up the spermatic cord.
Violent and long-lasting erections.
80. Great falling off of the hair of the genital organs.
Women. Nymphomania of lying-in women, with great sensitiveness of the genitals.
Menstruation too late.
Suppressed menstruation, with painfulness of the breasts and genitals.

Lochia and the secretion of milk are suppressed.
85. Sore nipples.

Respiratory Organs.
Spasmodic oppression of breathing.
Constrictive sensation around the chest, with pain in the chest, as if cut to pieces.
Shortness of breath from flatulence after eating.
Accumulation of mucus in the chest.
90. Burning in the chest. Coldness in the chest.
Stitches in the chest (left side) and heart.
Palpitation of the heart; irregular beats of the heart; occasionally one violent thrust of the heart.
Tension in the sternum.
Burning and soreness in the pharynx.
95. Hoarseness.
Roughness and dryness in the chest.
Sensation of emptiness in the chest.
Debilitating spasmodic cough from tickling in the larnyx, extending to the middle of the chest, with expectoration of yellow, purulent, blood-streaked, tenacious mucus, tasting disagreeably, sweetish-putrid, metallic; or of pure blood in the morning or during the day.
The cough is worse after eating, during rest, sitting, standing, from milk, sweets, spirituous liquors, during menstruation.

Back and Neck.
100. Pain in the small of the back on walking or sitting.
Stiffness and tension of the neck.
Itching herpes on the back.
Tension and stinging between the shoulder-blades.

Extremities.
Upper. Rheumatic pains and stinging in the shoulders, arms, elbows, wrists, hands and fingers.
105. Lameness and deadness of the hands.
Weakness and trembling of the hands when writing.
Dryness and cracked skin of the hands.
Cracks between the fingers.
Dry herpes on the hands and fingers; they are rough and itch.
110. *Lower.* Rheumatic pains in the legs, knees, ankles and feet.
Varicose veins on the upper and lower legs.
Tension in the knee.

Formication in the calves.
Erysipelatous inflammation and swelling of the tendo-achilles.
115. Stiffness of the ankles after sitting.
Weakness and trembling of the feet.
Paralysis of the feet.
Coldness of the feet at night.
Pulsating stitches in the toes.
120. Painful chilblains on the feet.

Sleep.

Continuous desire to sleep, especially in the morning or after meals, with yawning.
Unrefreshing sleep, disturbed by unpleasant dreams, with talking and loud crying out.

Generalities.

Violent trembling twitching of the whole body.
Pulsations through the whole body.
125. Sensation of soreness in internal and external parts.
Twitching of children.
St. Vitus' dance.
Convulsions after a fright.
Rheumatic pains in the extremities, aggravated from becoming heated and from exertions of the body.
130. The pains seem to be between the skin and flesh.
Tearing in the middle of the bones; the limbs lose their hold, from the pain.

Fever.

Pulse small and rapid in the evening, slower in the morning and during the day.
Pulse at times intermitting.
Violent pulsations in the veins during the heat.
135. Chill begins generally after eating and continues till late in the evening and during the night.
Chilliness in the open air and when touching a cold object.
Chills run down the back.
Chilliness on the approach of stormy weather.
Internal heat, with sensation of coldness in the abdomen and on the feet.
140. Flushes of heat, with trembling and short, hot breath.
Profuse perspiration during the whole night, with inclination to uncover oneself.
Perspires easily during the day, on exercising.
Badly-smelling perspirations.

ZINGIBER.

Skin.

Itching in the bends of the joints.
145. Violent itching at night in bed, disappearing as soon as one touches himself.
Formication between the skin and flesh.
Sensation of coldness in the bones.
Rhagades.
Suppurating herpes.
150. Varicose veins.

Conditions.

Most ailments appear after dinner and towards evening.
Aggravation after having eaten, from small quantities of wine, in the warm room.
Amelioration, in the open air, while eating. Chamomilla and Nux vomica cause restlessness at night and constipation; and if they do so, Zincum will remove them, frequently.

ZINGIBER.

Head.

Congestion of blood to the head, especially the temples.
Pressure over the left eye.
Drawing, aching pain over the eyebrows.
Hemicrania; nervous headache.

Eyes.

5. Sensitiveness of the eyes to the light, with stinging pain in them.
Weakness of sight; dimness of the cornea.

Nose.

Dryness and obstruction of the posterior nares.
Ozœna.

Face.

Hot, red face.
10. Dry lips and mouth.

Mouth and Throat.

Bad slimy taste in the mouth.
Breath smells foul to herself.

Dryness of the throat and difficulty of swallowing, as from an obstruction, with dryness of the posterior nares.

Stomach and Abdomen.

Much thirst.
15. Complaints from eating melons.
Weak digestion.
Belching, with diarrhœa.
Nausea; vomiting of mucus in drunkards.
Acidity of the stomach.
20. Heaviness, like a stone in the stomach.
Stitches in the spleen.
Unbearable sore pain on a small place in the right side of the abdomen.
Sharp pain in the left iliac region.
Flatulency in gouty persons.

Stool and Anus.

25. Diarrhœa from drinking impure water.
Belching, with constipation.
Diarrhœa in the morning, followed by nausea.
Redness, inflammation, burning-itching at the anus.

Urinary Organs.

Increased secretion of urine.
30. Thick, turbid urine.
Retention of urine (after typhus).
Acute pain in the orifice of the urethra while urinating.

Sexual Organs.

Itching on the prepuce, which feels cold.
Painful erections.
35. *Women*. Menstruation too early and too profuse; blood dark, clotted.

Respiratory Organs.

Smarting sensation below the larynx, followed by a cough, with rattling of phlegm.
Asthma humidum.
Dry, hacking cough, with pain in the lungs and difficult breathing; in the morning expectoration.
Violent stinging-pressing pain in the left side of the chest, in the region of the heart.
40. Stitches through the chest.

Back and Neck.

Stiffness of the back of the neck, with headache and nausea.
Dull aching in both kidneys, with frequent desire to urinate.

Dull aching and sensation of heat in the left kidney; worse while sitting, with frequent desire to urinate.

Sleep.

Great sleepiness; coma.

Fever.

45. Chilliness, beginning in the lower limbs, going upwards.
Chilliness and sensibility in the open air.
Hot and chilly at the same time.

LITHIUM CARBONICUM.

Head.

Pain over the eyes and tension, as if bound in the temples; diminished while eating, but returning soon after eating, and remains as a pressure in the temples until in the night, and only goes away after falling asleep.
Pains in a small spot in the right temple.
Pressure in the temples from without inwards, with a pressing pain in the middle of the chest.
Tension as if bound in the temples, with half vision.
5. Early on awaking, violent headache in vertex and temples (after sudden cessation of the menses), with nausea.
Heavy weight upon the vertex with pressure upon the left temple.
Headache worse when lying down; it pains everywhere; better when sitting; relieved by going out.
Looking at any thing makes the headache worse; can hardly keep the eyes open; they pain as if sore from morning till noon.
Trembling and throbbing in the head, the pains in the heart extend to the head.
10. Head seems too large.
Head externally sensitive.

Eyes.

Stitches in the right eye.
Eyes pain as if sore.
Sensation of dryness and pain in the eyes after reading.
15. Sensation as if sand were in the eyes.
Pain over the eyes, with half vision.
The sunlight blinds him.

Uncertainty of vision and an entire invisibility of the right half of whatever she looked at (during second day of menstruation).

Ears.

Earache, left side, from the throat, with prosopalgia.
20. Pain behind the left ear, in the bone, extending towards the neck.

Nose.

Nose obstructed, above and in the forehead, in the morning and forenoon.
Blows his nose very much in the evening, much mucus remains behind in the choana.
Dropping from the nose in the open air.
Nose swollen, red, especially on the right side, sore internally—shining crusts form in it; it is dry and as if inflamed (at the same time frequent urinating at night, disturbing the sleep).

Face.

25. Pain in the right side of the face (afternoon) from the root of the tooth that has been sawn off, extending to the temple, followed next day by the same pain in the left side, passing from the throat to the left ear, causing earache and moderate brief pain in the left temple.

Throat.

Sore throat extending into the ear.
Expectoration of mucus from the choana and out of the fauces in solid lumps, especially morning and forenoon.

Stomach and Abdomen.

Gnawing in the stomach worse before a meal, it goes away while he eats.
Nausea and gnawing in the stomach.
30. Nausea, with fulness in the temples; with headache.
Acidity in the stomach.
Fulness in the pit of the stomach, cannot endure any pressure of the clothes.
Pressure in the hepatic region.

Stool and Anus.

Diarrhœa after fruit.
35. Very offensive stools (during the night).
Very stinking discharge of the flatus.
Violent, painful, dull stitch in the perineum near the anus, from above downwards, from within outwards.

LITHIUM CARBONICUM. 713

Urinary Organs.

Sensitive pain, sharp pressure, in the vesical regions, more on the right side, after urinating.
Tenesmus vesicæ and micturition (evening while walking).
40. Flashes of pain in the region of the bladder, inferiorly, more towards the right before passing water; pain extends into the spermatic cord after urinating.
Quick strong tenesmus.
Frequent and copious micturition (disturbing the sleep).
Turbid urine with mucous deposit.
Urine scanty and dark, very acrid.
45. Dark, reddish-brown deposit.
On rising to urinate, a pressing in the region of the heart, which did not cease till after urination (morning).

Sexual Organs.

Men. Erection after urination at night.
Burning in the urethra.
Women. Menses too late and too scanty.

Respiratory Organs.

50. On inspiration the air feels so cold that it seems to be felt unpleasantly even in the lungs.
Pressure in the middle of the chest.
Constriction of the chest when walking (after breakfast), followed by expectoration of mucus.
Violent cough in the evening, while lying down, compelling to rise, without expectoration; the irritation to cough is in a little spot, posteriorly and inferiorly in the throat.
Rheumatic soreness in the region of the heart.
55. Sudden shock in the heart.
Throbbing; like a dull stitch in the region of the heart.
Pains in the heart after pains in the bladder.
Pains in the heart before and at the time of the commencement of the menses.
Trembling and fluttering of the heart (after mental agitation of a vexatious character).

Back.

60. Stitch in the sacrum.
Pain in the sacrum, when standing, with confusion of the head.

Extremities.

Upper. Burning stitch in the ball of the hand, in the left thumb.

46

Itching-throbbing, very sensitive pain in all the fingers, as if it were in and upon the bones, extending from the hands to the ends of the fingers, only during repose; it ceases upon pressure, when grasping, and during motion.

Soreness at the margin of the nail, with pain and redness.

65. *Lower.* Pain in the right hip, later in the left.

Rheumatic pains in the lower extremities.

Pain of the knees, above the knees, especially when going up stairs.

Prostrated feelings in the knee-joints, weakness of the knees, on going up stairs.

Rheumatic pains in the right foot on awaking at night, they pass away on rising.

70. Painfulness of the feet, ankles, metatarsus, all the toes, especially of the border of the foot and the sole, as if it were gouty.

Pain and weakness of the feet.

Burning in the great toe, especially around the corns.

Great soreness of the corns.

Itching of the sole of the (left) foot on the inner margin.

75. Pain in the little toes.

Generalities.

Paralytic stiffness in all the limbs of the whole body as if beaten; stiff and sore over the whole body, in all the bones, joints and muscles.

Pressing, as if with a dull point, here and there, internally, as if it were near the bone, most in the left side.

Burning stitch which goes from within outwards, and ends in an itching.

Contracting sensation, with shudder.

Sleep.

80. Sleepiness early in the evening; late in the morning.

Sleep at night disturbed by urination.

Voluptuous dreams, tenesmus vesicæ, and erections, which subside after urination.

Fever.

Shudder starting from the thorax.

Very copious perspiration.

85. Perspiration on the back of the hands.

Skin.

Itching, at the anus, in the middle finger around the margin of the nail, on the side of the thigh, in the sole of the foot, in the palm of the hand.

INDEX.

Aconitum napellus	5	Cicuta virosa	143
Aethusa cynapium	10	Cimex lectularius	146
Agaricus muscarius	11	Cina (Semen santonici)	148
Agnus castus (Vite)	13	Cinnabaris	152
Allium cepa	16	Cistus Canadensis	156
Aloe	17	Clematis erecta	159
Alumina	21	Coccus cacti*	163
Ambra grisea	24	Cocculus (Menispermum cocculus)	166
Ammonium carbonicum	27	Cochlearia armoracia	170
Ammonium muriaticum	31	Coffea cruda	170
Anacardium orientale	33	Colchicum autumnale	172
Angustura	36	Colocynthis (Cucumis)	176
Antimonium crudum	38	Conium maculatum	180
Apis mellifica	40	Copaivæ balsamum	185
Argentum	44	Corallium rubrum	186
Argentum nitricum	46	Creosotum	188
Arnica montana	48	Crocus sativus	193
Arsenicum album	52	Croton tiglium	197
Arum triphyllum	57	Cubebæ	199
Assafœtida	58	Cuprum	200
Asarum Europæum	60	Cyclamen Europæum	203
Aurum	61	Daphne indica	207
Baryta carbonica	63	Diadema (Aranea)	208
Belladonna (Atropa)	66	Digitalis purpurea	209
Benzoicum acidum	73	Dolichos pruriens	213
Berberis vulgaris	75	Drosera rotundifolia	214
Bismuthum subnitricum	78	Dulcamara (Solanum dulcamara)	128
Borax	79	Elaps corallinus	222
Bovista (Lycoperdon bovista)	81	Elaterium (Momordica elaterium)	226
Bufo	83	Eupatorium perfoliatum	226
Bromine	85	Euphorbium officinarum	228
Bryonia alba	87	Euphrasia officinalis	231
Cactus grandiflorus	92	Evonymus Europæus	234
Cadmium sulphuricum	95	Eupion	235
Caladium seguinum	96	Ferrum	235
Calcarea carbonica	97	Filix mas	239
Calendula officinalis	104	Fluoricum acidum	239
Camphor	104	Fragaria vesca	243
Cannabis sativa	107	Gelseminum	243
Cantharides	110	Glonoine	248
Capsicum annuum	113	Graphites	251
Carbo animalis	115	Gratiola officinalis	257
Carbo vegetabilis	118	Guajacum officinale	260
Cascarilla	122	Gummi gutti (Gambogia)	263
Castor equorum	123	Gymnocladus Canadensis	265
Causticum	123	Hæmatoxylum campechianum	267
Chamomilla vulgaris	128	Helleborus niger	269
Chelidonium majus	133	Hepar sulphuris calcareum	272
Chenopodium (Chenopodii glauci Aphis)	135	Hippomane mancinella	279
		Hippomanes	283
China (Cinchona officinalis)	137	Hydrophobin	285

* By a clerical error it was erroneously given as Coccionella Septempunctata.

INDEX.

Hydrocyanii acidum	286	Petroselinum	520
Hyoscyamus niger	288	Phellandrium aquaticum	521
Hypericum perfoliatum	292	Phosphorus	524
Ignatia amara	294	Phosphoricum acidum	528
Indigo	300	Phytolacca decandra	453
Ipecacuanha	302	Platina	535
Iris versicolor	305	Plumbum	539
Jacaranda caroba	307	Podophyllum peltatum	543
Jatropha curcas	309	Pothos foetidus (Putorii)	545
Jodium	311	Prunus spinosa	546
Kali bichromicum	315	Psorinum	548
Kali carbonicum	324	Pulsatilla pratensis	553
Kali chloricum	333	Ranunculus bulbosus	562
Kali hydriodicum	335	Ranunculus sceleratus	565
Kalmia latifolia	339	Raphanus sativus	567
Kino (Gummi kino)	342	Ratanhia	568
Kobaltum	342	Rheum	569
Lachesis (Trigonocephalus)	346	Rhododendron chrysanthemum	572
Lachnantes tinctoria	351	Rhus toxicodendron	576
Lactuca virosa	356	Rumex crispus	584
Lamium album	359	Ruta graveolens	586
Laurocerasus	360	Sabadilla (Veratrum sabadilla)	589
Ledum palustre	364	Sabina (Juniperus sabina)	592
Lithium carbonicum	711	Sambucus nigra	594
Lobelia inflata	368	Sanguinaria Canadensis	596
Lupulus (Humulus)	370	Sarsaparilla	601
Lycopodium clavatum	370	Secale cornutum	607
Magnesia carbonica	379	Selenium	610
Magnesia muriatica	384	Senega (Polygala)	613
Magnesia sulphurica	389	Senna	616
Manganum aceticum	393	Sepia	617
Marum verum (Teucrium)	398	Silicea	626
Menyanthes trifoliata	400	Spigelia (Spigelia anthelmia)	633
Mephitis putorius	403	Spongia tosta	637
Mercurius vivus	406	Squilla (Scilla maritima)	604
Mercurius sublimatus	416	Stannum	641
Mercurius proto jodatus	420	Staphysagria (Delphinum staphysagria)	645
Mercurius sulphuricus (Turpethum)	423	Stramonium (Datura stramonium)	649
Mercurialis perennis	426	Strontiana carbonica	653
Mezereum (Daphne mezereum)	427	Sulphur	656
Millefolium (Achillea millefolium)	433	Sulphuricum acidum	666
Moschus	435	Symphytum officinale	669
Murex purpurea	438	Tabacum (Nitotiana tabacum)	669
Muriaticum acidum	439	Tanacetum vulgare	670
Natrum carbonicum	443	Taraxacum (Leontodon taraxacum)	671
Natrum muriaticum	449	Tartarus emeticus (Stibiatum)	673
Natrum nitricum	457	Tellurium	676
Natrum sulphuricum	458	Terebinthina (Oleum)	677
Niccolum	462	Thea sinensis	678
Nitrum	466	Theridion curassavicum	679
Nitricum acidum	470	Thrombidium muscæ domesticæ	681
Nux juglans	477	Thuya occidentalis	681
Nux moschata	479	Thlaspi bursa pastoris	681
Nux vomica	484	Tilia Europæa	688
Ocimum canum	493	Urtica urens	690
Oleander (Nerium oleander)	494	Uva ursi (Urbatus)	690
Oleum animale	496	Valeriana officinalis	690
Opium	499	Veratrum album	692
Oxalicum acidum	503	Verbascum thapsus	698
Osmium	508	Vinca minor	700
Pæonia officinalis	509	Viola odorata	700
Palladium	510	Viola tricolor	702
Pareira brava	513	Zincum	704
Paris quadrifolia	514	Zingiber	709
Petroleum	516		

ERRATA.

Page 60. "Asarum Europæum" instead of "europ."

Page 87. "Bismuthum" should be page 78.

Page 163 should be "Coccus Cacti," instead of "Coccionella Septempunctata," which was a palpable error.

ERRATA.

Page 80. "Asarum Europæum" instead of "europ."

Page 97. "Blumenthum" should be page 78.

Page 163 should be "Crocus Gæcit" instead of "Cocolonella Вересянис-ras," which was a palpable error.